# Nighttime Breastfeeding

# Fertility, Reproduction and Sexuality

**GENERAL EDITORS:**

*Soraya Tremayne,* Founding Director, Fertility and Reproduction Studies Group, and Research Associate, Institute of Social and Cultural Anthropology, University of Oxford.

*Marcia C. Inhorn,* William K. Lanman, Jr. Professor of Anthropology and International Affairs, Yale University.

*Philip Kreager,* Director, Fertility and Reproduction Studies Group, and Research Associate, Institute of Social and Cultural Anthropology and Institute of Human Sciences, University of Oxford.

For a full volume listing please see back matter.

# NIGHTTIME BREASTFEEDING
## An American Cultural Dilemma

Cecília Tomori

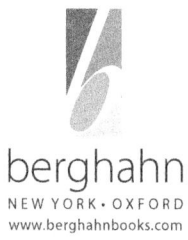

berghahn
NEW YORK • OXFORD
www.berghahnbooks.com

First published in 2015 by
Berghahn Books
www.berghahnbooks.com

© 2015, 2017 Cecília Tomori
First paperback edition published in 2017

All rights reserved. Except for the quotation of short passages for the purposes of criticism and review, no part of this book may be reproduced in any form or by any means, electronic or mechanical, including photocopying, recording, or any information storage and retrieval system now known or to be invented, without written permission of the publisher.

**Library of Congress Cataloging-in-Publication Data**

Tomori, Cecília, author.
  Nighttime breastfeeding : an American cultural dilemma / Cecília Tomori.
     p. ; cm. — (Fertility, reproduction and sexuality ; volume 26)
  Includes bibliographical references.
  ISBN 978-1-78238-435-9 (hardback) — ISBN 978-1-78533-346-0 (paperback) — ISBN 978-1-78238-436-6 (ebook)
  I. Title. II. Series: Fertility, reproduction, and sexuality ; v. 26.
  [DNLM: 1. Breast Feeding—United States. 2. Sleep—United States. 3. Anthropology, Cultural—United States. 4. Health Knowledge, Attitudes, Practice—United States. WS 125]
  RJ216
  649'.33—dc23

2014016239

**British Library Cataloguing in Publication Data**

A catalogue record for this book is available from the British Library.

ISBN 978-1-78238-435-9 hardback
ISBN 978-1-78533-346-0 paperback
ISBN 978-1-78238-436-6 ebook

*To my children, Jakob and Adrian*

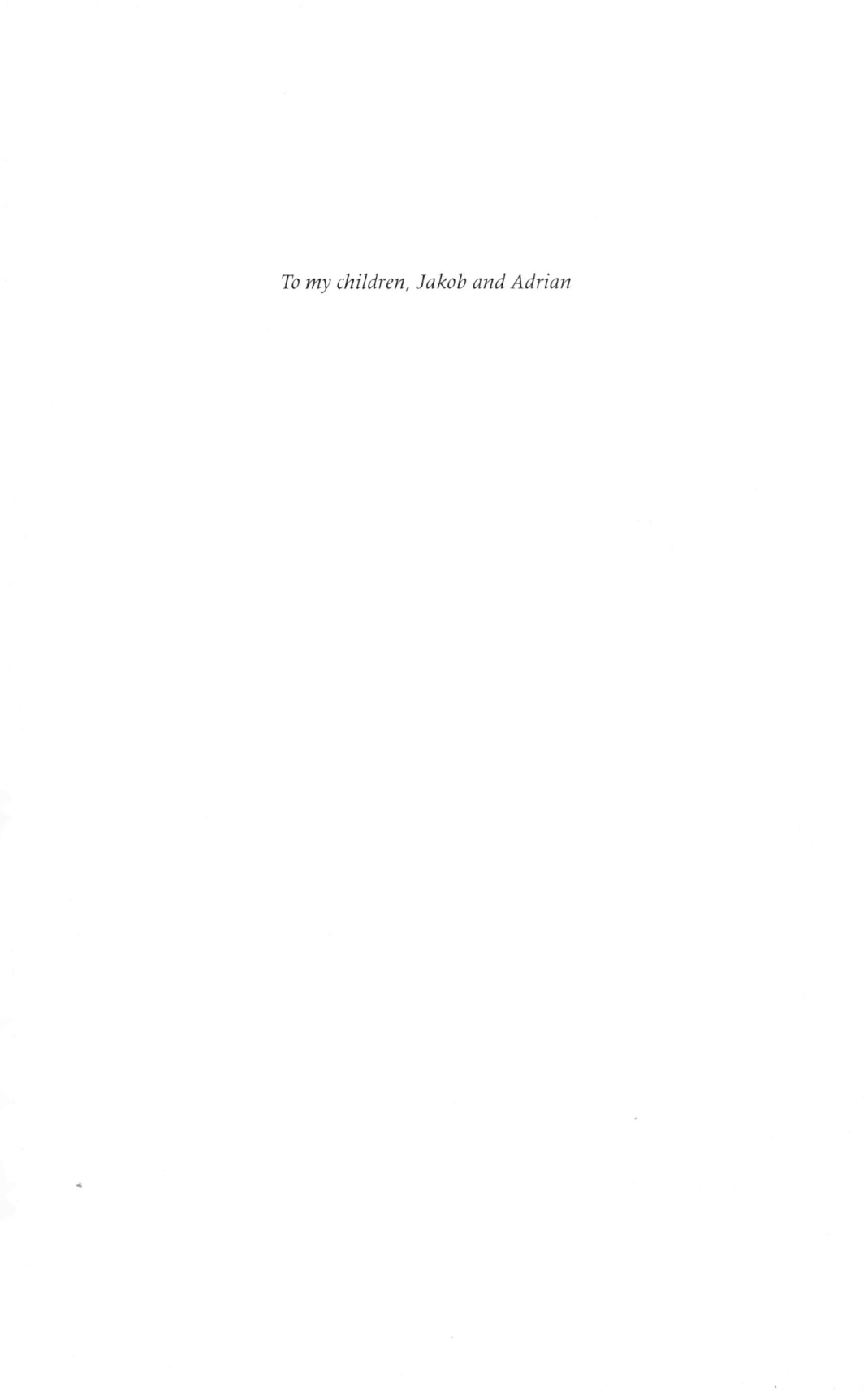

# Contents

| | |
|---|---|
| List of Illustrations | viii |
| Preface and Acknowledgments | ix |
| Introduction | 1 |
| **Chapter 1.** Embodied Cultural Dilemmas: An Anthropological Approach to the Study of Nighttime Breastfeeding and Sleep | 25 |
| **Chapter 2.** Struggles over Authoritative Knowledge and "Choice" in Breastfeeding and Infant Sleep in the United States | 55 |
| **Chapter 3.** Making Breastfeeding Parents in Childbirth Education Courses | 89 |
| **Chapter 4.** Dispatches from the Moral Minefield of Breastfeeding | 120 |
| **Chapter 5.** Breastfeeding as Men's "Kin Work" | 144 |
| **Chapter 6.** Breastfeeding Babies in the Nest: Producing Children, Kinship, and Moral Imagination in the House | 171 |
| **Chapter 7.** Time to Sleep: Nighttime Breastfeeding and Capitalist Temporal Regimes | 208 |
| Conclusion | 240 |
| Appendix I. Sleeping/Feeding Log | 245 |
| Appendix II. Table of Demographic Characteristics of the Couples Involved in the Study | 247 |
| Appendix III. Biographical Sketches of the Core Participants | 249 |
| Bibliography | 261 |
| Index | 289 |

# Illustrations

**Figure 6.1.** Rachel's and Nathan's nursery with their crib for Maya.    178

**Figure 6.2.** Pack 'n Play portable play yard.    184

**Figure 6.3.** Snuggle Nest placed in the middle of the parents' bed.    186

**Figure 6.4.** Carol's and Justin's Co-Sleeper being used as storage unit.    193

# Preface

This book explores the fraught cultural landscape of nighttime breastfeeding and sleep in the United States. Although breastfeeding and infant sleep practices are the subject of significant medical attention and feature prominently in conversations about parenting practices, few scholars have focused on how these issues figure in the experience of nighttime parenting. Yet, as the book demonstrates, nighttime for many new parents is filled with intense challenges. During the night, parents often confront conflicting medical guidelines about breastfeeding and infant sleep as well as larger questions about middle-class personhood and the social relations among children and their parents entailed in these reproductive processes. Through careful attention to the lived, embodied practices of breastfeeding and sleep and their significance within and across different cultures, this book offers a unique anthropological perspective on these complex negotiations and the cultural and moral dilemmas in which they are embroiled.

This work emerged out of many years of interest in and study of the embodied experiences of reproduction. My interest in breastfeeding was first piqued while working as a health services researcher at Northwestern University. During my research at an obstetrics/gynecology clinic staffed primarily by physicians who were completing their residency, I observed women express their breast milk using electric pumps during their lunch breaks. I later sat through meetings with some of my colleagues there, which took place during these pumping sessions. I was intrigued by these women's dedication, the equipment involved, and the lactation process itself. I did not yet know that I would soon be joining these women's ranks when I became pregnant with my first son.

As a college-educated woman who worked in health care settings and who had attended the recommended hospital-based childbirth education courses, I was surprised to find how little I actually knew about childbirth or breastfeeding. In fact, without support and encouragement from my husband, Kerry Boeye, I would have stopped breastfeeding within just days after our son's routine hospital birth. Without my husband's active participation and unfailing support throughout the years of breastfeeding our two children, neither breastfeeding nor this book could have been part of our experience.

At the University of Michigan's Department of Anthropology, my wide-ranging interests were nurtured by Gillian Feeley-Harnik, Marcia Inhorn, Tom Fricke, Elisha Renne, Raymond De Vries, Judy Irvine, A. Roberto Frisancho and by many others. I am particularly grateful to Marcia Inhorn for her support and enthusiasm for this project from its inception through its completion and for her sage advice, encouragement to develop my research into this book, and continued support for my work and interests. Marcia's own work and guidance have been exceptional sources of inspiration for me. I could not ask for a better mentor.

The Alfred P. Sloan Center for the Ethnography of Everyday Life, the Ruth L. Kirschstein National Research Service Award Training Grant from the Eunice Kennedy Shriver National Institute of Child Health and Development (T32 HD007339 & T32 HD007339-23) awarded by the Population Studies Center at the Institute for Social Research, the Rackham Graduate School, the Department of Anthropology, and the Center for the Education of Women at the University of Michigan have provided funding support for research for this book.

Joanne Bailey and Lisa Kane Low, as well as with lactation consultants, midwives, childbirth educators, physicians, and doulas whom I cannot name due to confidentiality reasons. I have learned a great deal from them and appreciate their support. I received some crucial encouragement from the members of the planning committee and many participants of the Breastfeeding and Feminism Symposium at the University of North Carolina, Chapel Hill. Specifically, I would like to thank Miriam Labbok, Paige Hall Smith, Bernice Hausman, Jacqueline Wolf, and Kristin Klingaman for their interest in my work. James McKenna's, Helen Ball's and their colleagues' work has helped spark new insights and stimulated my enthusiasm for this work.

Since arriving in Maryland, David Celentano has offered me a new academic home at the Johns Hopkins Bloomberg School of Public Health. I am grateful for his mentorship and support throughout the process of completing this manuscript and for his encouragement to find new ways to engage my anthropological knowledge and approaches in public health.

Throughout my work on this project I have been supported by a tremendous network of friends and colleagues of whom I can only name a few here. I cherish their friendship and generosity, and I am inspired by their own outstanding work in anthropology. I am especially grateful to Britt Halvorson, Jessica Smith Rolston, Jessica Robbins-Ruszkowski, and Laura Heinemann for reading my work and providing thoughtful and constructive comments. Sallie Han's work and support has inspired me throughout my research and writing. Jessica Robbins-Ruszkowski's insightful and encouraging comments on the penultimate draft helped me cross the finish line on this marathon project. I have also been very fortunate to be supported in very concrete ways through excellent food and even better company from Fernando Andrade, Anna Shahinyan, and their son, Andreas. Laura Starita and Amita Dahra helped me articulate my goals for the book and offered crucial encouragement for the completion of the final manuscript. Most of all, I am grateful to all of my participants, who have welcomed me into their lives and offered to share their breastfeeding experiences and dilemmas with me. I hope that I have stayed true to them in my accounts and that they will enjoy seeing the fruits that our time together has born.

# Introduction

When I visited Kate[1] and Joshua at their home for our first meeting a week and a half after their daughter's birth, we had a lot to catch up on. I had met Kate, a schoolteacher, and Joshua, an ecologist, a married couple in their late twenties, at a local childbirth education center several months earlier. Together with a group of other middle-class pregnant women expecting their first child, their partners, and an instructor, we spent two and a half hours together each week during the long Midwestern winter for the seven sessions of the course and the additional sessions of breastfeeding and infant care courses. This couple, like the others I worked with during my research, chose to participate in my study because they intended to breastfeed for at least six months, they were interested in my research, and they wanted to help out a student. Kate and Joshua welcomed me into their lives and approached my research on nighttime breastfeeding—much of which concerned aspects of their lives they rarely shared with others, let alone with a complete stranger—with the same openness and sense of humor that I observed during my initial interactions with them in childbirth education classes. Throughout the year that followed the birth of their daughter, Anna, we would spend many hours together as I learned more about their breastfeeding and sleep experiences and how these experiences fit into the fabric of their everyday lives.

During this particular meeting, Kate and Joshua were thrilled to introduce me to their new daughter. Amidst carrying, changing, and breastfeeding Anna, they shared their experiences with labor and childbirth at one of the local hospitals. I learned that although they did manage to achieve their goal of not using anesthetics during their daughter's birth, they nevertheless experienced several unwanted medical interventions. I also learned that, despite their extensive preparations, breastfeeding and infant sleep had both presented unanticipated challenges. Kate's breasts became extremely sore, raw, and "scabby" shortly after they returned to their home. Thanks to help from the visiting nurse on how to position the baby during breastfeeding and from an ointment prescribed by their nurse-midwife, breastfeeding was going much better in the few days prior to our meeting. Still, the soreness was returning as Kate was learning to breastfeed while lying down—a skill that she found challenging, although far less tiring and more comfortable than breastfeeding while seated and propped up with pillows. In the haze of exhaustion from the trials of the lengthy birth process compounded by breastfeeding difficulties, Kate and Joshua also found that Anna "did not want to" sleep when put down on her back in the three-sided bassinet, called a Co-Sleeper, that attached to their bed. When they tried putting her in the Co-Sleeper, Anna woke up after five minutes, and continued to do so each time they tried again. Thus, Kate and Joshua spent the night alternating between long breastfeeding sessions and sleeping for an hour or two with Anna sleeping on one of their chests.

Although sleeping with their daughter in this way allowed Kate and Joshua to get some much-needed rest and to breastfeed her with relative ease, this arrangement raised several concerns. Kate worried about the safety of falling asleep with Anna on her chest and the potential of not being aware of her location in relation to her and the bed. In turn, Joshua was concerned that Anna would learn only to sleep on a parent and therefore would not be able to sleep without being on a parent's body. In response to these concerns, Kate and Joshua developed a new way of sleeping, building on Kate's recent discovery that after breastfeeding her while lying down in bed, both she and Anna could stay asleep for two to three hours at a time. Using words and gestures, Kate described how the three of them now slept in the same bed, with Anna laying on her side at Kate's breast level, her body encircled by Kate's arm from above and her knees pulled up from below. Joshua continued to take Anna and sleep with her on his chest when she did not stay asleep after breastfeeding. While this discovery ultimately facilitated both their breastfeeding plans and sleep for Kate, Joshua, and Anna, it would take considerably more negotiations, assistance, and effort to comfortably settle into their nighttime feeding and sleep arrangements.

For Kate and Joshua, as well as many other couples in my study, the problematic status of breastfeeding infants sharing their parents' bed in the United States presented a major obstacle to attaining a sense of ease about their nighttime practices. Initially motivated by their desire to follow medical recommendations for the best way of feeding babies, many of the couples in my study suddenly found themselves at odds with medical advice about safe sleep, which prompted questions about endangering or even killing their child. Moreover, bringing their babies into bed and continuing to breastfeed them over the course of the year raised additional concerns about the implications of their nighttime practices for their children as well as for themselves. Would these practices cause their baby to be unable to sleep on her own in the future and fail to become an independent and self-reliant person? Would nighttime bed sharing and breastfeeding disrupt their marriage or somehow harm their child? Alternately, if they decided not to bring their babies into bed with them, how would they get their children to sleep and how could they manage to sustain nighttime breastfeeding? Couples were also ambivalent about when and how nighttime breastfeeding sessions would give way to continuous blocks of sleep, preferably in a crib in a separate room that they had lovingly prepared as a nursery, often months before their babies' birth. Developing an approach to nighttime breastfeeding and sleep often became a central issue for couples and formed a cornerstone of their parenting practices. Far beyond decisions about nourishment and rest, nighttime breastfeeding and sleep constituted a quandary that each family approached differently.

These dilemmas of nighttime breastfeeding and sleep are the subject of this book. For an anthropologist, such dilemmas highlight an area of tension and ambivalence that, when unraveled through careful research, can shed light on larger cultural concerns. While controversies around infant feeding and sleep decisions abound in the media and have generated scholarly discussions, comparatively little anthropological research exists on how those who plan to breastfeed actually negotiate these embodied processes. Furthermore, aside from the notable efforts of biological anthropologists, sociocultural anthropologists and other qualitative researchers have devoted little attention to nighttime breastfeeding and sleep. Drawing on insights from a longitudinal ethnographic study of middle-class breastfeeding families in a Midwestern U.S. city, my book addresses this scholarly lacuna. The volume explores how the quandaries of nighttime breastfeeding and sleep can provide insight into cultural expectations for babies and their relationship with parents, concepts of health and medical authority, and unequal sociocultural, political, and economic social relations that are the hallmarks of late capitalist America.

## The Cultural Problem of Nighttime Breastfeeding and Sleep in the U.S.

The couples in my study embarked on their breastfeeding journey at a time when the U.S. and similar wealthy industrial nations have witnessed a resurgence of breastfeeding due mainly to international and government-led health initiatives that promote breastfeeding in an effort to improve maternal and child health and reduce health care costs.[2] Although these efforts have led to a sharp rise in breastfeeding shortly after birth, significantly fewer mothers follow medical recommendations of exclusive breastfeeding for six months and continuing to breastfeed while supplementing with other foods for at least one year. Nevertheless, these rates represent a slow but steady increase. In 2011, the year for which the latest data are available in the United States, 76.5 percent of women began breastfeeding, a rate that dropped to 49 percent by six months (and a much lower rate of 16.4 percent for exclusive breastfeeding) and then to 27 percent by one year postpartum (CDC 2013a). Despite significant progress over the last decade, aggregate breastfeeding rates conceal considerable racial, ethnic and class differences among women (CDC 2013b, 2010c). The U.S. stands out among wealthy industrial nations for its resistance to implementing structural changes that support breastfeeding, such as access to health care, paid parental leave, subsidized and on-site childcare, and tighter regulation of the infant formula industry.[3] These discrepancies put parents in a paradoxical position where they must make infant feeding decisions in a climate that valorizes breastfeeding but does little to facilitate it.

Indeed, a growing body of scholarly literature criticizes breastfeeding advocacy for characterizing breastfeeding as a matter of individual responsibility and a morally superior form of infant feeding.[4] Feminist scholars and journalists have been particularly vocal in articulating their objections to the patriarchal implications of such a strategy and have expressed serious concern about breastfeeding promotion based solely on the biomedical properties of breastmilk.[5] Some critics, such as women's studies scholar Joan Wolf (2011), have questioned the scientific basis of breastfeeding advocacy and argued that such efforts have established a climate where breastfeeding is a moral imperative, ultimately contributing to an ideology of "total motherhood" that is characterized by a single-minded focus on minimizing risks for children while subsuming women's agency in this familial labor.

Yet media controversies surrounding breastfeeding reveal a much more complex cultural terrain wherein breastfeeding continues to elicit considerable anxiety.[6] Breastfeeding mothers are routinely asked to leave restaurants, art museums, airplanes, and other public spaces because of concerns over others' exposure to their nude breasts and the sight of children nursing at the breast, which is viewed as sexual.[7] Reports of breastfeeding children beyond one year generate concern about the mother's inappropriate, potentially incestuous, relations with her child.[8] Even breastmilk, the substance that ostensibly possesses precious biological qualities, generates suspicion and disgust—for instance, when breastmilk is expressed in the workplace and put in a communal refrigerator.[9] Moreover, breastfeeding and breastmilk are also considered potential threats to health. Breastfeeding has been portrayed as inadequate or insufficient, causing malnutrition, disease (e.g., rickets), starvation, and even death.[10] Breastmilk is considered a conduit for dangerous pharmaceuticals, illegal drugs, alcohol, environmental toxins, and potentially lethal infections, including HIV and the West Nile virus.[11] Thus, the moral status of breastfeeding is a complicated matter that warrants greater attention.

Many of these concerns were recently captured by reactions to the May 2012 *Time* magazine cover featuring a woman breastfeeding her three-year-old son. In the photo the white, blond, thin, and attractive mother, dressed in skinny jeans and a dark blue camisole, stands with one hand on her hip, looking straight into the camera, as she breastfeeds her son. Her son, wearing camouflage pants and a grey long-sleeved shirt, stands on a small chair and looks tentatively at the viewer as he breastfeeds from his mother's exposed breast. Below the woman's elbow, the caption reads "ARE YOU MOM ENOUGH?" with the latter two words highlighted in bold red lettering, and below, in smaller letters: "Why attachment parenting[12] drives some mothers to extremes—and how Dr. Bill Sears became their guru." Co-sleeping, which in colloquial language refers to sharing a bed with one's child,[13] was mentioned in the *Time* magazine article along with breastfeeding beyond one year in the list of unusual and "extreme" behaviors espoused by those following the attachment parenting philosophy, which is ostensibly "more about parental devotion and sacrifice than about raising self-sufficient kids" (Pickert 2012).

The photo selected for the cover produced a firestorm of reactions, the majority of them condemning breastfeeding a child at such an advanced age. A large number of comments on various sites that discussed the controversial cover reacted with visceral disgust, with comments suggesting that the mother was breastfeeding the child for her own (sexual) pleasure and was harming the child. Some suggested that it was time for the mother to let her husband take a turn at her breast. As others have pointed out, the cover was likely set up to draw this kind of reaction, since it highlighted the mother's gender and sexuality through her dress, pose, and exposed breast and accentuated the size of the child through the use of the chair on which he stood, as well as his masculinity through wearing camouflage pants.[14] Indeed, breastfeeding mothers are highly unlikely to adopt such a bodily pose for breastfeeding. The cover was designed to incite controversy by positioning women who breastfeed their children past one year as "extreme" with the subtext of incest lurking barely below the surface.[15]

By addressing the discomfort surrounding breastfeeding in the context of nighttime sleep arrangements, my study provides a unique window into this and similar other controversies. While bed sharing with infants is commonly practiced and accepted in many areas of the world, in the U.S. bed sharing magnifies cultural fears associated with breastfeeding and is presumed to hinder children's independence, disrupt parental sexual relations, interrupt parents' sleep, and even provoke incest. Consequently, as in the *Time* magazine article, bed sharing is often portrayed as "extreme." Yet, there is considerable cultural variation in the perception and practice of bed sharing even within the U.S.[16] Moreover, there are growing indications that, like Kate and Joshua, breastfeeding parents frequently bring their babies into their beds at night to ease breastfeeding and enhance both mothers' and babies' sleep.[17] Biological anthropological and biomedical research indicates that nighttime breastfeeding with proximal sleep arrangements mutually support the physiology of breastfeeding and human infant sleep.[18] Although this form of co-sleeping has not returned in step with rising breastfeeding rates, the recent National Infant Sleep Position Study has revealed that between 1993 and 2000 the portion of infants who slept with their mothers for all or part of the night doubled, reaching nearly 50 percent (Willinger et al. 2003). Experts attribute this increase at least in part to rising breastfeeding rates.[19]

Mainstream medical advice reinforces fears about bed sharing with added concerns about the increased risk of Sudden Infant Death Syndrome (SIDS) in early infancy[20] and the necessity of lengthy, uninterrupted sleep for optimal health for both children and adults.[21] Due to the stigma attached to bed-sharing, breastfeeding parents are left without guidance on how to sleep safely near their children and often conceal their bed-sharing practices. Only a small group of experts advocate a different approach that would support breastfeeding parents and provide evidence-based guidance that attends to the specific context of infant sleep arrangements.[22] Parental concern over how to approach nighttime breastfeeding and infant sleep is evidenced by the enormous amount of discussion of these issues on internet parenting sites, in news media, and in childcare books and magazines. As more parents attempt to breastfeed, more are also likely to confront cultural prohibitions and contradictory mainstream medical advice, intensifying debates about breastfeeding and sleep.

In *Nighttime Breastfeeding*, I show that such debates comprise a part of the challenges and tensions that arise from the global trend toward increasing medicalization or, more specifically, biomedicalization[23] of the body and of reproduction, in particular.[24] As the body has come under intense medical scrutiny, experts have become medical and moral authorities on every aspect of producing children.[25] Furthermore, in U.S. society, bodily processes are increasingly considered domains of health, wherein risk of illness and death can be monitored and managed.[26] Much of the expert attention is focused on maternal bodies and behavior that are seen as particularly important in shaping the health of children and ultimately the nation.[27] Scholars have documented that mothers themselves have actively participated and continue to participate in bringing about, resisting, internalizing, and negotiating medical authority, their positions shaped by their own sociocultural and economic position.

Moreover, the heated debates that surround topics we now consider health issues, including breastfeeding and infant sleep, reflect the specific structural challenges, complex social relations, and moral debates in which these bodily processes are embroiled. Drawing on in-depth ethnographic research, my book reveals that these reproductive processes are not only central to ever-expanding regimes of health, but also are at the heart of key cultural concerns about what it means to be a mother, partner, child, and family; what really matters in the relationships between parents and children; and how these relationships participate in far-reaching political economic webs that reproduce inequalities.

## The Ethnographic Study

This research arose from my findings in a previous pilot project that I undertook in 2003[28] to learn about the experiences of breastfeeding in Green City, a small Midwestern city that I will describe in greater detail below. In that pilot study of breastfeeding mothers, participants repeatedly returned to the topic of sleep in relation to their breastfeeding practices, which prompted me to design a larger ethnographic study to investigate these issues in greater depth. Although my research had a strong focus on nighttime breastfeeding, I aimed to situate my findings in this area within the larger context of breastfeeding. Thus, while my nighttime emphasis is apparent throughout the book, several chapters have a broader focus.

In contrast to public health studies that have focused on the barriers to breastfeeding in poor communities and among racial and ethnic minorities with low rates of breastfeeding, I chose to explore how middle-class families negotiate these experiences. The attention to middle-class families served multiple purposes. First, middle-class families provided a sample that would possess the resources necessary to breastfeed in accordance with medical recommendations, enabling me to observe how breastfeeding is incorporated into the experiences of everyday lives and relationships over a sustained period of time.[29] I had hoped, and indeed found, that this length of time would also enable me to develop closer relationships with participants, which would yield deeper insights into how they negotiated sleep in relation to breastfeeding, especially in light of the controversies that surround infant sleep practices that might make participants reluctant to discuss these arrangements. Second, I wanted to examine elements of social class that otherwise might be left unexplored in relation to breastfeeding, such as how these families mobilize their resources and divide labor in order to breastfeed and how these negotiations figure into the makings of social class as well as gender. Making these processes more visible would shed light on the subtle privileges middle-class parents might take for granted, thereby exposing the larger inequalities of which disparities in breastfeeding rates are a part. Finally, I sought to explore middle-class families as trendsetters.[30] My research into the history of childbirth in the U.S. has taught me (see chapter 2) that wealthier families played an important role in inviting physicians into the domain of childbirth, a transition that eventually transformed childbearing for all women in the U.S.[31] In a similar fashion, families' negotiations of the conflicting medical approaches to breastfeeding and sleep would potentially have implications for many others.[32]

## Research in Green City

Green City is a city of approximately 110,000 people located within commuting distance of a large Midwestern city that was a major center of the auto industry as well as other industry earlier in the twentieth century but that has since gone into significant economic decline. According to the 2000 census, the population of Green City was three-quarters white, about 12 percent Asian, and 9 percent African American, with a median household income of approximately $46,000[33] (U. S. Census Bureau 2000). Green City and its immediate vicinity is home to many higher educational institutions, including two large public universities, a large community college, as well as some smaller private institutions, and its population is highly educated.[34]

Green City was well suited to examine the relationship of breastfeeding and sleep arrangements because of its comparatively high breastfeeding rates,[35] the presence of a large community of alternative birthing practitioners and supporters, and a significant number of breastfeeding support organizations, some of which support co-sleeping. Green City had two large health systems—a university-affiliated system and a private system with approximately 4,000 annual births each. Green City was known locally as well as throughout the state for its resources in childbearing that cater to different philosophies of childbirth and approaches to breastfeeding and parenting. Both hospitals had affiliated certified nurse-midwifery practices in addition to the traditional obstetrics/gynecology practices. Furthermore, Green City had a strong community of home birth midwives. This is particularly notable, since home births are extremely rare in the United States, composing only approximately 0.6 percent of all births (MacDorman, Menacker, and Declercq 2010). Previous research indicated that those participating in alternative birth practices might also consider co-sleeping with their babies, contributing to a diverse sample of sleep practices in the study.[36]

To complement these local resources, families could attend several different childbirth education courses that were reimbursed by major insurers, choose from a large selection of trained professional birth support personnel (doulas) who assisted both low- and higher-income populations, hire pregnancy massage providers and lactation consultants, and shop in stores that supply a variety of goods relating to childbearing as well as other related services. Finally, in addition to hospital-based lactation consultant programs, Green City possessed a large chapter of La Leche League International (LLLI), an international non-profit breastfeeding support organization. During the period of my research, five local LLLI groups met on a regular basis in various locations across the city. My previous research revealed that in addition to Green City residents, parents from surrounding areas frequently utilized these groups. Since LLLI supports co-sleeping as an approach for accommodating infants' frequent need to breastfeed at night,[37] this resource is often considered helpful to those exploring alternative sleep arrangements that differ from mainstream recommendations. The wealth of these services reflected the presence of educated middle-class consumers in the area who were adequately covered by health insurance and could locate and purchase additional resources that they perceived to be necessary.

In sum, Green City was ideally suited for investigating parental practices such as long-term breastfeeding[38] and a variety of sleep arrangements that are relatively less common in the greater U.S. population, as well as for learning how middle-class parents incorporate these practices into their lives. Green City provided the center of the majority of my fieldwork activities, as it was the center for childbirth education resources, hospitals, and work for most of my participants. Following my participants also took me out of Green City to neighboring areas, primarily to Neighbor City, where three participating families—including Kate and Joshua—lived, and to three other communities that were located closer to the larger metropolis I described above. Nevertheless, families in Neighbor City had substantial work and educational ties to Green City, and the three latter families regularly relied on various Green City services, particularly in the realm of health care. In subsequent chapters I provide more detailed information on how these families were connected to Green City through childbirth education services, and I discuss details of the neighborhoods and communities in which my study participants resided.

*Ethnographic Fieldwork*

A key question in pursuing this research was how to gain knowledge about practices that occurred during the night, in participants' bedrooms. Biological anthropologists have employed laboratory research that included videotaping mothers and infants sleeping together and apart as well as the collection of physiological data during these periods.[39] These researchers have also conducted videotaping in hospitals and families' homes, complemented by survey questionnaires and interviews. As a sociocultural anthropologist, many of these techniques were neither possible nor necessarily desirable for developing a better sense of the sociocultural context in which nighttime breastfeeding and sleep arrangements were practiced. Other ethnographers, such as Alma Gottlieb (2005), learned about nighttime practices by living in the same community with their participants and overhearing and witnessing how they dealt with nighttime awakenings, and later discussed these arrangements in greater depth during the daytime.

Similar to the majority of my participants, I lived in Green City with my own family, but due to far less proximal housing arrangements and differences in the social practices of sleep, I could not interact with participants during the night. One option would have been to live with a specific family or alternate living arrangements among families. This option was not feasible due to my own family commitments. While this approach would have offered certain advantages, it would have also limited my ability to gather ethnographic data about a larger group of families over a longer period of time. By selecting childbirth education courses as the focal points for my recruitment, I was able to simultaneously situate my study in important local sites where groups of expectant parents gather while also entering into long-term participant-observer relationships with my core group of participants. Although these study methods prevented me from physically sharing the experiences of nighttime, the richness of interactions during the remainder of the day nevertheless enabled me to gather unique insights into the night. I complement my ethnography with research from biological anthropological studies in order to compensate for my lack of physical observations of nighttime interactions.

Fieldwork relationships were foundational to my ability to learn about breastfeeding and sleep practices, especially in light of fears of negative judgment about controversial sleep practices and various challenges to breastfeeding. I learned that it was primarily during the day that participants reflected on their nighttime experiences, discussed them with their spouses, and devised various plans for what they were going to do. These activities were not simply prompted by my presence or questions, although this additional sharpening of reflection was certainly a part of our interactions. But more often, participants reported their reflections along the way and their conversations with others that shaped their own understanding. This kind of reflexivity is itself a characteristic of middle-class conduct and is shaped by my participants' educational experiences, wherein reflexivity is encouraged, as well as by middle-class self-help literature and therapeutic discourses. Although I paid close attention to the conversations I had with my participants, I also devoted considerable time to learning about other aspects of their practice, including where and how participants slept and fed their children, how they conducted themselves in our interactions, and the material cultural practices in which they engaged.

Upon gaining Institutional Review Board approval, I conducted two years of fieldwork between 2006 and 2008, with brief follow-up work at a one of the local hospitals ("University Hospital") in 2009. During the fieldwork period, I attended courses at two large childbirth education centers that also served as my recruitment sites for core participants. I centered my study on pregnant women who were becoming first-time mothers[40] and who planned to breastfeed six months or more, their partners, and later their children. My focus on first-time mothers enabled me to document women's first bodily encounters with the practice of breastfeeding. Depending on the timing of these courses during their pregnancy, I followed participants from the second or third trimesters through at least the end of their child's first year of life. Since breastfeeding mothers constituted my primary participants, I met with them much more regularly than with spouses. Spouses participated in different ways. Some were able to and wanted to be part of our meetings on a regular basis, while others could not do so or were not as interested in setting up more regular meetings. I always met participants at their level of interest, staying attuned to their wishes. Consequently, I spent considerable time with some spouses, while I met others less frequently, during their lunch break or at a weekend or evening meeting.

During the fieldwork period, I undertook extensive participant observation, supplemented by additional methods described below. Participant observation was based primarily in the participants' homes, although some meetings took place at local cafes and restaurants, at workplaces, as well as in participants' neighborhoods. Participant observation included spending time with and participating in activities with the family. During these occasions we shared food and conversation, and participants attended to their regular activities. Much of this time included participants caring for their children, including breastfeeding, bottle-feeding, feeding of other foods (later), diapering, changing, burping, bathing, playing, and soothing (among others). I went for walks, held babies, washed dishes, and otherwise tried to be a helpful participant in these daily activities.

In order to make sure that I kept track of participants regularly over the course of the year, I conducted semi-structured interviews loosely scheduled around the targets of within a few weeks of birth and at three months, six months, nine months, and twelve months. Nearly all of these interviews were audiotaped.[41] However, I remained flexible in order to honor personal needs for recovery from childbirth as well as the vicissitudes of everyday life—primarily sickness, conflicting schedules, and work demands. I tried my best to impose as little as possible on participants' lives so that they did not feel like our meetings were yet another chore amidst the many others engendered by caring for small children, work, family obligations, and other demands.

During our first meeting, I collected basic sociodemographic data and elicited information about participants' plans for birth, breastfeeding, and sleep arrangements, and their reasons for making these plans. Furthermore, I asked about participants' families, employment practices, and plans for after their babies' birth. In these conversations I cast my net broadly to get a sense of the context of participants' plans. Over the course of later meetings I also elicited information about the experiences of the previous night, assessed present breastfeeding and sleep arrangements, and discussed plans for the future. I incorporated a sleep/feeding log documenting parents' and children's location in the house and any feedings and awakenings during the previous night in some of these discussions, depending on whether participants wished to fill one out (see Appendix 1).[42] Of the larger group, a smaller group of participants were willing to have more frequent meetings and conversations. These participants tend to feature more in my discussions, although I draw on examples from others and incorporate what I learned from every participant in the main arguments of the book. Within this smaller group, I also carried out some videotaped observations.

Over time I came to know my participants and their families quite well and even interviewed some of their extended family members. During fieldwork I listened to many difficult and heartbreaking experiences and shed tears as well as celebrated joy and laughter together. Many participants have kept in touch with me since the study's conclusion and have sent me their birth announcements for their second child as well as updates about their lives, and several former participants said that they missed our conversations and wished that we would be able to continue our meetings even after many months passed since our last study meeting. In turn, I also found that I grew quite accustomed to meeting with participant families and felt a part of them, albeit to different degrees. Despite this sense of connection, fieldwork remained quite challenging, due to both the pragmatic challenges of juggling visits to many different families at once as well as the work of learning about each person and family and their unique pattern of engagement with me.

Beyond following the core participants, I interviewed and talked informally with local childbirth educators, doulas, midwives, and lactation consultants, trained as a postpartum doula, observed local hospital childbirth and breastfeeding practices, attended local birth- and breastfeeding-related events, and kept informed of media coverage of childbirth, breastfeeding, and infant sleep issues. In all these ways, I sought to learn as much as I could about the experiences of breastfeeding for the core participants while also situating this knowledge in larger contexts. At the same time, by anchoring the study to the core participants' lives, I hoped to provide a contrasting and complementary perspective to those of medical professionals and public health researchers who may only encounter families for short periods of time, often in the brief and specific context of medical interactions.

## A Brief Overview of Core Participants

The core participants of the study were eighteen middle-class first-time mothers, fifteen of their spouses, and their children. An overview of the couples and the characteristics of their births, breastfeeding, and sleep arrangements over the course of the study can be found in the appendixes (see Appendix 2 and 3). Although all spouses were supportive of the study and were happy to talk to me in childbirth education classes as well as in informal interactions during the course of the study, three spouses chose not to formally participate due to their extensive work commitments. Nearly all participants were Euro-American, highly educated, heterosexual married couples and resided in or near Green City. The one same-sex couple in my study married in a ceremony not recognized by the state. All but one couple in my study gave birth at the above two local hospitals and many experienced typical medical interventions for childbirth, with the significant exception that participants used much lower than expected rates of epidural anesthesia (only eight of eighteen mothers received epidural anesthesia, which is given in over 90 percent of births at local hospitals). This result likely reflects the high percentage of couples in the study, and in many of the childbirth education courses I attended throughout my fieldwork, who desired an unmedicated birth and systematically sought out resources in order to pursue this goal.

All expectant mothers planned to breastfeed for six months to a year and all succeeded in doing so.[43] All but two of the eighteen mothers continued to twelve months and many beyond. Of these two women, one stopped at eight months due to a serious medical condition that required taking prescription medication with potentially serious side-effects for her baby. The second received pediatric advice for the cessation of nighttime breastfeeding, which contributed to her stopping breastfeeding by nine months. All but one family brought their babies into their bed during the night at least for short periods of time. Nearly all families practiced more sustained bed sharing over the course of the study, by itself or in combination with other sleep arrangements. At twelve months postpartum, ten couples still practiced partial or complete bed sharing. Compared with the U.S. population, most of these couples were part of the minority who breastfed at one year postpartum, and of an even smaller group who slept in bodily proximity to their children.[44]

### Positionality and Fieldwork Interactions

My own position in fieldwork was complex, as is the nature of ethnographic research. In many senses, I build on a long legacy of feminist ethnographers who have studied reproduction in the U.S. after encountering various aspects of reproduction through their own experience.[45] At the same time, I did not grow up in the U.S. and therefore did not return to examine reproduction there with fresh eyes, nor have I conducted previous ethnographic research elsewhere, as is common in the discipline. My own trajectory originates in Hungary, where I was raised until I entered high school on the East Coast of the U.S., learning English in the course of those years, during which I still spent considerable time in Hungary. By the time I entered fieldwork, however, I had gone to college in the U.S., married a U.S. citizen, birthed, breastfed, and cared for two young children with my husband, and had become a permanent U.S. resident. Throughout this process I had increasingly become not only a Hungarian living in the U.S., but a Hungarian American.

This brief account reflects the growing diversity of persons and life experiences ethnographers bring to anthropology. Unlike in the times of the discipline's origins, women (including mothers) now constitute a significant voice in anthropology, although they continue to face many gender-based barriers, especially as related to their responsibilities of caring for children.[46] With anthropology's growing incorporation of feminist approaches and reflexive ethnography, women have also increasingly incorporated their experiences of motherhood into their research.[47] Furthermore, ethnographers also increasingly represent a diversity of sexual, racial, ethnic, class, religious, and geographic histories. This diversity, as well as greater attention to the various ways in which similarity and difference is evoked in social interaction, has prompted anthropologists to question dichotomies between "native" anthropologists who have been described as studying "their own" culture and other anthropologists, who have followed disciplinary traditions to study "other" cultures.[48] Following this work as well as that of others who have reflected on the politics and experiences of fieldwork experiences,[49] I begin with a few reflections about my engagement in the research I undertook.

My own personal history figured into my ethnographic interactions in multiple ways. First, I was already a mother of young children when all the mothers and all but one of the spouses were expecting their first children. Second, I was an anthropologist studying reproduction. These are clearly interlinked domains; my own experiences were foundational for developing my commitment to study breastfeeding as an anthropologist. Furthermore, I was a mother-anthropologist with an explicit position that breastfeeding is an embodied process worth caring about and supporting. While I did not advocate breastfeeding, I was clear in my interactions with participants that I supported breastfeeding. At the same time, my own perspective on breastfeeding is a socially situated one—I was fully aware of the many obstacles to breastfeeding, empathized with participants' challenges in breastfeeding, their use of formula, and decision to stop to breastfeeding. I took a similar approach to sleep arrangements, again empathizing with the various difficulties participants encountered regardless of where they all slept each night.

The above orientations positioned me as someone who was knowledgeable about an area of life that my participants looked forward to with great anticipation, but to which most had little exposure in their everyday lives. Even those familiar with children through babysitting had not had a great deal of exposure to very young children. There was also a sense in which I was treated as an "expert," someone who possessed scholarly knowledge that included certain aspects of medicine related to childbirth, breastfeeding, and sleep, as well as embodied experience through having my own children. In this sense, I was probably regarded most similarly to a "breastfeeding expert," someone knowledgeable and supportive about breastfeeding and related challenges. I was aware of these roles and was careful to position myself as a friendly, supportive observer, rather than an expert. I am aware that these efforts mitigate, but do not erase this element in our interactions. Nevertheless, I did not share my own experiences of motherhood nor my anthropological knowledge without explicitly being asked to do so. Participants did inevitably ask many questions about both these realms of my life (as well as others), and during these occasions I answered honestly but without offering more than what I felt was necessary. Throughout, I was most careful to be supportive and caring and to avoid judgment. I believe that the results of this careful engagement are reflected in the openness of my participants to share their difficulties, dilemmas, and worries without fearing my disapproval.

Despite the potentially limiting effects of being seen as an expert, my own reproductive history greatly facilitated these field interactions. Most prominently, we shared experiences of having children and breastfeeding them. While my having "succeeded" in breastfeeding could be a source of anxiety for struggling mothers, several participants noted that they felt that knowing such a mother helped them feel more reassured about their ability to breastfeed. My physical comfort with breastfeeding was an important part of enabling my fieldwork. In a cultural climate where breastfeeding in public is shunned, mothers did not have to worry about exposing their breasts during breastfeeding in my presence (as affirmed by the lack of covering during these feedings as well as their comments). Furthermore, many mothers spent their early weeks and months at home, partly due to the difficulty of nursing discreetly in public when just learning how to breastfeed as well as the challenges of bundling up young babies in the cold winter and putting them in and out of car seats for transportation. For these mothers, I was welcome company and conversation partner. Consequently, I spent a great deal of fieldwork with mothers breastfeeding babies right next to me, from the beginning moments when they were just learning how to breastfeed and often struggled to latch on their babies to times when babies became increasingly interested in their surroundings and would happily unlatch in the middle of feeding and smile at me with breastmilk dripping down their cheeks. Such moments are rare in public spaces in the U.S. and would have been impossible to witness without participants' comfort with me. This sense of closeness was further facilitated by our similarity in race, age, education, and my fluency in English, which did not reveal my foreign roots.

There was a complex gendered element to these interactions. Since my study centered around breastfeeding mothers, I spent most of my time with mothers and shared many aspects of my embodied experiences with them, all of which enhanced our mutual sense of closeness. At the same time, I was cautious not to assume that my own embodied breastfeeding and sleep experiences were the same as those of my participants. While my early breastfeeding experiences with my first son were challenging, leading me to nearly abandon breastfeeding altogether in the first days, I did not encounter many of the difficulties my participants faced and breastfed both of my sons for several years. My own sleep arrangements were also similarly quickly worked out, with our children co-sleeping in our bed for similar lengths of time. These relatively uncommon practices in the U.S. were supported among my anthropologist colleagues and supervisors, who encountered similar arrangements in their work in other cultural settings. Furthermore, embodied experience always takes place within specific cultural and interpersonal contexts, making even what might appear to be similar experiences to be open to radically different interpretations. I paid close attention to participant accounts in order to avoid misrepresentation based on my own embodied assumptions.

In many regards, I was also a stranger in my participants' world. I grew up in a different culture, speaking a different language, in a different part of the globe that experienced dramatic transformations of the fall of the Soviet-linked socialist regime and the establishment of a new form of democratically elected, capitalist government. Both my native country and my own family within it possessed considerably fewer economic resources than the families in my study. I had children at a much younger age, with far less preparation and fewer financial resources than participants in my study. I approached childbirth and breastfeeding with the same set of expectations I had developed in Hungary, where most women simply went to obstetricians for their care and were told what to do. I did not know about Lamaze classes or any other classes outside hospital courses that physicians recommended nor did I understand why anyone would want to take them. While I assumed that I would breastfeed, as I had heard—although rarely seen—others do in Hungary, I had neither a specific goal for breastfeeding, nor was I aware of the "health benefits" of breastfeeding. At the time of our first son's birth, I did not know what the acronym of SIDS stood for and had never heard of parents sleeping in the same bed with their babies. I acquired more of this knowledge over time, largely through academic study. These experiences distinguished me from my participants and helped to position them in the role of experts as I learned about aspects of middle-class U.S. culture that I had not personally encountered or had only read about in books while taking graduate seminars.

With the passage of time, both men and women participants' perceptions of me shifted from a more expert-stranger positioning toward a kind of kinship brought about by the intensity of my participation in participants' family lives. These kinds of relationships and the appreciation I developed for both differences and similarities between my participants and myself constitute some of the most treasured aspects of fieldwork.

## Overview of the Book

The book is divided into seven chapters, followed by a brief conclusion. Each chapter offers a specific set of arguments that draw on a diverse set of literatures in order to illuminate different aspects of my research. These chapters can be seen as bits of mirrored glass that, while they each provide a unique vantage point, when placed together constitute a larger mosaic of one particular perspective on the cultural dilemmas of nighttime breastfeeding and sleep in the United States.

The seven body chapters are loosely organized into four parts. The first part comprises a single chapter that lays the groundwork for my anthropological approach to nighttime breastfeeding. Drawing on a diverse body of sociocultural and medical anthropological scholarship I develop the concept of "embodied moral dilemmas" raised by nighttime breastfeeding as a lens through which we can glean unique insight into the complex dynamics of American personhood, family relations, biomedicine, and the far-reaching effects of capitalism. While I have attempted to make my discussion of the relevant concepts accessible, readers unfamiliar with the discipline of anthropology may find this chapter challenging. These readers may wish to move forward to the next chapters, in which I pursue the above themes through historical and ethnographic examples. I welcome readers to dip back into this chapter based on their interest.

The following two chapters address the role of biomedicine and capitalism in breastfeeding and infant sleep in the U.S. using historical and ethnographic approaches. In chapter 2 I examine struggles over who possesses authoritative knowledge about breastfeeding and sleep to illuminate the complex and contradictory ways in which women and biomedicine are implicated in these processes. I explore the consequences of these complexities for U.S. feminist discussions of breastfeeding and create the framework for the analysis of the dilemmas that participants encounter in their experiences of breastfeeding. The third chapter explores the role of childbirth education courses in mediating biomedical approaches to breastfeeding and infant sleep practices through a comparative ethnographic analysis of two childbirth education sites. I suggest that childbirth education that includes breastfeeding courses is a privileged good that comprises a part of middle-class consumption practices, which constitute cultural ideals of parenting. Moreover, I show how the consumption of specific kinds of childbirth education courses provides different frameworks for parents' and children's personhoods and family relationships with one another within the context of a capitalist political economic system. Through their negotiations of biomedical authority in breastfeeding and infant sleep practices, parents engage with these frameworks based on their own histories and experiences.

The fourth and fifth chapters address the gendered negotiation of the dilemmas posed by breastfeeding, keeping nighttime concerns in focus. In the fourth chapter I provide ethnographic insight into middle-class breastfeeding mothers' experiences of the moral contradictions between the simultaneous valuation of the health effects of breastfeeding and the concern over its actual praxis. Mothers' accounts reveal that these contradictions engender modes of stigmatization, which can have profound embodied consequences even for those who achieve relatively greater success in meeting biomedical breastfeeding recommendations. In the fifth chapter I examine men's contributions to breastfeeding and document their manifold support without which breastfeeding would not have been sustainable for most mothers in the study. I show that men's vital support for breastfeeding constitutes an important kin-making process that simultaneously helps overcome structural and cultural barriers to breastfeeding and mitigates the effects of stigmatization. Furthermore, this "kin work" plays an important part in the construction of fathers' personhoods and the fashioning of social class.

The final two chapters bring nighttime concerns to the forefront of analysis. The sixth chapter investigates the house as a primary site for consolidating and renegotiating middle-class cultural models of personhood and family relationships. My ethnography illustrates how the process of negotiating nighttime breastfeeding and sleep disrupts cultural expectations for children's personhood and kin relations that are built into the very structure of the house. In a similar vein, in the seventh chapter I address the radical disjunctures between cultural models of nighttime, which are heavily influenced by capitalist labor practices, and the disruptive modes of temporality posed by the experiences of nighttime breastfeeding. Parents' experiences of moral ambivalence that arose in the struggles of navigating these conflicts renegotiated these modes of space and time, reshaped their models of personhood and relations with one another, and subtly reworked the effects of capitalism in families' everyday lives.

In the conclusion, I share my key insights into the cultural, historical, and structural reasons behind the controversies that surround breastfeeding in the U.S. Ultimately, I hope to show readers that careful anthropological research can transcend divisive media debates and reveal mothers' and their partners' struggles to negotiate the cultural dilemmas that arise from negotiating an embodied practice that is at once revered, unsupported, and stigmatized. These families' efforts to breastfeed reproduce social inequities even while they simultaneously challenge some of the pervasive effects of neoliberal capitalism, linking their local embodied practices to global political economic and cultural forces. Finally, I draw on these insights to suggest more effective ways to support breastfeeding families.

## Notes

1. All names in the book, including that of the city itself, and any details that would potentially identify specific persons have been changed in order to protect participants' confidentiality.
2. Wright and Schanler 2001; Crowther, Reynolds, and Tansey 2009; Grummer-Strawn and Shealy 2009.
3. Galtry 2000, 2001, 2003; Galtry and Callister 2005; Li et al. 2005; Calnen 2007, 2010.
4. See, for instance, Wolf 2007, 2011; Hausman 2003, 2011; Stearns 2010, 2009; Rosin 2009; Kukla 2006, 2005; Blum 1999; Carter 1995; Murphy 2004, 2003, 2000, 1999; Lee 2007, 2011; Lee, Macvarish, and Bristow 2010; Knaak 2010; Wall 2001; Schmied and Lupton 2001; Lupton 2000.
5. See chapters 1 and 2.
6. Hausman 2003, 2011.
7. See Gram 2009; Foster 2010; Hess 2011; Knowles 2012. The fact that breastfeeding and breastmilk can also generate sexual arousal and play a role in pornography as well as in other sexual practices contributes to perceptions of the sexual qualities of breastfeeding as inappropriate or transgressive (Foss 2012; Giles 2003; Bartlett 2005; Bartlett and Shaw 2010).
8. Gowen 2009; Cook 2010.
9. Jojo329 2009.
10. Hausman 2003.
11. Hausman 2003, 2011.
12. Attachment parenting is a philosophy of parenting based on psychological research on the significance of early, secure attachments to caregivers in child development and later adult well-being. This approach emphasizes that being responsive to the child's needs and providing

consistent loving care enables children to form secure attachments (Attachment Parenting International 2008). I discuss Sears and attachment parenting in greater detail in chapter 2.
13. "Co-sleeping" is the term my participants as well as most media reports on this subject use to describe bed-sharing sleep arrangements. McKenna, Ball, and Gettler (2007) have argued that because sleeping in a proximal configuration—within arms' reach—is possible on other surfaces, the two terms "co-sleeping" and "bed sharing" should be separated in order to specify the context of each arrangement. I follow his suggestion in my own usage throughout this paper, specifying the configuration of co-sleeping, but retain participants' original language in quotations.
14. Lowen 2012; M. Williams 2012.
15. Jamie Lynn Grumet, the mother featured on the *Time* magazine cover, has been critical in her blog about her portrayal both on the cover and in the accompanying article (Grumet 2012) as well as in news interviews. She has recently appeared on the cover of *Pathways to Wellness* with an accompanying article that clarifies her position, her aim to reduce stigma for breastfeeding, as well as her larger goal of raising awareness about orphans and HIV among children in Ethiopia (Reagan 2012). Unlike in the *Time* magazine cover, where she did not have the right to select the image for the cover, she retained this right for the *Pathways* cover. On this latter cover, Grumet is depicted breastfeeding her now four-year-old son, lovingly embraced by her husband and other child, who is adopted from Ethiopia.
16. Ball and Volpe 2012.
17. Kendall-Tackett, Cong, and Hale 2010.
18. McKenna, Ball, and Gettler 2007.
19. Willinger et al. 2003; McCoy et al. 2004; Kendall-Tackett, Cong, and Hale 2010.
20. AAP Task Force on Sudden Infant Death Syndrome 2005, 2011.
21. Fallone, Owens, and Deane 2002; Zimmerman and Bell 2010.
22. Ball and Volpe 2012.
23. Throughout the book I use the term "biomedicalization" and "biomedicine" to refer to the rise in global prominence and local manifestations of a particular system of medicine that arose in Western Europe in the seventeenth and eighteenth centuries. Lock and Nguyen (2010:57–82) describe these changes, their antecedents, and contemporaneous modes of medicalization elsewhere in the world and use the term "medicalization" in these descriptions. Throughout their text, however, they carefully distinguish "biomedicine" as a specific medical system. Clarke and colleagues (2003) employ "biomedicalization" to distinguish a more recent period in medicalization characterized by the rise of technoscience in contemporary medicine. In contrast, I use the term biomedicalization even in the context of earlier historical periods to specify the medical system to which I refer in an effort to distinguish

it from the professionalization of medicine undertaken in ancient Egypt or nineteenth century Japan, for instance.
24. See Ginsburg and Rapp 1995; Davis-Floyd and Sargent 1997; Clarke et al. 2003; Browner and Sargent 2011; Lock and Nguyen 2010.
25. For instance, see Apple 2006; Murphy 2003.
26. See, for instance, Metzl and Kirkland 2010; Lupton 1995; Rose, O'Malley, and Valverde 2006; Murphy 2000 on the neoliberal governance of risk in health.
27. On the relationship of reproductive bodily processes and the reproduction of the nation, see Ginsburg and Rapp 1995; Lock and Kaufert 1998; Browner and Sargent 2011.
28. This study was carried out with Institutional Review Board approval from the University of Michigan.
29. This stands in contrast to the brief weeks or few months of breastfeeding carried out by the majority of Americans.
30. Several authors have explored this concept in relation to reproduction. See Orit Avishai (2007) for a contemporary discussion of breastfeeding, Judith Walzer Leavitt (1986) on the history of childbirth and Jacqueline Wolf (2001) on the history of breastfeeding in the U.S.
31. See chapter 2.
32. Initially, I had planned to undertake a comparative study of two groups of parents: one that planned to bring their babies into their beds and another that did not. These goals were shaped by indications in my preliminary research that such groups might exist in the Green City area. However, I was not able to find parents who planned to bring their children into their beds. While four couples included the possibility of such arrangements within their plan, and one couple made these plans more explicit, none made a full commitment to such a plan and all purchased additional sleep equipment. Therefore, I altered my study to accommodate my participants' plans and practices. My attempts at finding a group of participants who planned to bring their babies into their beds are also reflected in the greater number of participants I recruited from one particular childbirth education site ("Holistic Center"). Based on my research, I anticipated finding more couples with explicit bed-sharing plans in courses at this site and therefore attended additional childbirth education sessions there to carry out my objective.
33. The median income was approximately $44,500 in the state and $42,000 in the U.S. at the same time (U. S. Census Bureau 2000).
34. Nearly nine out of ten Green City residents possessed some level of education beyond high school (compared with 51 percent in U.S.), with four out of ten having master's, professional, or doctorate degrees (8.9 percent in U.S.) (U. S. Census Bureau 2000).
35. Approximately 85 percent initiation rate v. 67 percent in the state and 72 percent in the U.S. at the time of my research (CDC 2010a, 2010b).
36. Bobel 2001.
37. See Elias et al. 1986; La Leche League International 2007.

38. Considered by U.S. standards.
39. See McKenna, Ball and Gettler 2007 for a review.
40. Here I mean "mothers to living children." The term "mother" is a problematic distinction, since several participants had suffered pregnancy losses prior to their first live births.
41. A few interviews were not recorded because of initial discomfort with the recorder and due to recorder malfunction.
42. The potential use of the log originated from Ball and colleagues (Ball, Hooker, and Kelly 1999) study, but it was not systematically implemented in my own work. Indeed, the log yielded different kinds of ethnographic insights, explored in chapter 7.
43. Although the 2005 recommendations suggested exclusive breastfeeding for the first six months and continuing with breastfeeding through the first year of the baby's life, on-line resources and in-person interactions with medical staff often gave parents different messages that failed to highlight the importance of exclusive breastfeeding and the total duration of breastfeeding.
44. See comparative statistical information in CDC 2010a, 2010b; Willinger et al. 2003; McCoy et al. 2004.
45. Rapp 2001; Ginsburg and Rapp 1995; Davis-Floyd 2004; Layne 2003, 1996.
46. Brondo et al. 2009; Wasson et al. 2008.
47. Brown and de Casanova 2010; Barlow and Chapin 2010; and previous note.
48. See Narayan 1993; Jacobs-Huey 2002; Bunzl 2004.
49. See Armbruster and Laerke 2009 for a recent review of these discussions.

*Chapter 1*

# EMBODIED CULTURAL DILEMMAS
## AN ANTHROPOLOGICAL APPROACH TO THE STUDY OF NIGHTTIME BREASTFEEDING AND SLEEP

One of the main objectives of this book is to show how anthropological ways of thinking can help illuminate points of conflict or tension that are often treated in a simplistic and polarized fashion in popular media. Specifically, while it is tempting to attribute the tensions over nighttime care of babies to conflicts over the ostensible superiority of breastfeeding or formula feeding, or solitary sleep versus co-sleeping, a more thorough engagement reveals that these bodily activities are entangled in a series of sociocultural domains that may not be readily apparent to a casual observer or even to new families attempting to navigate this embattled terrain. My goal is to offer an alternative perspective to these debates and reposition both dominant and more marginal models of nighttime infant care in the U.S. within the context of the rich sociocultural, historical, and interpersonal relations in which they exist. In this chapter, I bring these theoretical concerns to the forefront of analysis in order to uncover the reasons why nighttime infant care constitutes a cultural dilemma in America.

I propose an understanding of breastfeeding and sleep as *embodied*—simultaneously biological and cultural processes that are enacted and experienced through the body. First, I show how seemingly "natural" bodily activities are culturally constituted and fundamentally social, relational processes. This relationality has a specific inter-bodily dimension in the case of breastfeeding and co-sleeping, which involve the coordination and direct proximity of at least two bodies. Next, I delve deeper into the social relational aspects of the embodied processes of nighttime breastfeeding and sleep by examining how these interactions participate in the making of persons and family relationships (kinship or relatedness, in anthropological terms). I introduce the concept of embodied moral dilemmas as an important site for understanding the reproduction and potential transformation of cultural patterns. In the following section, I extend this discussion to show the multiple ways in which these embodied processes participate in larger political economic relationships that reflect and reproduce different aspects of capitalism. This theoretical framework ultimately enables me to use my ethnographic findings to show how the dilemmas posed by the embodied experiences of nighttime breastfeeding and sleep not only reveal and reproduce existing cultural patterns, but create opportunities for change.

## The Embodied Social Practice of Nighttime Breastfeeding and Sleep

Marcel Mauss ([1935] 1973), in his essay "The Techniques of the Body," suggested that bodily "habits" or *habitus* that may seem exclusively biological, such as the way people walk, "do not vary just with individuals and their imitations; they vary especially between societies, educations, proprieties and fashions, prestiges" ([1935] 1973:101). By establishing that "body techniques," or the ways in which people use their bodies, are acquired through socialization, Mauss opened the way for the investigation of bodily practice as a "social fact" (Durkheim [1895] 1982). Mauss's approach is particularly remarkable in its multi-dimensionality, since he considered embodied experiences, the processes by which people acquire body techniques, and their social uses and effects within the same framework. Since Marcel Mauss's seminal essay, considerable attention has been devoted to bodily practices and embodiment in anthropology and related disciplines.[1] Breastfeeding, sleep, and their interrelationships, however, have figured only marginally in these discussions.

Despite the burgeoning literature on embodiment, Talal Asad (1997) argued that anthropology could further benefit from a reexamination of Mauss's original arguments. Asad returns to Mauss's concept of the "habitus," suggesting that through this concept Mauss sought to "define an anthropology of *practical reason*. The human body is not to be viewed simply as the passive recipient of 'cultural imprints' that are 'clothed in local history and culture,' but as the *self-developable* means for achieving a range of human objects—from styles of physical movement ... through modes of emotional being ... to kinds of spiritual experience" (1997:47–48). Asad's emphasis helps direct attention to the social, relational way in which people acquire *habitus*, and his emphasis on practical reason opens Mauss's work to diverse analysis that includes a moral component.[2] To investigate the dilemmas engendered by breastfeeding and sleep, I follow Asad's call and first examine the ways in which these body techniques contribute to differentially enculturated modes of being.

A growing body of literature, written primarily by feminist sociologists and women's studies scholars, focuses on the complex and contradictory embodied experiences of breastfeeding in Europe, North America, and Australia. In these settings, breastfeeding is a body technique learned primarily in hospitals under the supervision of medical personnel and then practiced primarily at home in the first few weeks after birth. Medical supervision then shifts to the baby, primarily through monitoring elimination patterns and weight gain.[3] Furthermore, most women in these areas experience breastfeeding as a relatively short-term practice, lasting a few weeks or months, with artificial milk feeding quickly integrated and becoming the dominant mode of feeding by around three months postpartum (CDC 2013a). These studies suggest that while women often expect their embodied experiences to mimic the idealized maternal sentiments depicted in breastfeeding promotional materials, many experience ambivalent, negative, painful, revulsive, and mechanized/disembodied sensations that often lead to cessation of breastfeeding.[4] There is growing attention to how women experience expressing their milk using breast pumps, which are becoming increasingly important in scientifically managed breastfeeding, especially in cases of premature and ill babies and when women return to work.[5] Sexual feelings during breastfeeding can be particularly disruptive to the maintenance of the separation between the sexual and nurturing aspects of the maternal body.[6] At the same time, women can also experience sensual and welcome sexual pleasure, comfort, empowerment, and a sense of closeness and connectedness to their children.[7] Avishai (2007, 2011) has recently argued that women do not necessarily experience breastfeeding in dichotomous positive or negative frames; instead they may encounter several different, often contradictory experiences at the same time and over the course of the breastfeeding process.

Considerably less attention has been paid to women's experiences of breastfeeding in other cultural settings, albeit with some notable exceptions.[8] Perhaps most famously, Nancy Scheper-Hughes (1993) described *nervoso*, a state of stress and anxiety, which left women in a poor Brazilian shantytown feeling spent, exhausted, and unable to make breastmilk for their children—with enormous consequences for the children's health and survival. Scheper-Hughes' ethnography remains exceptional both in its attention to the embodied dimensions of experience as well as in its astute historical and political economic analysis. Scheper-Hughes described the appropriation of land for the growing of sugarcane that resulted in the mass eviction of poor people, who used the land as their primary source of sustenance. The poor were then forced to live in shantytowns with little opportunity for earning money for food and with limited access to clean water. The stresses of hunger, illness, and high levels of violence, combined with the promotion of infant formula by Nestlé that followed the path of USAID distribution of powdered milk, led mothers to believe that they were not capable of producing adequate breastmilk for their children. Scheper-Hughes' work, therefore, serves as an important guide for a social and relational study of embodiment grounded in political economy, which I take up below.

The embodied dimensions of sleep have been gaining recognition thanks mainly to the work of a small number of scholars, most especially historian Roger Ekirch (2005) and sociologist Simon Williams (2011, 2007, 2005; Williams and Crossley 2008) and some others (Steger and Brunt 2003; Brunt and Steger 2008). Ekirch's (2005) masterful study of the culture of sleep in Western Europe between circa 1500 and 1750 provides a much-needed historical dimension to this work. Through the use of diverse sources, Ekirch shows that early western European experiences of sleep differed dramatically from contemporary Euro-American ones in several key ways, of which I highlight just a few. First, Ekirch shows the widespread polyphasic practice of sleep, wherein sleep took place in multiple chunks, some during the daytime and some during the night. Similar polyphasic sleep patterns are documented in cross-cultural studies, such as in the case of Mediterranean practices of "siesta" and Japanese practices of napping. Second, Ekirch documents the complex social interactions during the night, including sexual relations, interactions with children, and bodily elimination. Ekirch is careful not to romanticize historical accounts of sleep as somehow more "peaceful" or closer to "nature," showing that nights were filled with many disruptions as well as dangers (including sickness, violence, and fire).

Simon Williams (2005) asserts that sociologists have neglected the study of sleep because they considered it to be a time away from social life. Instead, Williams argues that sleep should be regarded as an important social practice that can be examined on three mutually intersecting levels of analysis: the individual/(non)experiential,[9] social/interactional, and societal/institutional levels. Although Williams' effort to reposition sleep as an important domain of social analysis is foundational, I argue that in the realm of sleep that I describe, the individual/(non)experiential level and the social/interactional levels cannot be separated. More recent sociological research on sleep has shifted toward a more relational perspective that incorporates a life course perspective,[10] and addresses children,[11] the burdens and gendered negotiations of nighttime caretaking of children and elders,[12] and couples' interaction in sleep.[13] My own anthropological approach, drawn from the comparative perspective of shared sleep as a common social practice across many cultures, as well as the anthropological emphasis on social relations through which persons are produced, takes this relationality as foundational. As such, I consider the embodied qualities and experiences of sleep both in the context of and as producers of these social relationships and the personhood of children and parents. This approach also accommodates insights from biological anthropology about the physiological interrelationship of mothers' and infants' bodies during sleep and breastfeeding,[14] incorporating the material qualities of the interactions of slumbering and nourishing/feeding bodies that move between different degrees of awareness.

Thus far, biological anthropologists have undertaken the bulk of research in breastfeeding and sleep practices and have incorporated some ethnographic dimensions to their work.[15] A growing literature examines the interrelationship of breastfeeding and sleep, led by biological anthropologists James McKenna, Helen Ball, and their colleagues. These scholars have drawn on physiological data from sleep laboratories and participant homes, survey and interview data, cross-cultural evidence, as well as non-human primate data and other evidence from studies of human evolution, to argue that the evolution of breastfeeding and sleep are interlinked processes. According to this research, mother-child co-sleeping is a highly adaptive behavior that entails a complex set of physiological relationships between the child's and the mother's body and that plays a critical role in facilitating breastfeeding as well as in the thermo- and respiratory regulation of the infant.[16] These studies document the mutual regulation of sleep, wherein babies' and mothers' sleep is coordinated and mothers respond to subtle cues of babies and breastfeed them without either one fully awakening (McKenna, Ball, and Gettler 2007). Ball and Klingaman's (2007) recent work suggests that breastfeeding mothers who practice bed sharing adopt a specific physical position without any instruction. This side-lying position, with the arms encircling the baby who is facing the mother's breast, creates a sleep environment that maximizes breastfeeding and other physiological contact between the mother and the child, while also protecting the child from external hazards, including those common in western sleep environments, such as pillows and blankets. McKenna suggests that breastfeeding with co-sleeping may reduce Sudden Infant Death Syndrome (SIDS) and has other psychosocial benefits for mothers and children.[17] McKenna, Ball and colleagues have used their findings to challenge prevailing medical advice about infant sleep and have advocated for an integrative approach toward breastfeeding and sleep.[18]

Through their integrative approach, these scholars have shown the subtle ways in which bodily interactions are both shaped by and influence their cultural and material environments. Ball and colleagues (2006) have also documented substantial effects of even seemingly minor differences in postpartum sleep arrangements on breastfeeding. They found that infants in the U.K. randomized to sleep in free-standing hospital bassinets breastfed significantly less frequently than infants randomly assigned to side-car cribs attached to the bed or in the bed with an attached rail during their hospital stay. Importantly, those assigned to the hospital sleep arrangements that offered unhindered interaction between mothers and babies had significantly higher rates of exclusive breastfeeding even after sixteen weeks, indicating that early sleep arrangements play an important role in the establishment and maintenance of breastfeeding. These findings, in turn, may also help explain women's reports of insufficient milk, a main reason women stop breastfeeding (Ball and Klingaman 2007). This work provides an excellent example of the ways in which the very biology of human bodies is constituted in particular local circumstances, creating "local biologies" that reflect their cultural, political economic, and historical circumstances.[19]

At the same time, there is also evidence that the increase in breastfeeding rates can shift cultural perceptions about sleep practices. Ball, Hooker, and Kelly's (1999) prospective study of sleep arrangements in Britain suggests a similar intended pattern of sleep to Morelli and colleagues' (1992) findings: nearly all parents planned to have their babies sleep in the same room but not in the same bed as them for a few weeks, followed by moving them to a separate room. Contrary to expectations, however, although very few parents shared a bed with their babies habitually every night, the authors documented that a large number of infants slept with their parents regularly for part of the night or at least occasionally. Thus, co-sleeping was more common than both what parents planned and what researchers expected based on Euro-American ideologies of solitary sleep for children. Significantly, this study also documented the strong association between breastfeeding and co-sleeping (Ball 2003). Both mothers and fathers in the sample reported that it felt "right" for them to bring their baby to bed for breastfeeding and that this practice reduced the fatigue of nighttime feedings (Ball, Hooker, and Kelly 2000). Similar trends have been documented by others (Willinger et al. 2003; Kendall-Tackett, Cong, and Hale 2010), demonstrating how the very practice of nighttime breastfeeding and shared sleep can have powerful effects in shaping cultural ideologies.

Alma Gottlieb's (2004) ethnography of the culture of infancy among the Beng in West Africa captures some of these sensibilities from a cultural perspective as she considers the interactions between infant feeding and sleep practices. Gottlieb demonstrates her ethnographic strength in both drawing upon her own experiences of parenting to illuminate a particular domain of life that is usually left unexamined, while simultaneously subjecting her experiences to a rigorous comparative ethnographic analysis that enables her to see both Beng and her own approaches in their full cultural depths. Furthermore, as Gottlieb draws on the work of Margaret Mead, her lens is sharpened by attention to mothers, grandmothers, and other caregivers as well as the children themselves in their interactions. Although mothers are the focus of my own study, Gottlieb's sensitive approach to children and their social lives informs my work.

In Gottlieb's account, it is through the comparative analytical framework that we learn about different embodied dimensions of Beng babies' lives, including their nighttime co-sleeping and breastfeeding. Gottlieb shows that in the context of religious ideologies wherein parents must convince and entice their children to fully leave the afterlife and remain with them, the challenges of nighttime disruptions, including crying and frequent nursing, are addressed in a simple, matter-of-fact way, with little concern. In contrast, Gottlieb suggests that within the context of Euro-American middle-class ideologies, separate spaces similarly convey important values. Gottlieb states, "At the sociological level, the lesson conveyed by a bassinet, cradle, or crib that is placed in its own room at some point in the infant's first year is in keeping with the American-capitalist morality lesson that individuals ought to make their own way in the world on the basis of their own courage and efforts" (2004:184). Ben-Ari (2008) offers an analysis of some of these middle-class lessons based on an overview of previous ethnographic work and parenting books, which similarly attends to relationships between parents and children and expectations for children's personhood. A full-scale ethnographic investigation of these themes, however, has not been undertaken. My study could be considered the comparative ethnographic investigation of just such an "American-capitalist morality lesson," its confrontation with the embodied experiences of nighttime breastfeeding and sleep, and the transformative consequences for personhood, family relationships, and capitalism.

## Making Persons and Kinship through Breastfeeding and Sleep

On the surface, neither infant feeding nor sleep belong to the study of kinship, since they do not figure into mainstream American conceptualizations of relatedness. After all, contemporary Euro-American discourses emphasize breastfeeding solely between biological mothers and their children, people already conceptualized as kin. Furthermore, sleep in this cultural context is considered a time of removal from social life,[20] thereby limiting its potential social role. Yet, upon closer examination, these assertions reveal highly specific cultural ideologies about kinship, personhood, breastfeeding, and sleep that limit our conceptualization of these processes. Recent work in kinship studies highlighted the mutual constitution of kinship and personhood; that is, persons are produced through their engagement with others as well as their material surroundings (e.g., houses, food, land, etc.), and kin relations simultaneously arise from these engagements.[21] Investigations of new reproductive technologies have played a particularly important role in these discussions, since the intersection of global movements of technologies and ideologies with local understandings often reveals previously hidden understandings of taken-for-granted relations as well as new possibilities for making personhood and kinship.[22] While breastfeeding and co-sleeping may appear to be rather "old" reproductive technologies, with ancient roots going back to the origins of mammals, the new kinship studies enables them to be viewed as reproductive technologies that play an equally active role in the constitution of personhood and kin relations.

Janet Carsten (2004) astutely described how anthropologists have tended to set up a dichotomous analysis of Western, Euro-American bounded conceptions of personhood and kinship determined by biology against non-Western notions of personhood that are constituted through relations.[23] Indeed, historical and ethnographic research in Euro-American settings demonstrates that what is understood by "biology," "biogenetic substance," or "shared blood" is far more complex than it initially appears.[24] Carsten argues that such dichotomies derive from the reliance on legal and philosophical constructions of personhood and kinship instead of closer ethnographic study. Carsten acknowledges that both bounded individualism and biogenetic kinship have a strong presence in everyday lives in the West, but that careful ethnography reveals that these ideologies co-exist with other, more relational and processual ones.[25]

Viewed in this light, breastfeeding and sleep provide a heretofore-unexplored perspective on American person- and kin-making practices. Moreover, in the context of historical changes that have nearly eliminated and thoroughly transformed its practice in the U.S., breastfeeding may be quite a new reproductive technology for women who lack the cultural knowledge to facilitate it. Together, these perspectives suggest important possibilities for the exploration of kin- and person-making through the new/old reproductive technologies of breastfeeding and sleep. Let us consider these arguments in further detail.

Cross-cultural studies indicate that breastfeeding can play a critical role in establishing kinship relations. Katherine Dettwyler (1988), for instance, shows that women in Mali in a patriarchal setting are not considered related to the children to whom they give birth until they breastfeed them. Those women who do not breastfeed their children risk forfeiting their maternal relationship. Milk kinship is well known in Islamic settings, where women who nurse children become related to them and the children who breastfed from one woman become milk siblings who cannot marry.[26] On the island of Langkawi in Malaysia, breastfeeding is one component of an intricate set of feeding relations—including feeding food cooked at the hearth and nourishment gained from the mother's blood during pregnancy—through which children are incorporated into kin groups.[27]

The historically documented instances of closeness between wet-nurses and children, as well as concerns about the passing on of a wet-nurse's undesirable characteristics through the act of breastfeeding,[28] suggest that in the past breastfeeding has also played an important role in the construction of kinship and personhood in the United States. These sentiments linger in contemporary concerns about emotional states being passed on to children through breastfeeding. Recently, some women in the U.S. and in similar settings where wet-nursing has been replaced by formula feeding have returned to the practice of nursing one another's babies and/or sharing their breastmilk (Pleshette 2008; Eats on Feets). There are hints in the emerging literature that some of these exchanges are conceived of in terms of kin relations both among women and among women and children, such as in the case of "milk mamas"—a term used by some to refer to women who have shared their milk with children other than their own biogenetic offspring. Donating breastmilk can also be a part of the process of forging a form of relatedness to children who receive this milk—some women describe that they feel a special emotional bond to the children who are recipients of this milk, even if the recipients are constructed in their imaginations because meeting the children is not a possibility. Once relatedness is no longer simply assumed as given but as made, the tensions surrounding nighttime breastfeeding and sleep offer similarly important opportunities for investigating the role that these embodied processes have in the configuration of kin relations and the production of persons.

Although the social characteristics of sleep are well documented historically and across cultures, the role of this sociality in producing persons and relatedness and its relationship to nighttime breastfeeding has only been given attention in select ethnographic settings.[29] Cross-cultural comparisons reveal that in most cultures children sleep with adults (usually mothers) and siblings.[30] Sleep plays an important role in forging and reinforcing kin as well as community relations.[31] For instance, Caudill and Plath (1966) argued that in Japan children are considered separate beings at birth that need to be brought into kin relations through the act of sleeping together. In this case, co-sleeping produces important kin ties as well as a social, interrelated person.[32] Although pediatric advice in Euro-American cultures has emphasized the importance of solitary sleep in the last 150 years, there is considerable diversity even in these cultures in parent attitudes and practices of infant sleep.[33] For instance, frequent room sharing has been documented in Italy (A. Wolf et al.

1996), and bed sharing into the school years is common in Sweden (Welles-Nystrom 2005). Ethnographic studies also document the prevalence of the close interrelationship and matter-of-fact acceptance of night-nursing and co-sleeping.[34] In many settings when children are weaned, often when the mother is pregnant with the next child, the child moves to sleep with another adult or sibling.[35] The relationship between breastfeeding and sleep in Euro-American settings has not been adequately explored in ethnographic studies, but is also variable and includes bed sharing practices.[36]

The U.S. stands out as one of the only places surveyed where there are particularly strong cultural prohibitions against co-sleeping and even against babies staying in the same room with parents.[37] Here, solitary sleep practices also seem to play a significant role in shaping the personhood of children and their relationship with parents, but with a different goal in mind—to produce a self-reliant, "independent" child.[38] Despite the prominence of pediatric advice that condemns co-sleeping, there is evidence that some American cultural groups adhere to alternative ideologies of sleep.[39] Abbott's (1992) study of Appalachian families in Eastern Kentucky, for instance, documents a long history of socially valued bed sharing and room sharing that remained in place at the time of her research. Abbott argues that these practices play an important role in producing a sense of connectedness and belonging in the community. African Americans also practice higher rates of proximal sleep and bed sharing with children, and, in this case, the cultural value of independence is not opposed, but instead emerges through a sense of community (A. Wolf et al. 1996). Nonetheless, the ethnographically documented relationship of breastfeeding and co-sleeping seems mostly absent in these examples. Abbott does not discuss breastfeeding in relation to sleep arrangements, and among African Americans bed sharing often takes place without breastfeeding.[40] Viewing these findings in a historical context, it appears that the domains of proximal sleep and breastfeeding have become culturally separated in most of the United States.

Comparative studies provide insight into the difficulties nighttime breastfeeding poses for established norms of sleeping in the United States. In Morelli and colleague's (1992) study of middle-class American mothers and Mayan Guatemalan mothers, the latter co-slept with their children until weaning, while most of the U.S. women did not feel comfortable with feeding their babies in the parental bed. Among American breastfeeding mothers, nighttime feedings were considered disruptive and inconvenient, and mothers diminished or discontinued them by six months of age. These findings may reflect the particular historical moment when breastfeeding was once again becoming more common but was practiced in new sociohistorical circumstances of prevailing solitary sleep practices as well as highly scheduled feedings (see chapter 2).

The sexual relationship between parents and the fear of potentially incestuous sexual relations between mother and child is one documented aspect of kin relations that also appears to play a role in avoiding co-sleeping and breastfeeding.[41] In many other settings, postpartum sex taboos prohibit sex between spouses during the period of breastfeeding.[42] During lactation, sexual relations with a man may be associated with harming the child through "spoiling" or the "drying up" of the mother's breastmilk.[43] Euro-American concerns about breastfeeding and incest, however, appear to depart from those in other cultural settings, and are partly fueled by the sexualized perception of breasts.[44] Co-sleeping when combined with breastfeeding appears to reinforce the incestuous potential of breastfeeding, especially when practiced beyond the first few months of the child's life. Crook's (2008) historical study, for instance, documents Victorian-era English concerns about the incestuous intermingling of working class bodies in shared sleeping spaces. He argues that these moral concerns about inappropriate sexuality between parents and children was a major motivation for designing housing that provided separate bedrooms for children that were also segregated by sex. In England as well as in the United States, shifts in marital relations toward a prioritization of romantic love to the exclusion of children may have played an important role in the development of these concerns (J.H. Wolf 2001; Abbott 1992). Finally, the spread of Freudian psychoanalytic frameworks highlighted problematic sexuality in personal development, especially in relation to familial interactions, leading to growing concern about the potential witnessing of sexual acts in the parental bed and consequent incestuous Oedipal fantasies (Lozoff, Wolf, and Davis 1984; McKenna and McDade 2005).

Contemporary ambivalence about shared sleep arrangements to facilitate nighttime breastfeeding, therefore, is not simply the product of changing medical advice, but rather reflects tensions between different cultural-historical models for the negotiation of kin relations between parents and children and for the socialization of infants into culturally acceptable persons. Each of these models carries a moral dimension that is not only buttressed by arguments, but also a sense of what "feels right"—sentiments that are deeply felt on a visceral level but are nevertheless tied to cultural ideologies. As new parents navigate the practical, bodily challenges of nighttime breastfeeding and sleep, they must also navigate the moral dilemmas raised by the very experiences of these intercorporeal relations.

*Embodied Moral Dilemmas and the Potential for Transformation*

Kinship scholar Michael Peletz (2001) has suggested that moral contradictions and ambivalence are not only central to the construction of kin relations, but also serve as excellent entry points for studying the emergent properties of human sociality.[45] Moments of ambivalence and their negotiation reveal the dynamic intersections of different domains that produce uncertainty, contestation, and potential change. Anthropologist Jarrett Zigon's (2011a, 2011b, 2010a, 2010b, 2009, 2008, 2007) recent work on moral personhood draws on Mauss's concept of the *habitus* to anchor these moments of tension and ambivalence in the lived body, highlighting moments of "moral breakdown" (2008:165) when a person is confronted with a particular situation that propels her to reflect upon and objectify largely unconscious, "embodied dispositions."[46] The challenges of nighttime breastfeeding and sleep offer an example of such moments of moral breakdown that are articulated in the bodily discomfort new parents experience with this aspect of nighttime care, which then offers them an opportunity to rework their moral (and ultimately larger cultural) framework for interacting with one another.[47]

Within the study of reproduction, there are many excellent examples of similar moral challenges, especially surrounding the new reproductive technologies. For instance, Rayna Rapp's (1999) work on amniocentesis examines the "moral breakdown" engendered by the new technologies of amniocentesis that force women to consider their fetuses in terms of statistical calculations of risk for genetic diseases and ultimately make decisions about whether they will terminate their pregnancy via abortion. Rapp's study stands out for its careful and wide-ranging consideration of the moral uncertainties entailed in every level of negotiating amniocentesis—by the laboratory, genetic counselors, physicians, and mothers themselves—while paying close attention to how these moral ambiguities are negotiated in culturally specific ways structured by social class, education, race and ethnicity, and gender. Rapp describes the participants in her study as "moral pioneers"—exploring the moral quandaries generated by emerging prenatal testing technologies. I suggest that the new biomedicalized frameworks for breastfeeding and infant sleep generate similar dilemmas that are sometimes considered matters of life and death, making parents and children in my study into moral pioneers as well.[48]

The negotiations of moral ambivalence about nighttime breastfeeding and sleep have far-reaching implications.[49] My study provides insight into how parents confront the dilemmas posed by the "novel" process of breastfeeding as well as related difficulties in configuring family sleep arrangements, and it documents these negotiations over the course of an entire year after birth. I argue that, in navigating these dilemmas over time, parents and their children ultimately reconfigure personhood and kinship in substantial ways and push against some of the boundaries of local-global political economic relationships.

## Reproducing Capitalism, Remaking Embodied Inequalities

An important aim of the book is to show that the bodily processes of nighttime breastfeeding and sleep not only participate in the reproduction of certain kinds of bodily habits and social relations within families, but that they also reproduce capitalist ideologies and systems of inequalities. Breastfeeding and related sleep practices take place in a society that is integrally linked to global capitalist systems of labor, production, and economy. Within this system, families participate in capitalist labor practices that attempt to maximize the labor potential of workers and make only minimal accommodations for women's reproductive labor, contributing to gendered inequalities in both the paid labor realm as well as in the household.[50] More subtly, capitalism is woven into the fabric of everyday life through space, time, and consumption practices.

Below, I highlight how breastfeeding and related sleep practices are part of biomedical approaches to the body that are themselves constituted by gendered capitalist ideologies, and how women's and families' abilities to negotiate the challenges of these bodily processes reproduce inequalities along racial and class lines. Second, I show how breastfeeding participates in global neoliberal capitalist systems both through breastfeeding promotion and through the growing interest in the biocapital of breastmilk.

### *The Embodied Reproduction of Inequalities*

In her book "The Woman in the Body," Emily Martin[51] (1987) famously described the powerful ways in which metaphors of the body as a machine, and women's bodies as deficient versions of male machine-bodies requiring constant regulation, have permeated our understanding of menstruation, childbirth, and menopause. Martin showed that these metaphors have material consequences in the biomedicalized approaches toward each of these bodily processes that result in the authoritative regulation of women's bodies, dehumanizing medical treatment, and an alienation of women's bodies from themselves. These consequences are experienced differently across divisions of social class and race, with poor women of color facing the compounding effects of oppression. At the same time, Martin also observed instances of struggle, contestation, and successful subversion of these power structures. For instance, she noted how some women evaded medical intervention in childbirth and how others responded with anger when they were mistreated by physicians or nurses. Martin was hopeful that through these experiences of oppression women could also gain a critical perspective that might be able to challenge the dominance of this capitalist system of biomedicalization that governs women's reproduction. Martin's work has been extended by other scholars to breastfeeding, most notably by Fiona Dykes (2005), who showed how the capitalist metaphors of "supply" and "demand" governed hospitals' approach to breastfeeding and was ultimately internalized both by midwives and by new mothers. These capitalist systems of understanding often undermined women's ability to breastfeed and contributed to their sense of being a failed machine, unable to meet the production quotas required of them. Furthermore, both Dykes (2009) and Millard (1990) address the importance of the clock in providing the temporal framework for these capitalist approaches to women's (and children's) bodies, providing benchmarks against which bodily indicators (e.g., milk production, number of minutes per feeding) are measured (see chapter 7).

Robbie Davis-Floyd's (2004) study of U.S. childbirth practices originates from a symbolic anthropological framework that lacks close engagement with political economic dynamics, but, when considered in relation to Martin's work, adds another important dimension to understanding women's lived experiences of highly capitalistic forms of medicine. Davis-Floyd's study, first published in 1992, examines how the cultural values of technology, science, patriarchy, and institutions embraced by what she terms the "technocratic model" of childbirth are communicated through biomedical practices. She argues that these practices ultimately constitute a rite of passage that transforms women into mothers. Later work has taken up this theme for the production of fatherhood as well. These studies have clear implications for how persons are constructed through embodied relations in capitalist systems.

Davis-Floyd's study, similar to my own, focused on middle-class mothers and built on Martin's insights about middle-class mothers' internalization and acceptance of patriarchal capitalist biomedical systems of reproduction. In fact, Davis-Floyd found that most of her participants believed that routine medical interventions in childbirth were not only acceptable, but necessary and beneficial. Only a minority of women struggled with these approaches, and even fewer delineated contrasting ideologies of childbirth. Although Davis-Floyd was not very optimistic about the potential of these alternative ideologies to subvert the technocratic model, she did note the presence of a group of women who recognized some of the problematic aspects of the technocratic model and hoped that through similar recognitions (and concerted activism) more holistic models would gain greater ground. When she revisited her earlier work in the second edition of the book (Davis-Floyd 2004), however, she found that many biomedical interventions had become significantly more acceptable (e.g., induction, epidural analgesia, Cesarean section) with the expansion of a humanistic model of medicine, wherein women are treated in a less obviously authoritarian fashion and there is a much greater emphasis on increasing women's comfort. In the next chapter, I explore the historical roots of this process whereby biomedical approaches to all aspects of childbearing have become normalized, arguing that wealthier women throughout this history were important agents in bringing about these changes. Furthermore, similar to Davis-Floyd, I document the differential ability of white middle-class parents to negotiate, contest, and subvert mainstream biomedical approaches in childbearing. Throughout the book, using the frameworks of stratified reproduction and intersectionality that I lay out below, I return to Martin's fundamental political economic concerns about how these middle-class parents' relatively successful ability to navigate the challenges of nighttime breastfeeding enables them to participate in the reproduction of privilege.

In their introduction to the pivotal volume "Conceiving the New World Order: The Global Politics of Reproduction," Faye Ginsburg and Rayna Rapp (1995) outlined their goal to reorient the study of reproduction to the center of anthropological theory. In this effort, the authors identified one major research direction as the study of "stratified reproduction," which they defined, following Shellee

Colen, as "the power relations by which some categories of people are empowered to nurture and reproduce, while others are disempowered" (1995:3). The framework of stratified reproduction encompasses close attention to the structural as well as cultural and political aspects of inequalities and has been adopted widely in the study of reproduction.[52] The concept of stratified reproduction dovetails with theories of intersectionality that argue for an integrated examination of the effects of class, race, and gender and their complex, interactive effects in daily life. Leith Mullings and colleagues (Mullings and Wali 2001; Mullings 1997; Schulz and Mullings 2006) have been particularly important in promoting this perspective to address the multiple, compounding dimensions of oppression on health.[53]

Together, the above works provide a frame for considering the production of inequality in the practice of breastfeeding and related sleep practices that I develop in greater detail in chapter 2.

The inequalities in these realms that are most pertinent to this study are the racial disparities in breastfeeding and SIDS rates. Although the rate of breastfeeding among African Americans has been increasing and recently made significant gains (Wright and Schanler 2001; Grummer-Strawn and Shealy 2009; CDC 2013b), African American women in 2008 still initiated breastfeeding at significantly lower rates than white U.S. women (58.9 percent compared with 75.2 percent) and these rates diminished to 31.1 percent (v. 46.6 percent) at six months and 12.5 percent (v. 24.3 percent) at twelve months postpartum (CDC 2013b). Furthermore, considerable variation exists among states, with lower rates of breastfeeding among African Americans in Southeastern states (CDC 2010c). These disparities contribute in substantial ways to poorer health outcomes among both mothers and children (Phillip and Jean-Marie 2007; CDC 2010c, 2012). The lack of breastfeeding may also play a role in the disproportionately higher incidence of SIDS among African American babies, who die of SIDS at twice the rate than their counterparts (Hauck, Herman, et al. 2003; McKenna and McDade 2005; U. S. Department of Health and Human Services 2011). An examination of the roots of these racial disparities in breastfeeding rates, as well as the often problematic public health campaigns that aim to reduce these disparities, will serve as a comparative analytical frame for investigating the practices of the primarily white, middle-class participants in my study.

While the framework of intersectionality has been traditionally used to explore the compounding effects of multiple sources of oppression for African American women, I suggest that it can also be employed to highlight the construction of privilege for white middle-class families.[54] Although I will argue that stigma surrounding the practice of breastfeeding and related sleep practices extends into privileged social groups, white middle-class parents' ability to navigate this stigma and other obstacles make their breastfeeding possible. In turn, these families materially benefit from the embodied health consequences of this privilege.

With regard to the racial aspects of this privilege, John Hartigan's research (1999, 2005) shows that the racial category of whiteness can be both marked and unmarked, depending on people's ability to follow middle-class gendered norms. Comparative studies of breastfeeding confirm that white working class women indeed have a more problematic relationship with breastfeeding due to various factors, including more hostile and demanding work environments as well as differences in family support for breastfeeding.[55] The implications of the complex intersections of race, class, and gender, such as those followed in Hartigan's (2005) work on "white trash," however, have yet to be adequately explored in relation to infant feeding and sleep practices. In the case of my participants, together with wealth, education, and predominately heteronormative family relationships, their whiteness constituted part of a constellation of privilege that enabled them to breastfeed and negotiate complexities that arose from this practice.

Hartigan's research points to some of the hidden class dimensions of cultural constructions of "whiteness." Sherry Ortner (2005) has argued that the concealments of the dynamics and effects of social class are pervasive both in popular U.S. discourses as well as in the social sciences.[56] Attention to social class informs my discussion of the history of childbirth, breastfeeding, and sleep (see chapter 2) and contributes to the documentation of the diversity within the "middle class" and differences in families' abilities to raise their children according their desires. Furthermore, my research provides insights into how parents' ideals for how to raise their children are themselves shaped by middle-class cultural norms and consumption practices. For instance, I describe the selection of a home, as well as the furnishings deemed necessary for purchasing prior to the baby's arrival,[57] and the class-based differences in the selection and use of maternity services, with a special focus on childbirth education classes. Using the insights of scholars of consumption and material culture, I argue that these material practices not only constitute class, but also have important implications for the relational constitution of personhood[58] (see chapter 3).

## Global (Bio)Capitalism

So far I have focused on the analysis of political economic relations, reproduction, and inequality in the specific local context of the United States. Yet, the capitalism that infuses my study is of a decidedly global character. Collier and Ong (2005) trace the origins of global forms of capitalism in Max Weber's writings, wherein he argued that although capitalism arose out of a very specific cultural context of ascetic Protestantism, it ultimately became a global phenomenon through "decontextualization and recontextualization, abstractability and movement, across diverse social and cultural situations and spheres of life" (2005:11). Collier and Ong argue that such global phenomena converge into "global assemblages" with other heterogeneous elements that enable their perpetuation across a variety of domains (2005:13). Multinational economic treaties, industry regulations, and state policies can all constitute global assemblages that sustain global political economic relations and enable the continued reliance on capitalist forms of economy. My participants in the American Midwest participate in these global assemblages through various means, most clearly through their employment in multi-national corporations, their consumption of goods produced through networks of multi-national corporations, and their political activities, as well as through the less obvious ways in which they engage with state policies, laws, and administrative regulations (e.g., budgetary policies that are linked to complex global relations). Some of these less apparent linkages have become somewhat more visible through the recent global financial crisis, especially in media analysis that highlighted the relationship of mortgage financing practices, banking systems, and global financial markets.[59] Ong and Collier's (2005) volume also highlights the study of technoscientific global assemblages and their relationship to human bodies as a particularly fruitful area of study.[60]

Within studies of globalization, scholars have devoted attention to the rise and impact of neoliberal economic reforms.[61] Collier and Ong describe neoliberalism as a highly mobile global form that has been incorporated into diverse global assemblages (2005:13). Originating in the U.K. and the U.S., neoliberal reforms involve new fiscal policies that have undercut social welfare initiatives while putting increasing responsibility on individual citizens to succeed in a "free market" environment that is in fact structured by corporate interests.[62] These policies have had a profound influence on the practice of capitalism and have resulted in creating greater global inequalities.[63]

A major insight that neoliberalism scholar Nikolas Rose (1996, 2007) has made, drawing on Michel Foucault's work, is that neoliberal regimes do not simply bring about profound changes in how the economy is structured but that new forms of governance ultimately restructure the relationship of the state and its citizens. The shift in national and international approaches to health from a focus on disease to the maintenance of health through optimal practices has been a major part of this transition. Public health initiatives rely on bureaucratic state apparatuses that collect statistical data about various "risks" to health. Citizens are provided with guidelines so that they can make informed decisions about avoiding or minimizing these risks. By internalizing these forms of governance, citizens cultivate "technologies of the self" through which they apply internal monitoring and regulation and ultimately become morally responsible for their health. Rose argues that such technologies of the self have led to a growing focus on the body and its biological characteristics and have fundamentally transformed how people understand themselves. The intense focus on the body, or "somatization," is paralleled and enhanced by biomedical research that aims to improve health and create new possibilities for living (as well as products and profits, as we will see below).

Although my description highlights the unequal power relations between the state and its citizens, a key insight of Rose's work is the active participation of people within these regimes. Indeed, Rose and Novas's (2005; also Rose 2007) discussion of biological citizenship[64] emphasizes that people use these new biomedical technologies of the self to suit their own needs and realize their hopes for their own lives as well as those of others.[65] For instance, as Marcia Inhorn has shown (2010, 2003), the growth of infertility treatment clinics in the Middle East is motivated by couples' deep-seated desire for children. At the same time, there are other economies of hope involved in these processes, including the profit-seeking hopes of multinational corporations. Both public and private bodies—including government research institutions, universities, pharmaceutical companies, and biotech companies—participate in the extraction of value from biological materials, contributing to the development of "bioeconomies" and "biocapital" (Rose 2007).[66]

The implications of the global assemblages of neoliberal capitalism and biocapital have only recently begun to be explored in reproduction, and much less so in the realm of breastfeeding and sleep.[67] There is growing scholarship on neoliberal discourses of "risk" and moral responsibility in breastfeeding promotion efforts that I describe in subsequent chapters.[68] While I find these contributions valuable in many respects, I suggest that they do not adequately address other ways in which neoliberal regimes intersect with infant feeding practices. For instance, there are important indications that discourses of "risk" simultaneously portray breastfeeding as a way to reduce the risk of maternal and child illness, but also as contributing to increased risk by perceived inadequacies in women's ability to produce breastmilk that sufficiently nourishes children, by making possible the transmission of infection (particularly HIV) and environmental and pharmaceutical toxins to infants, and by violations of moral norms of sexuality.[69] In chapter 4, I show in greater detail how even as breastfeeding is increasingly promoted in public health, and not breastfeeding is becoming unacceptable in some circles, pervasive stigmatization of breastfeeding remains. In that chapter, I highlight how the cultural ambivalence toward breastfeeding, wherein breastfeeding is simultaneously perceived as a moral value and a source of moral danger, is internalized in the very bodily experiences of breastfeeding.

Furthermore, the neoliberal systems of the production of biocapital have not figured into the above discussions that emphasize the negative consequences of breastfeeding promotion efforts. I argue that this is a significant oversight in light of the deep historical connections between biomedicine and capitalism as well as extensive research on how global assemblages that facilitate biocapital follow in the footsteps of colonial legacies and make the world's poor significantly more vulnerable to exploitation.[70] It is increasingly apparent, for instance, that the recent scientific valuation of the properties of breastmilk has tremendous commercial implications. These new developments build on earlier systems of commercial wet-nursing as well as the more recent rise of the infant food industry, which has successfully marketed commercial substitutes for breastfeeding derived from cow's milk, and more recently soy beans, since the late nineteenth century.

First, commercial wet-nursing for fees ranging up to $1000 per week has made a recent reappearance in some wealthy circles (Stearns 2010; Nathoo and Ostry 2010). Second, there is growing interest in the marketing of human breastmilk for mothers who cannot or decide not to breastfeed (Shaw 2010). Technoscientific innovations increasingly enable multinational pharmaceutical companies to provide products that mimic various properties of human breastmilk. For instance, formula companies have recently added genetically engineered components to infant formula based on growing knowledge of the composition of breastmilk (Institute of Medicine 2004). Furthermore, other companies, such as Prolacta, have exploited the global humanitarian discourse of charity to solicit breastmilk donations for African orphans, most of which is then used to design expensive nutritional supplements sold to hospitals for premature and ill babies (Hassan 2010). Finally, researchers in China recently reported (Gray 2011) that they have successfully inserted human genes into cows so that they can produce milk with "the same properties as human breastmilk." The report includes quotations from the scientific report of this research, including the following: "Our study describes transgenic cattle whose milk offers ... similar nutritional benefits as human milk" and "The modified bovine milk is a possible substitute for human milk. It fulfilled the conception of humanising the bovine milk."

The commercial exploitation of the biological properties of breastmilk illustrates one of the consequences of the complex interaction of the global assemblages of capitalism and technoscientific biomedicine. The human bodies entailed in producing the knowledge and technologies necessary for this research are erased in both the case of manufacturing infant formula with genetically engineered components and in the case of transgenic cows producing "human-like" milk. Furthermore, the product that has now been transformed into a commodity has been reconfigured both as a triumph of technological innovation and simultaneously "renaturalized" to make it appear more human (e.g., the "humanization of bovine milk") (Collier and Yanagisako 1987; Hassan 2010). The products of this research participate in furthering already deep inequalities with wealthy consumers purchasing "human-like" milk while poor women are neither supported in breastfeeding nor can afford safe alternatives. Moreover, the focus on breastmilk as a biomedicalized and commodified "product," as Barbara Katz Rothman (2008) cautioned, extracts the substance of breastmilk from the context of the breastfeeding relationship and erodes the actual practice of breastfeeding for all families.[71]

### Room for Change?

The above discussion of capitalism sets the stage for my investigation of breastfeeding as a privileged practice that constitutes an important part of certain models of personhood/parenthood that parents can "choose" to consume and that ultimately reinforces and enhances unequal capitalist social structures. At the same time, I also show that the dilemmas posed by the embodied, relational practices of nighttime breastfeeding and sleep disrupt many interrelated dimensions of capitalist forms and practices—from biomedical approaches to women's and children's bodies, the gendered organizations of the family, and the cultivation of parents' and children's personhoods and relationships with one another, to the organization of spatial and temporal regimes underpinning labor practices, and the interests of multinational pharmaceutical companies that market infant formula.

## Conclusion

In response to the reductive, polarized portrayals of breastfeeding and nighttime infant care in mainstream U.S. media and the relative absence of ethnographic investigations of these issues, my study provides an in-depth, longitudinal, and relational view into families' negotiation of nighttime breastfeeding and sleep. While much of my study focuses on the intricacies of embodied interactions entailed in nighttime breastfeeding and sleep among a small number of middle-class participants, throughout the ethnography I employ a comparative lens using cross-cultural, historical, and intersectional studies to provide a broader view of how these bodily practices participate in cultural models of personhood, relatedness, and unequal political economic systems. Using this framework, in the following chapters I examine the historical and sociocultural origins of how nighttime breastfeeding and sleep became embodied cultural dilemmas in the U.S. I then use the moments of moral ambivalence that arise from these dilemmas in my own ethnographic study as a guide to reveal how the embodied relational practices of breastfeeding and sleep both reproduce and transform persons, family relations, and even certain aspects of capitalism.[72] Ultimately, I hope that these theoretical insights, coupled with close ethnographic study, can contribute to a richer understanding of nighttime breastfeeding and sleep in this setting.

## Notes

1. See Bourdieu 1977; Foucault 1990; Martin 1994, 1987; Scheper-Hughes and Lock 1987; Lock 1993; Csordas 2002, 1994, 1990; Turner 2008; Young 2005 for some key examples.

2. See this volume and Crossley 2007 for a recent sociological discussion of Mauss's work in sociological investigations of embodiment.
3. See Whitaker 2000 for an Italian example.
4. Beasley 1996; Britton 1998; Blum 1999; Murphy 1999; Schmied and Barclay 1999; Stearns 1999; Schmied and Lupton 2001; Van Esterik 2002; Shaw 2004; Bartlett 2005; Dykes 2005; Kelleher 2006; Avishai 2007, 2011; Crossley 2007; Gatrell 2007; Hausman 2007; Burns et al. 2009; Johnson, Williamson, et al. 2009; Stearns 2009; Bartlett and Shaw 2010; Johnson, Leeming, et al. 2012.
5. Avishai 2011, 2007, 2004; Stearns 2010.
6. Campo 2010; Traina 2000; Hausman 2003.
7. Schmied and Lupton 2001; Bartlett 2005; Avishai 2007; Avishai 2011; Stearns 2009; McBride-Henry and Shaw 2010.
8. See Maher 1992 and contributions therein; Scheper-Hughes 1993; Zeitlyn and Rowshan 1997; Gottlieb 2004; Mabilia 2005; Gottschang 2007; Hashimoto and McCourt 2009; Liamputtong 2011; Tsianakas and Liamputtong 2007; Yimyam, Morrow, and Srisuphan 1999.
9. Here Williams is negotiating the lack of conscious awareness of some of these embodied aspects of sleep.
10. Williams, Meadows, and Arber 2010.
11. Williams, Lowe, and Griffiths 2007; Wiggs 2007.
12. Bianchera and Arber 2007; Arber and Venn 2011; Arber et al. 2007; Venn et al. 2008; Burgard 2011.
13. Meadows et al. 2009; Meadows et al. 2008.
14. McKenna, Ball, and Gettler 2007.
15. McKenna, Ball, and Gettler 2007; Ball, Ward-Platt, et al. 2006; Klingaman 2009; Worthman and Brown 2007; Worthman 2011; Ball 2009; Ball and Volpe 2012.
16. McKenna 1986; Mosko, Richard, et al. 1996; Mosko, McKenna, et al. 1993; McKenna, Thoman, et al. 1993; McKenna, Mosko, and Richard 1999, 1997; Richard and Mosko 2004; McKenna, Ball, and Gettler 2007; Gettler and McKenna 2011.
17. See above references, and also McKenna and McDade 2005.
18. Ball and Klingaman 2007; Gettler and McKenna 2010; Ball and Volpe 2012.
19. Lock 1993; Lock and Nguyen 2010.
20. S. Williams 2005.
21. See Carsten 2004 for a detailed discussion.
22. Franklin and McKinnon 2001.
23. See also Carrithers, Collins, and Lukes 1985.
24. Feeley-Harnik 2001; Weston 2001; Heath, Rapp, and Taussig 2004.
25. For instance, in her own work on Scottish adoptees, Carsten (2004) found a sense of incompleteness and longing for the kin from whom they were separated (2004:103–107). Carsten argues that these sentiments indicate "a notion of personhood where kinship is not simply added to bounded individuality, but one where kin relations are per-

ceived as intrinsic to the self ... [a] sense that something was missing in their own personhood" (2004:106–107). Sallie Han's (2009a, 2009b, 2013) research on pregnancy in the American Midwest follows precisely this line of work, showing how middle-class fatherhood is constituted through a variety of kin-making activities, including working on the house and the nursery in preparation of the baby's arrival and engaging in "belly talk"—reading, singing, and talking to their baby-in-the-making in the womb, while touching and caressing their partners' bellies.

26. Dettwyler 1988; Khatib-Chahidi 1992; Parkes 2001.
27. Carsten 1995, 1997, 2004. See also Zeitlyn and Rowshan 1997; Wright, Bauer, and Clark 1993; Lambert 2000.
28. Golden 1996.
29. Worthman and Brown 2007; Worthman 2007.
30. Barry and Paxson 1971; A. Wolf et al. 1996; Jenni and O'Connor 2005; McKenna, Ball, and Gettler 2007.
31. Caudill and Plath 1966; Whittemore and Beverly 1996; A. Wolf et al. 1996; Yang and Hahn 2002; Gottlieb 2004; Worthman and Brown 2007.
32. See also Ben-Ari 1996 on Japanese naptime.
33. Ball 2007; Ball and Volpe 2012.
34. Super and Harkness 1982; Morelli et al. 1992; Dettwyler 1988, 1995; Gottlieb 2004.
35. Morelli et al. 1992; Whittemore and Beverly 1996.
36. Ball, Hooker, and Kelly 1999; Ball and Volpe 2012.
37. M.F. Small 1998; Ferber 2006; McKenna, Ball, and Gettler 2007.
38. McKenna, Thoman, et al. 1993; A. Wolf et al. 1996; Keller and Goldberg 2004; McKenna, Ball, and Gettler 2007; Worthman 2011.
39. See Ball and Volpe 2012 for a recent review.
40. Willinger et al. 2003; McCoy et al. 2004.
41. Lozoff, Wolf, and Davis 1984; Shweder, Jensen, and Goldstein 1995.
42. Gottlieb 2004.
43. Yovsi and Keller 2007; Yovsi and Keller 2003; Mabilia 2005.
44. Dettwyler 1995; Stearns 1999.
45. Several key tensions underlie current anthropological debates (Heintz 2009; Sykes 2009; Lambek 2010; Zigon 2008; Faubion 2011) concerning distinctions in terminology and theoretical assumptions about "morality" and "ethics that warrant attention in my own analysis. First, as Heintz (2009) points out, morality is associated with Durkheim's work, which many have argued tends to collapse categories of the social and the moral, and overemphasizes social rules. On the other hand, the terminology of ethics tends to be associated with Weber as well as with terminology in moral philosophy, which many find too abstract and overly focused on rational thought as opposed to action. Heintz uses the term morality, following Beidelman's (1986) direction, to reflect the construction of ways of being and distinctions between right and

wrong through social interaction. Jarrett Zigon (2008, 2007) also employs morality for his larger analytic project, but incorporates ethics within that scheme via Foucault, who distinguishes between a set of rules (morality) and a person's capacity to act on oneself (ethics). Others have found the terminology of ethics more useful and veer away from using morality altogether. For instance, Michael Lambek (2010) draws on Aristotelian notions of virtues to argue for an ethics that neither replicates the rigid objectification of social rules nor removes ethics from the realm of action, which would duplicate mind/body dichotomies. Lambek gives a more subtle reading of Durkheim as well, acknowledging both his totalizing tendencies as well as his recognition of struggle, ambivalence, and conflict (2010:12). Lambek sees Weber's (1958) use of ethics as especially helpful for understanding how particular orientations toward the world in one cultural and historical setting can spread to others, in this case facilitating the rise of a certain form of capitalism. At the same time, he finds that in articulating these orientations, Weber presents an overly dichotomous model of rationality and nonrational "affectual, traditional or habitual orientation" (2010:24). Lambek advocates for a(n Aristotelian) modification via MacIntyre and argues for an understanding of a concept of tradition that is "an historically extended, socially embodied argument, and an argument precisely in part about the goods which constitute that tradition" (MacIntyre 1984:222 cited in Lambek 2010:24). Similar to Beidelman and Heintz, I employ the term "morality" and "moral dilemmas," rather than ethics, in order to emphasize the social construction of morality. At the same time, my take on morality is similar to that of scholars who articulate theories of ethics. In particular, I resonate with Lambek's notion of ethics due to his emphasis on the construction of ethics in and through social praxis, his attention to agency and conflict, and his argument that ethics takes place at the intersections of conscious/unconscious, reflexive/embodied experience. Furthermore, I share Lambek's concerns about the lack of ethnographic grounding in Foucault's work that makes his concepts too easily applied across domains and ethnographic settings without adequate examination of the local circumstances. Finally, while I do not accept Zigon's sharp distinction of the ethical from other aspects of morality, I find his work useful for elaborating the embodied dimensions of a morality that strongly resembles Lambek's concept of "ordinary ethics."

46. Zigon (2008) argues for a multi-dimensional model toward morality that distinguishes between institutional, public discursive, and embodied dispositional domains. In Zigon's view, "embodied dispositions" (2008:164) of morality resemble Mauss's concept of the habitus in that these are largely unconscious, unreflexive ways of being that enable people to make moral decisions without having to think about them. Moments of "ethical dilemmas" (2008:165) engage all three different dimensions of morality and ultimately lead to transformations of per-

sonhood. While each of the three dimensions of morality constrain this process, a person's interactions with these realms reconfigures them as well. In this sense, through their social relationships, persons are continually "working" on themselves while also remaking public discourses and institutions. Although I will not adhere to the schematic distinction between morality and ethics, I find Zigon's effort to produce a relational, interactive, and processual perspective on morality that integrates the corporeal realm compelling and helpful for my own purposes.

47. In Zigon's (2011) own ethnography in Russia, people infected with HIV through injecting drugs participate in rehabilitation programs run by the Russian Orthodox Church and cultivate ethical stances through which they attempt to rework themselves as moral persons. Zigon describes the unanticipated larger consequences of this process of ethical labor, wherein the newly acquired moral qualities of personhood make participants more compatible with and better integrated into the neoliberal state to which the Church stands in ideological opposition.

48. Many examples of "moral breakdown" and ensuing ethical debates discussed by Zigon, including the ethnographic example from Rapp's work I cited above, are prompted by ethical dilemmas that arise from new regimes of biopolitics that I described in the previous section. Zigon's own approach is significantly more ethnographically grounded and elaborated than that of Nikolas Rose's in his articulation of "somatic ethics" and attends to a wider range of moral issues, some of which intersect with neoliberalism in specific ways. This broader scope, together with the greater attention to the specific local elaborations of morality, makes Zigon's orientation more useful for my own purposes. At the same time, Rose's use of "somatic ethics" seems less invested in the analytical separation of ethics from other modes of morality, and on that specific point I support Rose's direction.

49. Michael Peletz (2001) has shown that, while moral contradictions and ambivalence in kinship was long recognized and documented, recent work in kinship studies has developed a much more sustained interest in these issues.

50. Following Rubin (1975), Collier and Yanagisako (1987), Yanagisako (2002), di Leonardo (1987), Creed (2000), and others, I anchor my analysis of political economy in the everyday negotiations of kinship. These scholars insist that the gendered dynamics of kinship are foundational to understanding the division of labor and economic interrelationships that lead to inequalities both within and beyond the household. Recent scholarship, such as Jessica Smith Rolston's study of mining in the American Midwest (Smith 2008; Rolston 2010), has highlighted the ties between household and wage-labor economies through the simultaneous gendered production of kinship both at home and at work.

51. Martin (1994) has since documented how shifts in capitalist regimes of labor toward an emphasis on "flexibility" are also associated with dif-

ferent understandings of the body, specifically the immune system. The notion of "flexible bodies" remains to be explored in depth in the realm of childbirth/breastfeeding.
52. See Browner and Sargent 2011 for a recent discussion.
53. Mullings' analytical approach, originating from a historical materialist tradition associated with the writings of Karl Marx and infused with critical perspectives on gender and race, has served to illuminate complex problems, such as the issue of poor birth outcomes in Harlem (Mullings and Wali 2001) and other similarly challenging issues. In a similar vein, drawing on ethnographic insights from her work with the Syracuse Healthy Start Program, Sandra Lane (2008) has shown how the daily experience of structural violence produced by systematic discrimination and a multitude of social, economic, and environmental inequalities ultimately results in the devastatingly high infant mortality rates seen among the children of poor women of color in Syracuse. Complementing these approaches, Dorothy Roberts's (1997) work, originating from close study of American law, addresses the intimate interrelationship of reproduction, forms of production, and political power. Roberts's focus on the practice and consequences of slavery highlights the central role that controlling captive women's reproduction played in producing more slaves who in turn provided the labor (both reproductive and other forms of labor) that sustained the institution of slavery. Furthermore, Roberts' comparative historical analysis demonstrates the wide-ranging legal controls that continue to seek to regulate black women's reproduction after the value of their reproduction diminished once slavery collapsed. Finally, Khiara Bridges' (2011) recent work has combined insights from anthropology and law to paint a complex portrait of pregnancy as a site of racialization. In Bridges' research at a large public hospital in New York City, pregnant women on Medicaid were subjected to intensive state surveillance and were grouped together as a racialized, "at-risk" population despite their diverse racial and ethnic origins, social circumstances, and practices and beliefs. Through their interactions with the staff, who were themselves a racial and ethnically diverse group and who often cared deeply for their patients, they experienced systematic stereotyping and discrimination.
54. Indeed, in Bridges' work above, racialization of pregnancy at Alpha Hospital was constructed through comparison with the neighboring Omega hospital that did not accept payment with Medicaid, and therefore served predominately white, wealthier patients.
55. Blum 1999; Murphy 1999, 2003; Gatrell 2011.
56. Ortner draws on her ethnography of the trajectories of the Weequahic High School class of 1958 in New Jersey as well as other sources to elaborate upon Marx's pivotal insights about the relations of production in capitalism. Based on her findings, Ortner concludes that class continues to play a foundational role in the production of social differ-

ence and inequalities in the U.S. Ortner examines the concept of class at length and shows how the folk category of the "middle class," which includes the majority of Americans, includes considerable fragmentation resulting from economic changes in late capitalism that have significantly widened the gap between wealthier and poorer Americans. These inequalities are concealed by the strategic use of "middle class" to reduce stigma associated with certain forms of labor (labeled "blue collar" or "working class") and to avoid being labeled as overly wealthy ("upper-middle" or "upper" class). In her analysis of the class of '58, Ortner demonstrates the virtual disappearance of the working class, the considerable shrinkage of the middle of the "middle class," and the expansion of the professional-managerial "upper-middle" class. While the members of the class of '58 have moved up compared with their parents, these trends, coupled with the simultaneous expansion of poverty and inequities, reflect the erosion of possibilities for others. Ortner argues that while similar trends have been observed elsewhere, in the U.S. the growth of inequalities is hidden by cultural ideologies about opportunity and moral responsibility for success.
57. Layne 2000; Clarke 2004; Han 2009, 2013; Taylor 2000.
58. Miller 2001, 1998, 1987; Layne 2000, 1999.
59. See, for instance, Krugman 2010.
60. Although Lock and Nguyen (2010) do not employ the terminology of "global assemblages," their characterization of biomedicine dovetails with Ong's and Collier's discussion. Lock and Nguyen point out that biomedicine was, in fact, global from its early history, through its historical role in colonialism. They demonstrate that biomedicine played a critical role in responding to the threats of colonial epidemics, infertility, and hunger, resulting in an increasingly biologized understanding of these phenomena that could be managed through bureaucratic interventions. The authors suggest that global biomedicine continues to carry these historical legacies within itself in the postcolonial world, resulting in the perpetuation of global inequalities.
61. Collier and Ong 2005; Edelman and Haugerud 2005; Ferguson 2010.
62. See also Collins, Williams, and di Leonardo 2008.
63. Rose, O'Malley, and Valverde 2006; Rose and Novas 2005; Rose 1996; Navarro 2007; Collins, Williams, and di Leonardo 2008.
64. Rose's concept of biological citizenship draws upon and expands Petryna's (2002) analysis of the consequences of the Chernobyl nuclear disaster in Ukraine as well as Rapp and colleagues' (Rapp 2001; Heath, Rapp, and Taussig 2004) discussion of "genetic citizenship" in the context of prenatal testing technologies.
65. Rose is building on Sarah Franklin's (1997) use of "hope technologies" in her work on assisted reproduction in the U.K. and Carlos Novas's (2006) discussion of the economies of hope.
66. Rose asserts that the production of "biocapital" and the circulation of new technologies that facilitate it engender moral dilemmas and ethical

debates that have been primarily regimented through the field of bioethics and institutionalized within biomedicine and state administrative policies. But Rose contends that these debates extend far beyond the field of institutionalized bioethics and belong to the larger field of "somatic ethics" because they concern how we comprehend and negotiate our "corporeal existence" (2007:257). Rose builds on Weber's famous phrase "the Protestant ethic and the spirit of capitalism" to coin "somatic ethics and the spirit of biocapital" (2007:252–259) in order to demonstrate that intrinsic link between the moral and ethical questions that arise from navigating new regimes of biocapital and the emergence of biocapital itself. See also Franklin and Lock 2003 and contributions therein.
67. Although see Wolf-Meyer 2008 on sleep.
68. Blum 1999; Murphy 2003, 2000, 2004; Kukla 2006; Lee, Macvarish, and Bristow 2010; Lee 2011, 2008, 2007; Knaak 2010; J.B. Wolf 2011, 2007.
69. Hausman 2010, 2011.
70. Cohen 2005; Petryna 2009; Bharadwaj 2010.
71. The commodification of breastmilk has important implications for breastfeeding in the U.S. as well, which I address in greater detail in chapter 2.
72. Abu-Lughod 1990.

*Chapter 2*

## STRUGGLES OVER AUTHORITATIVE KNOWLEDGE AND "CHOICE" IN BREASTFEEDING AND INFANT SLEEP IN THE UNITED STATES

Contemporary perspectives and practices of infant feeding and sleep are inextricably entangled with biomedicine. This chapter seeks to unravel this involvement of biomedicine in infant feeding and sleep in the United States using the concept of authoritative knowledge, defined as a system of knowledge that is valued to the exclusion of other ways of knowing. Brigitte Jordan (1997, [1978] 1993) developed and later elaborated the concept of authoritative knowledge through her comparative ethnographic work on childbirth in the Yucatan, the Netherlands, Sweden, and the United States. According to Jordan (1997:57), authoritative knowledge is embedded in a system of power relations that make this knowledge appear natural and consensual.[1] In this chapter, I draw on Jordan's framework as a helpful, albeit partial and imperfect, guide to address the far-reaching influence of biomedicine in breastfeeding and nighttime family sleep practices. In a significant departure from Jordan's use of this concept, however, I do not wish to construe biomedical knowledge as seamless and hegemonic. Instead, I focus on points of tension in order to provide insight into the multiple forms of knowledge about these bodily practices, the social processes by which certain forms of knowledge become valued over others, and the contestations through which these valuations can change over time.

Drawing on the above insights, in this chapter I address struggles over authoritative knowledge about infant feeding and sleep between biomedical approaches and women, within biomedicine itself, and among feminist critiques of biomedical involvement in breastfeeding. First, I describe the dramatic historical transformation of infant feeding and sleep into separate cultural and biomedical domains, in which artificial milk feeding and solitary infant sleep became the norm, with breastfeeding only recently making a return. Next, I pursue the consequences of this transformation in contemporary pediatric advice about infant sleep through contestations of biomedical authority between breastfeeding and infant sleep experts. In the third section, I turn to feminist debates about the role of biomedicine in breastfeeding, once again focusing on the cultural complexities of biomedical authority in infant feeding. Finally, I offer an anthropological approach focusing on breastfeeding as part of social relationships that moves beyond these debates to enable us to better understand the complex dilemmas American families face when they embark on the journey of breastfeeding—during the day and, for the purposes of this book, especially during the nighttime.

## The Rise of Biomedical Authority in Breastfeeding and Infant Sleep in the United States

Until the middle of the nineteenth century, most women breastfed their children until the second summer in the child's life or at least for a year (Salmon 1994; Wertz and Wertz 1989).[2] The domain of infant feeding and care was part of a complex of childbearing-related knowledge that mothers shared among one another and that they learned from midwives who attended them in childbirth (Leavitt 1986; Wertz and Wertz 1989; Ulrich 1990). Midwives played a particularly important role since they cared for women throughout pregnancy, birth, and in the postpartum period in the mothers' homes, and often also served as local healers (Ulrich 1990; Wertz and Wertz 1989; Fraser 1998). Their knowledge of breastfeeding was set within the context of the larger continuum of women's reproductive lives, the raising of children, and family circumstances.[3] Throughout the early history of breastfeeding in the U.S., not every woman breastfed her biological child. Other lactating mothers breastfed babies whose mothers were unable to feed them due to illness or death (Ulrich 1990; Golden 1996; Schwartz 1996). More prosperous women often hired wet-nurses to feed their children, a practice that had a long history among the wealthy in Europe and that was associated with high infant mortality rates both for wet-nursed children as well as children born to wet-nurses (Golden 1996; Hrdy 1999). Slave-owning families in the South also used enslaved women of African ancestry to breastfeed their babies (Schwartz 1996).

Breastfeeding was associated with a wealth of perceptions and beliefs that not only recognized its importance in keeping children growing and healthy (Schwartz 1996; Ulrich 1990), but also regarded it as a moral obligation for women. Religious leaders, such as the Puritan minister Cotton Mather of the seventeenth century, often emphasized breastfeeding's moral and spiritual significance, considering breastfeeding (and childbirth) a sacred duty through which women fulfilled God's will (Golden 1996; McMillen 1997).[4] At the same time, breastfeeding was also fraught with danger since it was believed to confer the physical, moral, and psychological characteristics of the breastfeeding woman, particularly in the case of wet-nursing (McMillen 1997; Golden 1996). For instance, Puritans of the seventeenth century warned against the dangers of having red-headed women as temporary wet-nurses because these women could be witches, whose milk would harm the child (Cone 1981). Similar sentiments were later echoed in concern over the transmission of undesirable moral characteristics from immigrant and poor wet-nurses in nineteenth century America (Golden 1996).

Complex intersecting causes underlie the dramatic transformations in the patterns of infant feeding in the U.S. beginning in the mid-nineteenth century. During the nineteenth and early twentieth centuries, male physicians began to attend a growing number of middle-class women's births, offering forceps and other interventions in emergencies, and anesthetics for pain in labor[5] (Leavitt 1986; J.H. Wolf 2009). Since many women had a large number of children and many died in or shortly after childbirth (Leavitt estimates a lifetime mortality rate of 1 in 30), women increasingly accepted the presence of physicians during birth. The acceptance of physicians' supervision of childbirth in wealthier circles was also reinforced by the perception of upper-class women as fragile and weak, unable to tolerate the pain of labor, lacking the strength and endurance to give birth (Leavitt 1986) and to produce nourishing milk to breastfeed their children (Golden 1996). Physicians' growing involvement in birth facilitated increasing supervision of childbirth and childrearing, leading to increased medical management of infant feeding, which was further cemented by the transition to hospital birth beginning in the early twentieth century, especially after 1920, and ensuing protocols that interfered with breastfeeding (Wertz and Wertz 1989; Leavitt 1986).

Historian Rima Apple (1987) argues that physicians' interest in regulating infant feeding practices, coupled with commercial interest in manufacturing infant formulas, led to the steep declines in breastfeeding by the 1950s. Physicians advocated a rational, scientific approach to childbirth and breastfeeding, marked by strict time schedules, measurement, and an array of medical interventions, necessitating intensive medical supervision. Adding another dimension to this argument, Golden (1996) documented physicians' discomfort with wet-nurses and the challenges of regulating their moral qualities and health, which added further impetus to replacing breastfeeding with infant formula.[6] Apple suggests that physicians' approach to infant feeding emerged from changing social circumstances associated with increasing industrialization that led to the growing valuation of "scientific motherhood" (1987:99–100), wherein mothers could rationally and efficiently address tasks associated with their children and households.[7]

Although physicians' influence on replacing breastfeeding with formula milk derived from cow's milk is clearly significant, historian Jacqueline Wolf (2001) presents convincing evidence that women in the late nineteenth century already began weaning their children within the first three or four months, due to a variety of other reasons. First, the increasing sexualization of the breast in the rise of nineteenth century notions of romantic love among middle- and upper-class people may have made some women uncomfortable with the idea of breastfeeding and concerned that children's nursing would destroy the beauty of their breasts (2001:23–25). These concerns compounded growing concern, often cast in eugenic arguments, about wealthier white women's ability to birth and successfully breastfeed their children due to the stresses of urban life and by other social and environmental changes.[8] Illnesses, psychological states, and other potentially harmful characteristics of women were thought to pass to breastmilk, thereby threatening its quality (2001:92–99). Furthermore, immigrant women and other poor women who migrated to urban areas in search of work also weaned their children early if they initiated breastfeeding at all, due to labor conditions that did not accommodate breastfeeding (2001:19–22).

Paradoxically, while many physicians and public health officials continued to value breastfeeding, nineteenth century and early twentieth century efforts to address high rates of infant mortality associated with early weaning and increasing bottle feeding unintentionally contributed to further demise of the practice. Physicians became involved in programs to distribute "clean milk," pasteurized cows' milk in sealed bottles, at milk depots for the urban poor, as well as in efforts to produce an alternative to human milk (2001:42–73). The distribution of "clean milk" implied that human milk was easily replaceable with cow's milk, and the emphasis on cleanliness made human milk appear potentially unclean, and therefore dangerous, by comparison.

Historians agree that eventually, and especially with the rise of the ideology of "scientific motherhood" (Apple 1987), women embraced infant formula. Apple suggests that formula was highly suitable for the scientific management model for mothering, since it could provide an alternative source of nutrition that could be controlled by the physician, rather than accommodating the complex interactions of maternal and infant physiology and psychology. Formula was produced, measured, and provided in exact amounts and at specified times to the infant according to physicians' instructions, whereas determining the amount and composition of milk consumed by the breastfeeding child presented numerous challenges. Formula offered a modern, scientific, and rational method of feeding babies compared with the "irrational" patterns of on-demand nursing often practiced by immigrants and ethnic minorities.[9] In addition, formula presented an ideal alternative to the perceived dangers of wet-nurses (Golden 1996). With formula that was produced under scientific, hygienic circumstances, there would be no more worries about the transfer of disease, alcohol, and lower class or immigrant moral qualities to the child.

The growing consolidation of physicians' authority in childbirth also facilitated this shift. Despite early public health efforts following the 1921 Sheppard-Towner Act to improve maternity care services, these initiatives were soon overtaken by physician efforts to increase their clientele (Fraser 1998).[10] These efforts began to erode the authority of midwives in poor, immigrant, and African American communities. White physicians increasingly supervised the activities of these midwives through young, white, medically trained nurses, eventually limiting the care that they could provide altogether. Their activities also led to the elevation of biomedical approaches to birth as the golden standard, and the simultaneous stigmatization of midwifery and associated practices in these communities as "backward" and inferior, associated with racialized notions of poverty (Fraser 1998; Litt 2000; Golden 1996). Since breastfeeding was part of the midwifery model of care (Leavitt 1986), these efforts had tremendous implications for breastfeeding and contributed to its decline.

The scientific management of breastfeeding and childbirth created additional need for formula. Physicians encouraged long periods between feedings and a minimization of physical contact between mother and child in order to reduce the risk of infection, which led to inadequate stimulation of the breasts and production of an "insufficient milk supply," one of the very problems scientific management aimed to resolve (Apple 1987; Millard 1990; Hausman 2003). Thus, while physicians still considered breastfeeding a superior source of infant nutrition, the rational management model heavily undermined women's actual ability to breastfeed. This trend was reinforced and strengthened by the hospitalization of birth, necessitated by the use of anesthesia, medical equipment, and the large number of staff trained to use these tools, which relocated the first few days of infant feeding under the complete supervision of the medical staff (Leavitt 1986; Apple 1987). Finally, increasing commercial interest in formula production spurred heavy advertisement, growing physician endorsement, and mass distribution of samples of formula (Apple 1987). All of the above factors resulted in an ever-increasing number of women never initiating breastfeeding, and breastfeeding rates plummeting in the first three decades of the twentieth century. From the 1920s through the 1970s, even initiating breastfeeding was rare; by 1970, only about one in five women were putting the baby to breast in the hospital and even fewer in the weeks beyond (J.H. Wolf 2006).

Although the history of infant sleep has generated considerably less attention than that of childbirth and breastfeeding, we know that advice and practices related to infant sleep underwent similarly fundamental changes during the late nineteenth and early twentieth centuries. By the 1920s, children's sleep, which was mostly viewed as unproblematic in early U.S. history, became a subject of intense concern for middle-class parents (Stearns, Rowland, and Giarnella 1996).[11] As in the case of childbirth and breastfeeding, these changes were linked to the rise in the prominence of medical experts in every realm of childbearing as well as to other social changes detailed below. Medical experts directed considerable attention toward lengthening the sleep of young children in order to improve their health. Furthermore, physicians began to recommend that parents no longer place their infants in cradles next to their own or their nurses' beds. Instead, infants were to be laid in cribs—beds with railings to contain children—located in separate room (Stearns, Rowland, and Giarnella 1996). These recommendations for separate sleep were also extended to older children, who usually shared a bed with siblings. Stearns and colleagues (1996) argue that the change from shared sleep arrangements to solitary ones was perhaps the most important reason for the growing frequency and intensity of concern about "sleep problems" that appeared in popular magazines and pediatric advice.

In addition to the changes in medical attitudes toward children's sleep arrangements, Stearns and his co-authors identify several other factors that played a role in this transition, including changes in middle-class attitudes toward marriage and sexuality, which Jacqueline Wolf (2001) also noted: declining fertility rates that placed greater emphasis on the health of each child;[12] the rising cost of domestic servants, which made them far less available for middle-class families who previously relied on them; new sources of noise in urban centers where the increasingly concentrated population led to greater stress and disruptions during the night; and the need to conform children's rhythms to the schedules dictated by factory labor.

Prominent medical experts in the early twentieth century, such as Emmett Holt, who was also a major proponent of cow-milk based infant formula, emphasized the establishment of regular bedtime routines and the minimization of nighttime contact between parents and children (Stearns, Rowland, and Giarnella 1996). The most extreme versions of this emphasis derived from behaviorist theories of child development advocated by John Watson in the 1920s and 1930s, who argued that children needed to be trained to adopt a rigid schedule suitable for their parents and that human contact during nighttime hours should be minimized to ensure their future health. Although such approaches were not adopted by parents in their entirety, the importance of schedules left its mark on subsequent parenting advice, such as that of the influential Benjamin Spock, who emphasized solitary sleep and regularity but included greater flexibility and accommodation of the child's needs as perceived by her mother. By the mid-twentieth century, solitary sleep for children, surrounded by loving bedtime rituals, became the unquestioned norm for healthy child development. Nighttime separation accommodated a philosophy of minimizing nighttime feedings as well, facilitating the physical as well as ideological erasure of the previous relationship between breastfeeding and proximal sleep arrangements (McKenna, Ball, and Gettler 2007).

In sum, male physicians and women themselves both actively participated in medical experts' rising prominence, with significant consequences. First, authoritative knowledge about childbearing and childcare that previously resided with mothers themselves and in the hands of local knowledgeable women, now rested in the hands of primarily male physicians. Physicians' efforts to professionalize and to gain access to more patients virtually eradicated local midwives and enabled the rise of obstetrics and pediatrics as medical specialties. While wealthy women initiated these changes, middle-class and poor women also eventually shunned midwifery and associated practices, such as breastfeeding and proximal sleep arrangements, as they became associated with "backwardness" and with poverty. With the removal of childbirth from the home to the hospital, out of view of other women in the community, knowledge about childbirth and breastfeeding was no longer easily accessible. Solitary sleep and the emphasis on minimal interruptions during the night reinforced hospital routines that undermined breastfeeding and contributed to its demise. Artificial formula feeding and solitary sleep practices took root in the context of related social transformations that ultimately resulted in mutually reinforcing effects experienced on an embodied level. These new embodied norms provided the expectations for subsequent generations of parents.

## The Emergence of Breastfeeding Advocacy and the "Resurgence" of (Biomedicalized) Breastfeeding

Grassroots maternalist movements in the 1950s, most prominently marked by the formation of La Leche League (LLL) in 1956 as well as other organizations and public health groups, began to challenge dominant medical practices surrounding childbearing and formed the basis for a greater interest in breastfeeding (Weiner 1994). Many of these organizations contested the prevailing norms of scientific motherhood, its rigid schedules, reliance on expert advice, and the turn away from "natural" ways of bearing and raising children. In sharp contrast to the behaviorist developmental advice, breastfeeding for many months and multiple years—including during the night, facilitated by sleeping close to one's young children—were embraced by the League. According to historian Lynn Weiner, the overwhelming response to LLL's philosophy originated from the particular post-World War II U.S. historical climate. First, pronatalism became particularly prominent in the 1950s, resulting in a significant rise in the number of children per woman and an intensive focus on children. Thus, the strong maternalist sentiment conveyed by the League resonated with many others. The League's understanding of women's far-reaching influence through the rearing of children that ultimately had the potential to transform human beings worldwide bore the marks of nineteenth century ideals of "sacred motherhood" (1994:1370).

The League's discussion of women's "natural" role as mothers appealed to religious groups and others with more conservative moral beliefs about the family and who retained some of these older ideals (Weiner 1994). Simultaneously, this emphasis on the "natural" as something shared by all humans regardless of race or class differences also attracted those involved in the later 1960s and 1970s movements that challenged dominant cultural paradigms, e.g., the "hippie movement," which shared an interest in a return to the "natural" and an interest in social and political equality. Since its creation, the League has negotiated and continues to negotiate the series of inter-related tensions between maternalism and feminism, religiosity and secularism, and scientific evidence and maternal sentiment, which are all part of this historical legacy (Ward 2000; Weiner 1994). I will address the feminist dilemmas arising from the first set of tensions later on in the chapter.

The League captures the complicated relationship between challenging certain aspects of medical authority while also simultaneously relying on medical expertise to promote breastfeeding. The founding mothers of LLL frequently consulted and were influenced by physicians from the inception of the organization through familial connections as well as through physicians involved in the natural childbirth movement (Weiner 1994). Gregory White, founder Mary White's husband, and his mentor, Herbert Ratner, a Chicago health commissioner, both physician supporters of breastfeeding and childbirth without medication, played a particularly important role in shaping and working with the League. Thus, the founders, while also critical of inaccurate and uninformed advice about birth and breastfeeding from medical authorities, were always closely connected to medicine and male expertise, albeit with physicians who espoused the minority alternative perspective within medicine (Ward 2000). At the same time, the founders were also aware of the challenges of presenting such information because arguing for breastfeeding on the basis of scientific evidence presented the possibility of refuting their claims using alternative sources of evidence. The tension between presenting scientific information and support for mothering through breastfeeding remains embedded in the structure of the organization, especially since the rise of evidence-based medicine meant a massive proliferation of studies overwhelmingly in support of breastfeeding. Over the course of the second half of the twentieth century and up to the present day, the League has not only played a critical role in offering knowledge and mother-to-mother support through its free groups run by trained volunteers, but also educated physicians and other medical providers about breastfeeding (Weiner 1994). The organization maintains ties with and is recognized as an authority on breastfeeding by other national and international health organizations, such as the World Health Organization.

Beginning in the 1970s, following the accumulation of scientific studies highlighting the health differences between breastfed and formula-fed children, major international and national public health efforts began to bolster grassroots advocacy (Wright and Schanler 2001; Grummer-Strawn and Shealy 2009). The first major consolidation of international collaboration developed in response to growing concern about infant malnutrition and death caused by the introduction of infant formula to poor nations; it resulted in the 1981 International Code of Marketing of Breastmilk Substitutes. Although the U.S. Surgeon General held a workshop in 1984 on how to establish better breastfeeding support and promotion in multiple realms, no major structural changes or public health initiatives were implemented and the workshop was followed by a significant decrease in breastfeeding rates, whose origins remain unclear (Grummer-Strawn and Shealy 2009; J.H. Wolf 2003). International health advocacy took shape in 1991 in the World Health Organization/UNICEF Innocenti Declaration on the Protection, Promotion, and Support of Breastfeeding, which relied on extensive scientific research to recommend exclusive breastfeeding for four to six months, and breastfeeding to be continued through the second year of life (Wright and Schanler 2001).

While the U.S. was slower to act than many other wealthy industrial nations, the 1990s marked the first major efforts to raise its breastfeeding rates, beginning with establishing breastfeeding objectives in 1990 through Healthy People, then the 1998 National Breastfeeding Policy Conference that established the United States Breastfeeding Committee (USBC), and concluding with the Department of Health and Human Services establishment of the Blueprint for Action on Breastfeeding in 2000 (Grummer-Strawn and Shealy 2009). In the meantime, the American Academy of Pediatrics (AAP) released a policy statement on breastfeeding and human milk in 1997 and incorporated recent research to recommend six months of exclusive breastfeeding and an additional six months of continued breastfeeding along with supplementary foods (AAP Work Group on Breastfeeding 1997). Notably, although this recommendation left breastfeeding beyond the one-year recommendation an option for mothers, as long as it was mutually desired by them and their children, the guidelines did not adopt the WHO recommendation of breastfeeding for two years. This work was paralleled by a renewed rise in breastfeeding, especially in initiation rates (Grummer-Strawn and Shealy 2009).

From 2001 onward, there were more systematic efforts to implement the goals of the now decade-old Innocenti Declaration in multiple realms, including in the organization of the workplace, public education, professional education, the health care system, and in support services for breastfeeding (Grummer-Strawn and Shealy 2009). Within the health care system, the international Baby Friendly Hospital Initiative has made significant headway, with over 6 percent of U.S. births now taking place at BFHI-certified hospitals, which have undergone systematic evaluation for their implementation of standards established to support breastfeeding (CDC 2012). State legislation that ensures the protection of breastfeeding in public has also substantially increased. Significant changes have been implemented in the Women, Infants, and Children (WIC) program to support breastfeeding, although this work remains underfunded. Furthermore, the 2010 Patient Protection and Affordable Care Act includes provisions for employer-provided lactation breaks and spaces as well as an IRS deduction for the use of breast pumps (United States Breastfeeding Committee 2011). The largest changes have taken place in the area of public education and professional education, with the result that more people are aware that breastfeeding plays an important role in health and more health workers are trained to provide appropriate information about breastfeeding. Government-led initiatives that are tied into global public health efforts now lead the way in U.S. breastfeeding promotion based on scientific research. Although grassroots organizations continue their advocacy efforts, the majority of families learn about breastfeeding in the context of health, often from medical providers.

The cultural landscape of breastfeeding in the U.S. and the role of breastfeeding promotion remain complex (Grummer-Strawn and Shealy 2009). While advocates have been working for decades to provide structural and cultural support for breastfeeding, there is considerable reluctance to implement such changes on the legislative level and to fund even existing initiatives. Paid maternity leave, on-site childcare, and job security after an extended leave remain elusive for most women. Lactation spaces and breast pumps are also lacking at most workplaces, although there has been much more of an effort on this front in the workplace—due to significantly lower health costs for breastfed children—than in enabling women to actually breastfeed their children through the above-mentioned more expensive measures.

Although the number of lactation professionals has risen, especially in hospitals, lactation support is not available to most women after their hospital discharge (Grummer-Strawn and Shealy 2009). Physicians and nurses also continue to lack adequate knowledge about breastfeeding and are influenced by the formula industry's ongoing influence. Survey reports indicate that the majority of physicians now recommend the AAP endorsed timeline for breastfeeding, but many do not believe that the "benefits of breastfeeding outweigh the difficulties or inconvenience" (Grummer-Strawn & Shealy 2009:S36). These findings are echoed by larger cultural trends among U.S. adults, who reported an overall recognition that breastfeeding has beneficial health consequences (although lack more specific knowledge), yet nearly a third also agreed that formula feeding is as good as breastmilk. Furthermore, in 2004 over a third of those surveyed still indicated that breastfeeding should be carried out in a private space, reflecting ongoing moral concern about the visibility of breastfeeding in public.

Commercial interests of formula manufacturers, a four billion dollar industry in the U.S., continue to play a major role in shaping infant feeding decisions through direct marketing as well as their involvement in health care institutions, advocacy efforts, and legislation (Walker 2007). Although the U.S. endorsed the Code in 1994, it has not taken a particularly active role in enforcing it, enabling infant formula manufacturers to continue to violate it. Most women receive "gift bags" by formula companies that include highly problematic information about breastfeeding as well as free samples of formula upon their discharge that influence breastfeeding rates and disproportionately affect poor, minority women (Rosenberg, Eastham, and Kasehagen 2008; Declercq et al. 2009).[13] Such materials are not allowed in hospitals that have earned the Baby Friendly designation. Formula advertisement is pervasive in parenting magazines, internet sites, and stores that cater to pregnant women and new mothers. The formula industry also provides significant financial support to the AAP and is one of the most effective lobbies in Washington (Kassirer 2007; Brody 2010; J.H. Wolf 2006). These links have significantly undermined public health efforts to promote breastfeeding, as in the case of the National Breastfeeding Advocacy Campaign that focused on highlighting the risks of not breastfeeding, which was significantly curtailed due to the successful lobbying efforts of the formula industry (J.H. Wolf 2006).

The public health treatment of breastfeeding among African American women offers a complex contemporary case study for how even efforts that aim to reduce inequality by improving health outcomes can contribute to the reproduction of embodied inequalities through the legacies of pervasive racism. While earlier in the twentieth century African American women breastfed at higher rates than white women, these rates were reversed due to the expanding interventions of biomedicine as well as women's own decision to turn away from breastfeeding because of its association with poor, racial, and ethnic minorities (Apple 1987; Litt 2000). Comparatively lower rates of breastfeeding have made African American women a target of contemporary breastfeeding interventions (Phillip and Jean-Marie 2007). In one of the ads of the National Breastfeeding Advocacy Campaign of 2003–2005, for instance, an African American pregnant woman riding a mechanized bull was used to draw a comparison between avoiding risks during pregnancy to the risks of formula feeding. Although white women were also featured in similar activities in the campaign, the images of African American women build on and perpetuate stereotypic racialized images of African American mothers as irresponsible, ignorant, and dangerous (Roberts 1997; J.B. Wolf 2011; Hausman 2003; Kukla 2006). These images are then reinforced when breastfeeding is presented as a source of danger in racialized ways, through the use of drugs, alcohol, cigarettes, and through infections such as HIV (Reich 2010; Hausman 2003, 2011).

Several other factors contribute to these gendered, racial stereotypes in relation to African American infant feeding and sleep practices. In her sociological analysis of the SIDS public health campaigns, Martine Hackett (2007) shows how differences in the rate of reduction of SIDS between black and white women became reframed as racial disparities in public health efforts and sparked "targeted" intervention efforts to increase black mothers' "compliance" with recommendations to put their infants to sleep in cribs on their backs. Despite efforts to make these messages "culturally competent," there was little exploration of the reasons for infant sleep practices that differed from these guidelines, or the tremendous variation among those labeled "black" women, especially with respect to ethnicity and social class. Indeed, just as the expansion of infant formula use was linked to physician advice, Hackett's study traces placing children on their stomachs to earlier pediatric advice that dominated much of the twentieth century. Ultimately, black women experienced these "targeted" messages as highly insensitive to the history of racial discrimination in the U.S., where they have been systematically viewed negatively, and felt that these messages created a sense that black mothers were being held responsible for the deaths of their babies.

Thus, while white women's bed sharing practices might be seen as a matter of "choice" that is driven by the favorably viewed desire to breastfeed, bed sharing without concurrent breastfeeding lacks any potential redeeming qualities and is viewed as a matter of ignorance and even willful "defiance." Consequently, African American mothers are constructed as "deviant" and experience multiple sources of "targeted" health interventions that employ similarly racialized and problematic images, admonishing them to breastfeed on the one hand and to practice solitary sleep in cribs for their children on the other hand. In fact, the imagery used in safe sleep campaigns can be much more blunt and fear-based than that used in the breastfeeding campaigns, featuring butcher knives next to babies lying in bed and headboards that are used as tombstones (Kendall-Tackett, Cong, and Hale 2010; Gettler and McKenna 2010; Ball and Volpe 2012).

In the context of the history of slavery, including the practice of forced wet-nursing of white owners' children (Schwartz 1996), as well as the continued restrictions on African American women's reproduction and the stigmatization of African American families (Roberts 1997; Bridges 2011), it is not surprising that many African American women remain skeptical of public health interventions that promote breastfeeding (Blum 1999). Sharing concerns about public health efforts' perpetuation of racist, classist, and sexist ideologies, some scholars have argued against breastfeeding advocacy.[14] In contrast to these views, I draw on Leith Mullings' (1997) insights about using anthropological and related research in service of the systematic exploration and elimination of the embodied effects of inequalities.[15] I argue that supporting and enabling women to breastfeed and sleep safely close to their babies must be a shared priority in this process. I develop these insights further in the sections below.

The recent Department of Health and Human Health Services "Call to Action to Support Breastfeeding" (U. S. Department of Health and Human Services 2011) attempts to refocus public health advocacy to reduce barriers to breastfeeding rather than simply promoting its health "benefits"[16] or highlighting the "risks" of not breastfeeding. As Surgeon General Regina M. Benjamin stated in the press release, "Many barriers exist for mothers who want to breastfeed. They shouldn't have to go it alone. Whether you're a clinician, a family member, a friend, or an employer, you can play an important part in helping mothers who want to breastfeed." Dr. Benjamin focused on five key areas for enhancing breastfeeding support: 1) community mother-to-mother programs; 2) the healthcare system, especially through increasing the number of Baby Friendly Hospitals; 3) clinician training and provision of advice on breastfeeding; 4) employer-established paid maternity leave and lactation programs; and 5) the family. Although the shift toward supporting breastfeeding is significant, it remains to be seen how these directions will be implemented in actual policies, especially in light of recent budget concerns and the lack of a federal initiative on paid family leave.

In sum, while advocacy efforts resulted in significant increases in breastfeeding, breastfeeding today takes place within a thoroughly biomedicalized context. Although it is tempting to describe the "resurgence" of breastfeeding as a return to previous historical practices, the cultural conceptualizations of breastfeeding present a dramatic departure from its practice in the nineteenth century, making breastfeeding a novel reproductive process in many aspects. This transformation took place in the context of larger, global expansions of the role of biomedicine in all areas of life. Breastfeeding has figured into these transformations in multiple ways, through the biomedicalization of childbirth and through the biomedicalization of the care of children. At the same time, this transformation was never monolithic, and biomedicine continues to have a complex and contradictory relationship to breastfeeding.

At present in the U.S., nearly all breastfeeding is initiated after hospital births with very high rates of interventions, including a 32 percent Cesarean section rate that is expected to continue to rise (MacDorman, Menacker, and Declercq 2010). Despite efforts to transform medical practice, just as in the early history of the biomedicalization of childbirth, hospital routines and treatment continue to undermine successful breastfeeding (Declercq et al. 2009; U.S. Department of Health and Human Services 2011). Furthermore, due to the rise of medical experts and the near-disappearance of breastfeeding during the twentieth century that I documented in the previous section, families have little experience with the practice of breastfeeding compared with accumulated cultural experience with artificial milk feeding. Medical experts are the main sources of authoritative knowledge on breastfeeding, but they communicate their contradictory stance of promoting breastfeeding without necessarily believing that it is worth the effort, all the while maintaining ties to and enabling the formula industry to accrue high profits. Finally, public health efforts that aim to increase breastfeeding operate primarily within the biomedical framework and have had considerably less success at shaping government policies that would lead to the necessary structural changes that support and enable breastfeeding. Thus, although advocacy efforts have succeeded in greatly increasing breastfeeding initiation rates, breastfeeding rates plummet within just a few weeks after birth and formula feeding remains by far the dominant way of feeding children in today's United States (CDC 2013a). These trends place the U.S. far behind many other wealthy nations who have had greater success in protecting and promoting breastfeeding (U.S. Department of Health and Human Services 2011).

In addition to the above difficulties, the practice of breastfeeding continues to be hindered by pediatric sleep advice that encourages solitary, uninterrupted sleep for children. In the following section I shift my attention from the expansion and complexities of biomedical authority over breastfeeding and infant sleep to the contestations of authoritative knowledge within biomedicine itself prompted by conflict between breastfeeding and pediatric sleep medicine.

## Contestations of Authoritative Knowledge in Sleep Medicine, Breastfeeding Medicine, and Pediatric Advice

Compared to the recent efforts to promote breastfeeding, there has been no similar return to previous models of shared and proximal sleep arrangements for children. In fact, the solitary model of sleep has remained firmly in place and equated with "normal" and "healthy" development despite its relatively recent appearance in history and considerable cross-cultural evidence that such arrangements are unusual among human cultures. Pediatric sleep researchers have directed their attention to addressing the growing number of sleep disorders that they identified over the course of the twentieth century. Since the 1970s, much of this attention has focused on Sudden Infant Death Syndrome (SIDS), initially called "crib death," a syndrome identified by process of elimination from other sleep-related deaths and whose etiology remains shrouded in mystery. Research findings on the association of the prone sleep position (on the stomach) prompted public health campaigns beginning in the

1990s that encouraged parents to place their infants on their backs (McKenna, Mosko, and Richard 1997), an effort that significantly reduced SIDS rates. During this time, despite the initial name of the disorder, bed sharing was also identified as a "risk factor" for SIDS, further providing medical impetus for solitary sleep advice. The relationship between breastfeeding and bed sharing was simply not considered by these researchers, since the culture of formula feeding and solitary sleep were so deeply entrenched (McKenna, Mosko, and Richard 1997; McKenna and McDade 2005). As in the case of infant feeding practices, commercial interests also play a role here, through the children's furniture industry, which includes the makers of cribs and related accessories, who have a vested interest in promoting solitary sleep.

Although co-sleeping has not returned in step with rising breastfeeding rates, the National Infant Sleep Position Study has revealed that between 1993 and 2000 the percentage of infants who slept with their mothers for all or part of the night doubled, reaching nearly 50 percent (Willinger et al. 2003). This increase may be partly driven by the frequency of co-sleeping among breastfeeding parents (McCoy et al. 2004; Willinger et al. 2003; Ball and Volpe 2012). Mothers employed outside the home, who are away from their children during the day, may especially attempt to reduce fatigue by avoiding getting up to breastfeed at night (Harmon 2005; Kendall-Tackett, Cong, and Hale 2010). This shift in sleeping patterns has caused medical experts to consider the relationship of breastfeeding and sleep arrangements once again after the relationship between these two domains was virtually severed in the early twentieth century. So far, however, such reconsiderations seem to be fairly one-sided, with breastfeeding experts advocating for a more nuanced approach to sleep that incorporates the interrelated physiology of breastfeeding and mother-infant sleep, and sleep experts mostly remaining within the bounds of the dogma of solitary sleep.

The rift between breastfeeding and SIDS experts dates back to the beginnings of SIDS research, and it cuts to the core of the premier pediatric association, the American Academy of Pediatrics (AAP). From their inception, guidelines on infant sleep have been closely watched by those interested in breastfeeding. McKenna and colleagues, as well as other researchers, have identified a number of major problems in the ways in which SIDS data are collected and analyzed (McKenna, Ball, and Gettler 2007). Due to prevalent bias against proximal sleep arrangements between adults and children, deaths that took place when adults and children shared a sleep surface (or even after they had done so but the child was in a crib at the time of death) were often characterized as caused by bed sharing regardless of differences in the sleep surface or other circumstances, such as alcohol or drug impairment. As a consequence, rigid recommendations against bed sharing were issued. These guidelines failed to account for the substantially different physiological interactions between breastfeeding mothers and babies and formula-fed babies, and ignored the potential relationship between different infant feeding approaches and SIDS.

Over time, however, evidence was accumulating that breastfeeding as well as a proximal sleep environment between mothers and children also contribute to a substantial decrease in SIDS rates (Gettler and McKenna 2010). Research showed that breastfed babies are significantly more arousable than their formula-fed counterparts (McKenna, Ball, and Gettler 2007). Moreover, there are no indications that sharing a bed with an infant in the absence of smoking, alcohol, and other drugs, on a firm surface, and with care in avoiding the use of soft bedding, results in increase of SIDS (Blair 2010; Blair, Heron, and Fleming 2010). All of this evidence is consistent with biological anthropologists McKenna, Ball, and colleagues' (McKenna, Ball, and Gettler 2007; Gettler and McKenna 2010; Ball and Klingaman 2007; Ball and Volpe 2012) research suggesting that maternal-child nighttime interactions in the context of breastfeeding play an important role in the development of the architecture of human infant sleep.

While the relationship between breastfeeding and SIDS was discussed in the AAP's 2005 breastfeeding guidelines (AAP Work Group on Breastfeeding 2005), breastfeeding was still not explicitly recognized to play an important role in the reduction of SIDS in the AAP's guidelines on SIDS issued in the same year (AAP Task Force on Sudden Infant Death Syndrome 2005). Only the recommendation of proximate sleep arrangements, while continuing to discourage bed sharing, was incorporated into these latter guidelines. A flurry of letters to the editors and press releases questioned the 2005 SIDS guidelines. Writing on behalf of the AAP's Section on Breastfeeding, representing pediatricians with expertise and interest in breastfeeding, Eidelman and Gartner (2006) faulted the guidelines for failing to take into account the potential negative consequences of such a prohibition on breastfeeding.[17] Similar critiques were issued by other breastfeeding experts and advocates, including cautions against the AAP recommendation to provide pacifiers at bedtime, which can be potentially detrimental to breastfeeding. Nancy Wight, President of the Academy of Breastfeeding Medicine, wrote with James McKenna that the guidelines represented a "truly astounding triumph of ethnocentric assumptions over common sense and medical research" (Wight and McKenna 2005).

Six years after these guidelines, the AAP has revisited the evidence on the relationship of breastfeeding and SIDS, and the new guidelines now recommend breastfeeding in order to reduce the risk of SIDS (Hauck et al. 2011; AAP Task Force on Sudden Infant Death Syndrome 2011). The blanket recommendation against bed sharing, however, remains in place for all groups, including breastfeeding mothers who do not smoke and have not consumed alcohol, due to "insufficient evidence to recommend any bed sharing situation in the home or at the hospital as safe" (AAP Task Force 2011:e1351). Although there is significantly greater attention to the cultural variability of infant sleep practices in these guidelines, the authors do not address underlying cultural assumptions about the normative nature of solitary sleep for infants or the recommended equipment necessary to implement this practice. The guidelines recommend that infants sleep in "a safety approved crib, portable crib, play yard, or bassinet" (AAP Task Force 2011:e1349).

There are some signs that infant sleep studies are making attempts to incorporate some attention to the broader context of infant sleep safety. For instance, there are a growing number of qualitative studies investigating African American infant sleep practices that have yielded insight into parents' decision making about sleep location (Joyner et al. 2010), their reasons for bed sharing (Chianese et al. 2009), and their perception about the infant sleep environment (Ajao et al. 2011). Chianese and colleagues (2009), for instance, showed that poor inner city parents in Pittsburgh, the majority of whom were African American, perceived bed sharing as helpful in keeping children safe from environmental threats, such as house fires and pests, while also promoting better sleep for both the children and for themselves. Yet these studies remain hindered by their lack of adequate attention to problematic and often overlapping definitions of race, ethnicity, social class, and "culture," and continue to reinforce white middle-class cultural ideals of solitary infant sleep. Similarly, a recent meta-analysis that aimed to resolve the debate on bed sharing and the risk of SIDS (Vennemann et al. 2012) concluded that bed sharing "strongly increases the risk of SIDS" (47), although the authors acknowledged that neither the sleep surface (e.g., couch v. bed) nor feeding methods could be ascertained in the studies they reviewed. Although in this case the authors were more careful to point out that the appropriateness of a blanket public health recommendation against bed sharing or a more context-specific one remains unclear, such categorical advice remains the norm in the U.S.

Helen Ball and Lane Volpe (2012) have recently argued that in order to move the "discussion forward" (2012:84) on SIDS and infant sleep, campaigns that simply provide information without paying attention to the variation in parental practices and the cultural significance of infant sleep location will remain ineffective. Moreover, they can have detrimental effects when fear-based strategies, such as tombstones in the form of headboards or butcher knives appearing next to babies sleeping in an adult bed, are used. Instead, more nuanced research and culturally-specific and sensitive interventions are needed that build on previous studies that have taken these issues into account and have successfully reduced infant deaths.

In addition to conflicts over SIDS, considerable debate surrounds continued medical recommendations for long periods of uninterrupted sleep and for parents' role in actively "training" infants to "sleep through the night" at an early age. A recent article by Henderson and colleagues (2010) entitled "Sleeping through the Night: The Consolidation of Self-regulated Sleep across the First Year of Life," published in the premier journal of the AAP, *Pediatrics*, demonstrates the continued prevalence of these historically and culturally specific ideologies of infant sleep development. The papers' first sentences read as follows: "Infants' sleep/wake patterns consolidate from birth and throughout the first year of life. The developmental task of sleeping through the night is attained when sleep changes from an even, multiphasic, diurnal distribution at birth to consolidated, uninterrupted sleep during the night" (2010:1081). Having claimed, without citing any data, that such consolidation of sleep patterns is the normative pattern of infant development, the authors move onto problematizing infants who do not follow such a pattern in the next sentence: "The failure of an infant to sleep through the night, particularly in concert with their parents' own sleep, is a common parental concern" (2010:1081). The paper then uses data on infant sleep that do not distinguish between different kinds of infant feeding patterns or sleep location to argue that consolidation of sleep among infants begins at one month, and that this evidence can be used to guide parents' approaches toward infant sleep.

McKenna's and Ball's (2010) letter of response to the study reflects their frustration with the paradoxical stance of the AAP that claims to advocate breastfeeding but continues to ignore breastfeeding's important relationship to sleep in its sleep advice. McKenna and Ball argue that the assumption that human "infants can and should sleep 'through the night' from a very young age" (2010:e1081) undermines nighttime breastfeeding, which plays a critical role in both successful lactation as well as in nourishing infants, and ignores potential dangers associated with infant sleep environments that hinder arousal, which may be pivotal for infant survival. They also note that although the authors do not directly encourage sleep training, they shape parental expectations and plans that lead to the use of such methods. They cite a 2010 *Chicago Tribune* article entitled "When should an infant sleep through the night? Sooner than you think" (2010:e1081), which uses the study to recommend sleep training based on Henderson and colleagues' article beginning at one month. While breastfeeding experts and breastfeeding-sleep researchers continue to challenge the kind of research exemplified by the above article and the resultant sleep advice meted out to parents, pediatric sleep advice remains dominated by the paradigm of uninterrupted solitary infant sleep.

The kind of sleep advice reflected in the *Tribune* article mentioned above is amply represented by sleep advice books written by medical experts. Perhaps most well-known among these experts is Dr. Richard Ferber, whose book "Solve Your Child's Sleep Problems" (2006), first published in 1985, advocates leaving children in their cribs for increasing lengths of time without feeding them or responding to their cries. Ferber's advice relies on scientific work and professional experience derived from pediatric sleep medicine, a medical specialty that addresses sleep problems among children (he is director of the Center for Pediatric Sleep Disorders at Children's Hospital Boston). This specialty has thus far paid minimal attention to the relationship of breastfeeding and children's sleep or to the historical and cultural context out of which it emerged (McKenna, Ball, and Gettler 2007; Jenni and O'Connor 2005). In his discussion of co-sleeping in the recently revised edition of the book, Ferber argues that the evolutionary history of the wide-spread cultural practice of co-sleeping has little relevance in modern society. Furthermore, in contrast to biological anthropological work that demonstrates the intricate physiological relationship between breastfeeding mothers' and babies' bodies, Ferber (2006:41) claims that most children sleep nearly continuously throughout the night and are not "conscious of where they are or who else is or is not with them." It is little wonder that breastfeeding is only mentioned twice in the entire book, once in relation to the timing of the introduction of the pacifier, and the second time to discuss sleep disruptions caused by "too much feeding" by children under two who are "*still* breastfeeding or using the bottle" (2006:137; emphasis mine). Equating breastfeeding to the norm of formula feeding allows Ferber to omit any further discussion of potential physiological interactions between breastfeeding and sleep, making nighttime breastfeeding (along with any other feeding) a part of an undesirable, problematic behavior that must be eliminated.

By presenting solitary, continuous sleep as the norm for "modern" children, Ferber is able to advance his argument, which echoes Holt's and Watson's pediatric advice put forth nearly a century ago (Stearns, Rowland, and Giarnella 1996; McKenna, Ball, and Gettler 2007). For instance, Ferber (2006) advocates sticking with his approach even if the child vomits from crying. In such a situation, he recommends going in and quickly changing the sheet and pajamas but cautions, "But do so quickly and matter-of-fact, then leave again. If you reward him for throwing up by giving him too much attention, he will only learn that vomiting is a good way for him to get what he wants. Occasional vomiting will not hurt your child, so don't feel guilty. Like the crying, it will soon stop" (2006:102). Although passages such as these have led many parents to accuse Ferber of promoting a cruel approach to taking care of children, his book remains tremendously popular. Furthermore, major elements of the Watsonian approach continue to be promoted in the majority of sleep advice (Ball and Klingaman 2007), albeit in somewhat tempered forms. These approaches all use a form of habituation to extinguish nighttime crying and feeding.

At the same time, with the increases in breastfeeding rates prompted by medical findings of the benefits of breastfeeding for both children and mothers, parents are increasingly bringing their children into their beds (Willinger et al. 2003; McCoy et al. 2004; Kendall-Tackett, Cong, and Hale 2010; Ball and Volpe 2012). Some of these parents have turned for sleep advice to a minority group of medical experts who have taken a contrasting approach from the above prevailing trends. Most of these experts can be characterized as ascribing to the philosophy of Attachment Parenting (AP), a philosophy of parenting based on psychological research on the significance of early, secure attachments to caregivers in child development and later adult well-being. According to the principles of attachment parenting, being responsive to the child's needs and providing consistent loving care enables children to form secure attachments (Attachment Parenting International 2008).

The term "attachment parenting" was first used by Dr. William Sears, who has authored numerous books (as single author as well as with his wife and son), and is the current leading advocate of this parenting approach. Parents adhering to principles of "natural parenting" or "natural family living," a term used in *Mothering Magazine*, tend to embrace attachment parenting and often rely on Dr. Sears' publications for expert advice (Warner 2005). Breastfeeding is a centerpiece of this approach, although Dr. Sears argues that parents who do not breastfeed can also practice attachment parenting principles (Attachment Parenting International 2011). Nevertheless, Sears' work and attachment parenting are often associated only with breastfeeding advocacy, partly due to the La Leche League's use of this material (La Leche League International 2011).[18] This approach to parenting encourages breastfeeding on demand throughout the day and night, encourages carrying children close to mothers' and partners' bodies, and supports proximal sleep arrangements, including bed sharing, and child-led weaning. Sears does not advocate bed sharing as the only recommended sleep arrangement, but cautions against methods that leave children without any reassurance for long periods of time and raises the possibility of harmful effects from raised stress levels.

Just as mainstream pediatric sleep experts do, Sears derives his authority from his status as a physician and employs scientific research to support his position, although he also relies on his own and his wife's experiences of breastfeeding and sleeping with their six children. Attachment parenting has been subject to considerable criticism from feminists due to its implicit romanticization and "naturalization" of women's domestic roles, the assumptions of privilege that enable the maintenance of attachment parenting practice in daily life, and its questionable use of science to justify its approach (Warner 2005).[19] Despite the issues raised by critics, Sears continues to provide the most common alternative resource on caring for children from a perspective that thoroughly incorporates the embodied experiences of breastfeeding. It is difficult to assess the number of parents who practice attachment parenting, although the rates of breastfeeding and bed sharing indicate that this group constitutes only a small minority of parents.[20] This group, along with Sears, was the target of the *Time* magazine article which accompanied the controversial cover of Grumet nursing her toddler and which labeled AP parenting practices "extreme" (Pickert 2012).

As the above examples demonstrate, medical experts devote considerable attention to infant sleep and dominate sleep advice for children. Within the community of such experts, however, there are significant differences between those who approach breastfeeding and infant sleep as fundamentally related, and those who view infant sleep as a separate topic. Breastfeeding and breastfeeding-sleep researchers attempt to reorient paradigms for "normal" infant sleep as one that should be always examined in the context of infant feeding and sleep location, while infant sleep researchers tend to search for ways to address what they see as sleep problems and pathologies. Furthermore, pediatric sleep advice relies on the well-established authority of physicians to promote ideologies of solitary sleep with little consideration for the impact of such advice for breastfeeding. The most prominent voices among those who contest such mainstream sleep advice consider breastfeeding central to parenting, and similarly rely on medical authority to make their case, albeit with the important modification of personal experience that incorporates breastfeeding. The above discussion reveals that even within biomedicine, where breastfeeding is ostensibly considered important, there are heterogeneous and contradictory approaches toward infant sleep practices. Together with the insights gleaned from historical study, the divisions among breastfeeding and sleep experts provide a complex portrait of the role of biomedicine in breastfeeding and infant sleep practices. In the final section below, I discuss how feminists have wrestled with these issues and offer possibilities for moving beyond polarized debates about the role of biomedicine in breastfeeding and sleep.

## Feminisms, Biomedicine, and the Matter of Infant Feeding "Choice" in the U.S.

In the following discussion, I examine U.S. feminist responses to biomedical engagement in breastfeeding. No such parallel feminist debate surrounds infant sleep arrangements, primarily because infant sleep has not been conceptualized in relation to women's bodies in this setting, although there have been feminist critiques of parenting approaches that encompass co-sleeping practices.[21] Due to the lack of sustained feminist attention to co-sleeping, I center my discussion around breastfeeding and return to implications for sleep at the end of the chapter.

Although breastfeeding has not generated nearly as much feminist attention as other realms of reproduction, such as abortion rights, public health advocacy efforts have prompted a growing feminist response. In line with the historical focus of this chapter, I focus on U.S. feminist work, although these debates clearly circulate across national boundaries and have become prominent in Canada, the U.K., Australia, and New Zealand. Nevertheless, in attending to U.S. perspectives, I aim to "localize" these discussions and anchor them to the histories out of which they arise. These debates center on contestations of authoritative knowledge in biomedicine's relationship with breastfeeding. I argue that the diversity of feminist positions on biomedical approaches to breastfeeding reflects the heterogeneity of the history and contemporary involvement of biomedicine in breastfeeding. I will conclude with a discussion of the use of "choice" in feminist discussions and argue for a move away from this language toward an anthropological approach grounded in attending to embodied social relations.

La Leche League International embodies a particular kind of feminist voice, one that is built on maternalism, and arose out of the context of the 1950s Catholic Family Movement (Ward 2000; Weiner 1994; Hausman 2003:155–188). While the League specifically decided to form a secular movement that transcended religious divides, it continued to espouse ideologies of breastfeeding as part of a larger "sacred motherhood" narrative that had deep religious roots and that also promoted specific notions of the family unit based on a white, middle-class, married, heterosexual couple with a male wage-earner and a woman in a primarily domestic role. Although the League challenged many aspects of the domestic division of labor, due to its dominant maternalist narrative and difficulties of accommodating working women and different models of families, the League is at odds with many other feminists.[22]

As I discussed in the first section of the chapter, the La Leche League has had a heterogeneous and sometimes contradictory relationship with biomedicine from its formation due to its efforts to challenge prevailing medical norms while also relying on medical experts and, later on, growing scientific evidence to promote breastfeeding. Today, La Leche League International remains committed to the ideal of promoting the larger goal of mothering through breastfeeding, in which biomedical research plays an important role. At the same time, the League also relies on a range of other scientific materials as well as accounts drawn from personal experiences of breastfeeding to promote its agenda. For instance, the League has featured McKenna's research on nighttime breastfeeding and sleep as well as Katherine Dettwyler's evolutionary approach to hominid weaning patterns. These biological anthropological perspectives have been marginalized within mainstream medical guidelines. Furthermore, the League uses science, including biological anthropological research, to support a return to a "natural" or "instinctive" kind of parenting of which breastfeeding is an important part, thereby naturalizing its highly culturally specific model of breastfeeding, gender, and kinship (Hausman 2003:155–188).[23]

Social historians of childbirth, breastfeeding, and wet-nursing have taken pro-woman and pro-breastfeeding positions that are cautious about the involvement of biomedicine in breastfeeding based on the undermining of women's authority and detrimental effects on women's reproduction (Apple 1987; Golden 1996; J.H. Wolf 2001). Historian Jacqueline Wolf has taken a particularly active role in translating her historical insights for public health and health worker audiences (2003, 2008) as well as for feminist scholars (2006). Wolf argues that women should take a much more active role in lobbying for their right to breastfeed as well as for children's rights to be breastfed. She believes that women deserve to have access to full information about the health consequences of formula feeding for children as well as for women so that they can make an informed decision about breastfeeding. Furthermore, historical study can inform women about how artificial milk feeding became normative practice and assist feminist critique of commercial interests in infant feeding, such as in the industry's campaign to undermine the National Breastfeeding Advocacy campaign in the middle of the last decade. Finally, Wolf suggests that by advocating for breastfeeding, feminists can also open up other social issues for discussion, including employment practices, parental leave, and childcare, and undermine the pervasive sexualization and objectification of women's bodies. Neither Wolf's historically-informed nor the previous socially-enriched public health approaches wish to promote traditional gender roles or an uncritical stance toward biomedicine.

Other feminists are more explicit in their challenge of the biomedicalization of breastfeeding and potential biological reductionism, but maintain a biosocial view that recognizes the unique biological contribution of women to reproduction. Women's studies scholar Bernice Hausman (2003), drawing on anthropologist Penny Van Esterik's earlier work (1989), has advocated for a feminist position that values and recognizes breastfeeding as a potentially liberating opportunity to incorporate relationality into feminist ideals of a traditionally more individualist concept of autonomy. This concept of relationality not only encompasses the intercorporeal relationship between mother and child, but also espouses a broader, ecological approach that includes other social relationships and human-environmental interactions. Thus in her argument, Hausman walks a narrow line between a strong critique of biomedicalized approaches to breastfeeding—which reinscribe patriarchal gender roles, deepen inequalities along the lines of social class and race, and assert medical expert authority over women—and a reliance on scientific evidence to make a concerted effort to enable all women to breastfeed their children. Hausman (2011) has recently elaborated on her approach and on the concept of choice, to which I will return below.

Feminists who reject the use of biomedical research to support breastfeeding but wish nonetheless to advocate for breastfeeding find themselves in a challenging position. Thus, feminist sociologist Barbara Katz Rothman (2008) seeks to articulate a position that advocates for breastfeeding without buying into biomedicalized ideologies for doing so. For Rothman, biomedicalization is too intimately tied up in the unholy triumvirate of patriarchy, capitalism, and technology and their role in the construction of race and gender (including how feminist arguments about breastfeeding themselves are made through these relations). She ultimately argues that, similar to replacing unmedicated childbirth with surgical and interventionist birth, something important would be lost if breastfeeding was no longer practiced. Rothman argues that breastfeeding advocacy on the basis of health agendas masks these other relational aspects of breastfeeding, which resist easy characterization and cannot be replaced even if artificial supplements were perfected.

Sociologist Linda Blum's (1999) challenge of public health advocacy for breastfeeding builds on some of the same sociological analyses of biomedicalization and its gendered, classist, and racialized consequences that inform Rothman's work. Blum specifically attends to British sociologist Pam Carter's (1995) discussion of breastfeeding in her own study, which mounted a significant critique of breastfeeding on the grounds of essentialism. Blum's work sits at a critical juncture in the U.S. feminist literature, where the biomedicalization of breastfeeding is not only critiqued, but the use of artificial milk feeding seems significantly less consequential. Indeed, Blum critiques Scheper-Hughes (1993) for her analytic focus on the consequences of not breastfeeding for poor Brazilian children's lives (and deaths) that I discussed in chapter 1. Blum argues that Scheper-Hughes should have paid more attention to the larger context, in which most of these children would have died regardless of breastfeeding (Blum 1999:46).[24] Hausman (2003:189–223) suggests that this rhetorical move then enables Blum to regard the health implications of breastfeeding as fairly inconsequential in the U.S. Blum proposes that while breastfeeding can potentially serve as a feminist practice that challenges biomedical ideologies, it can also be a mode of acquiescing to governmental regimes of surveillance, coercion, and control. In the case of marginalized women, especially African American women who have been historically sexualized and exploited through the institution of slavery and subsequent racism, resistance to breastfeeding advocacy is both a logical and a feminist response.

Carter's and Blum's stances have been recently elaborated by philosopher Rebecca Kukla (2006), journalist Hanna Rosin (2009), and women's studies scholar Joan Wolf (2007, 2011).[25] Kukla (2006) questions the ethics of breastfeeding promotion on the basis of a series of arguments that concern the constraints on women's ability to "choose" breastfeeding. Kukla argues that the language of "choice" obscures the circumstance of women's decisions, wherein breastfeeding is a difficult, if not impossible, undertaking for many. Furthermore, Kukla argues that the risk-based approach of the National Breastfeeding Advocacy Campaign imposed moral responsibility for making the decision to breastfeed onto individual women. Kukla asserts that this advocacy strategy causes a "distortion in mothers' moral perception" (2006:176) that causes women to locate blame in themselves and ultimately limits their autonomy. As Hausman also observes (2011:78), Kukla employs the language of the "benefits" of breastfeeding that present breastfeeding as something "extra," beyond the norm, and implies that these "benefits" are only marginal and do not warrant the above moral impositions on mothers.

Hanna Rosin (2009) and Joan Wolf (2007, 2011) are also concerned with the moral obligation of breastfeeding and the consequences of this responsibility for women, but they do so by more explicitly challenging scientific claims that support breastfeeding. Rosin is primarily concerned with the patriarchal implications of imposing this responsibility on mothers, although she also makes claims about larger issues of inequality (see chapter 5). In contrast, Wolf (2007, 2011) argues that breastfeeding advocacy constitutes an important part of a neoliberal construction of biomedicalized risk culture that embraces an ideology of "total motherhood," where mothers operate as solely concerned with managing and minimizing risk for their children. Both Rosin and Wolf, the latter much more intensively, review the medical literature on breastfeeding and conclude that, in industrialized settings, the benefits of breastfeeding are minimal and therefore do not warrant public health advocacy.

Both authors suggest that medical efforts to promote breastfeeding rely on science that is not rigorous and vastly overstates the health effects of breastfeeding. They reject the significance of breastfeeding in women's and children's physiology and consider the decision of breastfeeding a "choice" that should be made by women and their families on their own, without the imposition of government-led advocacy.

In her careful analysis, Hausman (2003, 2009, 2011) finds that Blum's, Kukla's, Rosin's, and Joan Wolf's arguments each hinge upon the assumption of breastfeeding having only marginal health effects. Consequently, Hausman argues that if this assumption was found to be incorrect, it would make these feminist arguments significantly less tenable. It is beyond the scope of this book to enter into the specific details of research on breastfeeding, but in agreement with many others who have reviewed this body of research, my own reading leaves me quite convinced of the substantial health consequences of not breastfeeding.[26] I also agree with numerous critics of Rosin and Joan Wolf that these authors make significant errors and omissions in their approach to the literature and consequently reach incorrect conclusions (Hausman 2009; Heinig 2007; Hopkinson 2007).

Furthermore, a social historical assessment of the growing prevalence of artificial milk formulas makes it quite difficult to see these products simply as a triumph of "human ingenuity," as Joan Wolf suggests (2011:150). Indeed, it is striking to observe the ideological erasure of how breastfeeding came to be replaced with a substance manufactured from the body of another lactating animal with the addition of various bioengineered additives derived from diverse sources. While Joan Wolf's critique of the science is the sharpest among these feminists, I suggest that all of them embrace a rather uncritical, "technocratic"[27] perspective on infant formula. This perspective downplays the political economic, historical, and sociocultural forces that have made the manufacturing of infant formula possible and continue to enable its enhancements and global circulation. Moreover, this view does not adequately address biomedicine's complex relationship with infant feeding: the rise of science and biomedical research that underlies the production of infant formula, the science behind breastfeeding advocacy, and the substantial debates about breastfeeding within biomedicine. Therefore, I argue that although these critics aim to oppose biomedical authority, in fact they embrace a form of biomedical authority that is deeply entwined with neoliberal capitalism.[28]

This argument leads to my final discussion of the language of "choice" and "autonomy." These terms have been employed by proponents and critics of breastfeeding promotion. Bernice Hausman (2003:91–120) eloquently demonstrates how the notion of "informed choice" in breastfeeding has actually led to the conception of breastfeeding and formula feeding as essentially equivalent. Furthermore, Hausman, along with all feminist critics mentioned thus far, finds advocacy efforts that position women as individuals who can freely choose breastfeeding without any regard to their social circumstances unacceptable. Hausman draws on historian Rickie Solinger's (1998, 2001) work on reproduction in the U.S. to argue that the language of choice, instead of producing a greater set of possibilities, actually distinguishes those who possess the privileges of making these "choices," thereby contributing to greater inequalities.[29]

To further this argument, we need to examine the concept of "choice" in the context of ideologies of personhood that portray people as discrete, rational decision-making entities that have been propagated in the global spread of neoliberalism (see chapter 1). "Choosers," in this sense, are distinguished by their social position not only to engage in certain activities but also in patterns of consumption that are constitutive to their personhood. In this light, the use of the concept of choice is problematic both in breastfeeding promotion efforts and in the criticism of feminists who see breastfeeding advocacy as a constraint on women's autonomy and choices. A more holistic feminist critique of current infant feeding practices would not simply attend to the constraints imposed by breastfeeding advocacy, but also to the complex historical, cultural, and political economic elements shaping women's decisions. Critiques that only focus on breastfeeding advocacy as a limitation on freedom ignore the history of the biomedicalization of childbearing, including breastfeeding, and the significant commercial interests that shape infant feeding behaviors. Moreover, such critiques fail to consider that the patterns of consumption that include infant formula use, and the associated notion that infant formula use enhances women's freedom, are thoroughly immersed in local-global capitalism and the perpetuation of the inequalities of production and reproduction. Ironically, these patterns constitute some of the unexamined consequences of the neoliberal ideologies critiqued by Blum (1999) and Joan Wolf (2011).

One recent effort to overcome discourses of choice and individualist public health interventions that promote breastfeeding has emerged from the collaborative efforts of a group of interdisciplinary breastfeeding advocates led by public health scholars Paige Hall-Smith and Miriam Labbok and feminist scholar Bernice Hausman. In their recent edited volume *Beyond Health, Beyond Choice: Breastfeeding Constraint and Realities,* they seek to develop a new approach to breastfeeding that embraces the shared goals of feminism and public health to engage in "social action and social justice—practices to improve human experience and end inequalities that contribute to health disparities" (Hausman, Smith, and Labbok 2012:10). Moreover, they outline their desire for a feminist discourse that engages fully with the intersecting dynamics of race, class, and gender to better understand and reduce the many obstacles that hinder women's ability to breastfeed. The authors propose that public health practitioners incorporate these insights to develop breastfeeding advocacy that addresses these structural and cultural barriers and ultimately helps to improve women's and children's health. These scholars employ biomedical knowledge about the biological impact of breastfeeding but do so in a critical manner that is sensitive to the entailed history and power dynamics. Within this framework, women themselves (along with others) can use biomedical knowledge to advocate for social change that brings about better health not only for their own families but for all others.

## Conclusion

Through the three interrelated frames focusing on points of tension and contention, I have shown that a historically oriented sociocultural analysis of biomedicine's involvement in breastfeeding and infant sleep can help develop a nuanced perspective that resists simple dichotomies. An anthropological analysis is particularly well-suited to the study of complex problems, such as the multiple ways in which biomedicine has become involved in and has transformed our understandings and lived experiences of these bodily processes. It is essential for such an investigation to consider specific, local manifestations of biomedicine through ethnographic and comparative study of social relations instead of presuming its existence as a monolithic category.

The historical transformations in childbearing that I outlined above form the background for understanding the present-day dilemmas confronted by my participants. Whereas breastfeeding continues to be entangled in images of idealized motherhood, buttressed by new scientific claims for its superiority, the everyday aspects of practicing breastfeeding remain mired in the legacy of cultural ideologies that enabled artificial formula milk feeding to supplant breastfeeding during the twentieth century. Thus, families face a paradoxical situation in which the idea of breastfeeding is publicly valorized, but its practice—including nighttime breastfeeding—is nonetheless stigmatized and constrained by innumerable barriers.

Anthropologists can add a unique dimension to feminist discussions of breastfeeding and infant sleep practices. I see the joint framework proposed by Hausman, Smith, and Labbok (2012) as a promising path forward—one that incorporates many of the same perspectives that inform this book and that can be further enriched by anthropological perspectives. Grounded in careful study of humanity across time and space, anthropologists attend to the specificities of embodied experience in complex local sociocultural and political economic circumstances and examine their role in social relationships. In Penny Van Esterik's contribution to Smith and colleagues' edited volume, she reminds us that "breastfeeding is, after all, about creating social relationships" (2012:57). In the remainder of this book, I turn to my own ethnographic evidence to investigate these social relationships and ask what they can tell us about nighttime breastfeeding and sleep in the context of the broader cultural landscape of the United States.

## Notes

1. Jordan further argues that the global spread of biomedical systems of obstetrics, which she terms "cosmopolitical obstetrics" constitutes "biomedical colonization," in which technology plays a particularly important role. Jordan asserts that "technology, by determining what is to be taken as authoritative knowledge, in turn establishes a particular regime of power—a power that must be counterbalanced by a new respect for the legitimacy of indigenous traditions and indigenous ways of giving birth" (1993:215). Attention to authoritative knowledge has yielded many important insights about the global inequalities engendered and reinforced by biomedicine, demonstrating the stratification of reproduction in diverse ethnographic settings (Davis-Floyd and Sargent 1997). At the same time, recent work has highlighted the heterogeneity and multiple power relations within the local origins and manifestations of biomedicine, in indigenous systems of knowledge and social relations, and in their intricate interactions.
2. American Indian women breastfed longer than women of European ancestry, to at least two years (D'Emilio and Freedman 1998:8).

3. While initiating breastfeeding remained common throughout the century, patterns of breastfeeding differed from current medical recommendations since many breastfeeding women added thin gruels, mashed table foods, and later other foods to children's diet from the early months onward (J.H. Wolf 2001).
4. The religious significance of motherhood in the U.S. has its roots in Judeo-Christian traditions and was amplified in Christianity by the role of Mary, a human woman who gave birth to and breastfed the baby Jesus, considered to be the son of God. The figure of the Virgin Mary inspired a proliferation of devotional practices that continue to bear significance to many Christians today (Ward 2000).
5. See also Ulrich 1990 for an earlier example of such intervention and its consequences based on Martha Ballard's diaries from 1785–1812, who practiced midwifery in Maine.
6. The systematic vilification of wet-nurses parallels that of midwives in physicians' efforts to professionalize and displace these women (cf. Leavitt 1986, Borst 1995, Fraser 1998).
7. See especially Apple 1987:97–132.
8. See also Leavitt 1986 and Golden 1996.
9. See also Hausman 2003; Litt 2000; Fraser 1998.
10. Based on Wisconsin case studies from 1870–1920, Borst (1995) argues that the decline of midwifery there was driven by the acceptance of a scientific model of medicine that was emerging in the late nineteenth to early twentieth centuries rather than simply by physicians' efforts to push midwives out of practice. In Wisconsin, women increasingly called upon family physicians for childbirth, leading to a decreasing demand for midwives by the first decades of the twentieth century. It was obstetricians around 1920, rather than family physicians, who began a more concerted effort to delimit and eliminate midwifery on a national scale. This argument parallels that of Jacqueline Wolf's (2001) about the decline of breastfeeding.
11. See also Hardyment 2007.
12. See also Zelizer 1994.
13. The distribution of these bags has recently been prohibited in New York City, as part of the Latch On NYC campaign, inciting controversy and accusations of Mayor Bloomberg playing "Nanny" (Limbaugh 2012).
14. See, for instance, Joan Wolf's work (2011).
15. See also Nancy Krieger's (2010) similar use of the concept of intersectionality in a public health framework.
16. The emphasis of "benefits" has problematic implications since it assumes that formula feeding is the norm beyond which breastfeeding offers "extra," but not necessary, positive effects (Riordan 2005). Lactation consultants and others have worked to reorient this language to establish breastfeeding as the norm to which formula feeding is compared, pointing out that artificial milk substitutes have harmful effects compared with breastfeeding. Thus, while the emphasis on the benefits

of breastfeeding aimed to encourage breastfeeding, it has the paradoxical effects of undermining efforts to establish breastfeeding as the human norm for feeding babies.
17. See also Bartick 2006; Gessner and Porter 2006; Pelayo et al. 2006.
18. Despite these commitments, Sears has come under criticism from LLLI and other breastfeeding advocates in 2001 due to undisclosed commercial ties to formula manufacturers, including displaying banner ads for commercial formula on his website that violated the International Code on the Marketing of Breastmilk Substitutes (Granju 2001).
19. See also criticisms of La Leche League's use of AP in Faircloth 2010b; Bobel 2002; Hausman 2003; Ward 2000; and the following section.
20. Sears's *The Baby Book* (2013), which includes both breastfeeding and sleep discussions, maintains a high position on Amazon's parenting list, with nearly 600 positive reviews between its 2003 and 2013 editions. We cannot easily compare this position to Ferber's book, however, since *The Baby Book* is not only a book focused on sleep. There are considerably more popular books that follow a more "moderate" version of the controlled crying approach on the list, and nearly all of them aim to reduce/eliminate night feedings. Further research needs to be undertaken to evaluate the use of on-line sleep advice that is a growing source of information for parents.
21. See Warner 2005.
22. See Hausman 2003 and Blum 1999 for a discussion.
23. I have argued elsewhere (Tomori 2005) that in League discourses the language of the "heart" serves as an important way of channeling an embodied sense of morality that also encompasses these scientific and biomedical components.
24. See Hausman's (2003:189–223) full discussion of Blum's treatment of Scheper-Hughes.
25. See also Hausman's (2008, 2009, 2011) discussion of these authors.
26. See U. S. Department of Health and Human Services 2011 for an overview.
27. I am borrowing Davis-Floyd's (2004) term.
28. Here, I am specifically referring back to Collier and Ong's (2005) work on global assemblages that I addressed in chapter 1.
29. Anthropologist Christa Craven's (2010) ethnography of the homebirth midwifery movement in the U.S. indeed shows how deploying neoliberal consumerist choice rhetoric in a social movement can lead to reinforcing historical inequalities along the lines of social class and race.

*Chapter 3*

# MAKING BREASTFEEDING PARENTS IN CHILDBIRTH EDUCATION COURSES

Childbirth education courses have become a mainstay of preparations for middle-class couples expecting their first baby. The courses not only provide foundational knowledge about childbirth and infant care in a society where expectant couples often have minimal prior exposure to birth and the care of young children, but they also constitute an essential American rite of passage through which women and men become mothers and fathers, respectively (Davis-Floyd 2004; Reed 2005). This rite of passage, however, comes with a price tag. High quality childbirth education that includes breastfeeding and other aspects of infant care courses is a consumer good that middle-class expectant parents seek out and to which they devote considerable resources of time and money in an effort to ensure that they undergo the best possible preparation for having a baby. As such, these courses comprise a part of middle-class consumption practices that constitute "good" parents, who provide the best possible start for their baby.[1] Learning about breastfeeding in order to pursue the medically endorsed and morally superior option for infant feeding and acquiring other fundamentals of culturally salient aspects of infant care fit neatly into this package of goods.

Davis-Floyd's (2004) analysis of popular childbirth education courses has identified significant differences in the content of these courses as well as their transformative power to socialize expectant mothers into particular ideologies of childbirth. As I will show, I have also found that these courses have distinctive approaches to and profound influences on parental practices of breastfeeding and nighttime infant care. First, expectant parents are exposed to specialized knowledge about breastfeeding in the context of other realms of knowledge about birth and sleep, which intimately affects their understanding of breastfeeding. Second, in the process of sharing knowledge about the bodily processes of childbearing, childbirth education courses also offer models of parental personhood for participants into which participants are socialized by attending classes, participating in exercises, and purchasing the recommended materials. Using ethnographic evidence from two local childbirth education organizations in Green City that both supported breastfeeding, I will show how each organization constructed different approaches to breastfeeding and infant sleep through which couples negotiated competing ideologies of personhood, parent-child relationships, and capitalism. Couples selectively embraced different aspects of the models that they were offered, resisting reductionist characterizations. Nevertheless, these organizations themselves are part of a capitalist political economic landscape of stratified reproduction, where privileged "choosers" [2] can mobilize resources through the exercise of their consumer choices, while "beggars" who lack these privileges cannot do so (Solinger 2001; Craven 2010).

## Childbirth Education as a Privileged Good

Per the recruitment criteria of the study, all study participants enrolled in some form of childbirth education at two major local sites in Green City. All but one family partook in a childbirth education course series, and nearly all also completed a breastfeeding class as part of a package of courses that also included newborn or infant care. Childbirth education courses for most of my participants constituted the main source of in-depth knowledge about the process of having a baby. In addition, participants talked with maternity providers, read on-line or physical books and magazines, and talked with family and friends to learn more. However, few participants had access to the nitty-gritty details of giving birth or breastfeeding one's baby from others who experienced having a baby in the recent past. The few exceptions were those who had sisters to whom they were particularly close (e.g., Kate, Leslie, and Corinne). Even in these cases, the bulk of specific information originated from childbirth education courses.

These expert-led courses have replaced guidance from older, experienced kin because breastfeeding knowledge has been lost in the generations who practiced feeding with artificial milk substitutes (Avishai 2007; Hausman 2003). The knowledge gap is widened by U.S. patterns of age segregation, where prior to becoming parents couples often lack exposure to caring for young children. The difficulty of getting detailed information is compounded by cultural taboos that surround certain "polluting" aspects of having a baby (e.g., the parts of labor that involve blood or urine and feces, or breastfeeding in front of others, for instance) as well as by the intense moral scrutiny to which the process of having a baby is subjected (Battersby 2007). Finally, although maternity care providers do possess privileged knowledge about many aspects of birth and breastfeeding, they have little time to share this knowledge with expectant parents. Rather, couples are expected to take a childbirth education course recommended by the provider or by the informational materials the provider gives to the families. These courses then become key cultural institutions for acquiring knowledge about childbirth, breastfeeding, and infant sleep.

Participants in my study took part in childbirth education courses at one of two local organizations. These courses were the ones most commonly attended by participants who were planning a birth at the university-affiliated hospital in Green City, while the other local hospital, "Private Hospital," had its own childbirth preparation courses.[3] Participants who chose obstetricians at University Hospital were often referred to Family Center, whereas certified nurse-midwives frequently recommended Holistic Center. In addition to these larger organizations, Green City had several other childbirth education options, including local chapters of national organizations that promote childbirth with minimal to no medical interventions.[4] Furthermore, individual home birth midwives and doulas offered their own private educational sessions in the community. Thus, Green City residents who had sufficient resources to locate and pay for childbirth education had an abundance of options for these services.

The wealth of childbirth education resources in Green City stood in stark contrast to other nearby communities, reflecting their socioeconomic differences (see chapter 6). Neighbor City, for example, did not have the same community resources but because of its proximity, Green City's abundance of courses on weeknights as well as on weekends fulfilled these needs. Rachel and Nathan, Corinne and Jacob, and Kate and Joshua chose to attend Green City's courses. Their decision was partly based on their providers' recommendations and on their sense of the philosophy of the courses. All of these couples selected birth providers at Green City's University Hospital.

Rachel and Nathan and Kate and Joshua chose the midwifery service, while Corinne and Jacob chose an obstetrician there. Although the courses at Private Hospital were geographically closer to each of these couples, their choice to deliver at University Hospital made it less likely that they would attend the other hospital's courses. Rachel and Nathan chose Family Center, while Corinne and Jacob and Kate and Joshua chose Holistic Center because of their sense that it was particularly supportive of childbirth with minimal interventions. Despite the proximity of Neighbor City to Green City, those with transportation limitations, financial and time limitations, and those who did not have adequate educational resources would not have been able to participate in these courses.

Most other nearby cities and suburbs fared far worse, since in the absence of local childbirth education options, expectant parents were funneled into hospital-based courses. These courses have been critiqued in previous research on childbirth education for their emphasis on simply producing "good patients" instead of truly educating parents on optimal practices and the reduction of unnecessary medical interventions (Morton and Hsu 2007; Davis-Floyd 2004; Rothman 1981). The three expectant parents who enrolled in my study from neighborhoods beyond Green City and Neighbor City were aware of this lack of services in their communities and selected Green City's courses due to their belief in its superior quality even in the face of lengthier commutes to reach these courses. Each of these three couples drew on their own research of childbirth education options, along with their health care providers' recommendations and friends' opinions, in their decision-making process.

Two of these three couples in my study planned to deliver their children at one of the two hospitals in Green City instead of in their own communities because of their belief that these hospitals provided higher quality care. Kristen's and Daniel's choice of Green City's Private Hospital was partly driven by the fact that their community did not have a closer hospital and therefore driving to Green City did not require going out of the way. They chose to attend courses at Family Center based on their obstetrician's recommendation and because of Kristen's familiarity with Family Center's philosophy from her mother, who also attended similar courses and was a proponent of making informed decisions in childbirth and in breastfeeding. In contrast, for Paula and Matthew the decision to go to Green City's University Hospital necessitated a significantly longer drive, which they felt was necessary to receive the highest quality care in the area—care that supported their desire to give birth with midwives and with minimal interventions. The midwives' recommendation to attend Holistic Center as well as hearing that Holistic Center was supportive of "natural childbirth"—childbirth with minimal to no medical interventions—influenced their decision to attend this site. The third couple, Lynn and Gary, opted to deliver their child at a hospital closer to their home that offered an alternative birth center within the hospital, which was staffed by midwives for those intending to give birth with minimal medical interventions. Lynn was told by the midwives at that hospital to consider the courses at Holistic Center because they were the best in the area for those planning a "natural birth."

Each childbirth preparation site I attended in Green City offered traditional six- to seven-week series of evening childbirth preparation courses that lasted two to two and a half hours each. The structure of these courses presented significant challenges for expectant parents. Expectant parents with stable, daytime work and ample time in the evenings free of other necessary commitments had a far better chance of being able to participate in lengthy multi-week courses (Morton and Hsu 2007). In an effort to provide alternative options for busy parents, each site in my study also offered condensed courses that could be taken over the course of one of two weekends.[5] Of the seventeen couples in my study who attended the childbirth education series, all but one couple attended the six- or seven-week option rather than the condensed weekend series. Rachel's shift schedule as a health care worker, which included evenings and nights, and Nathan's coursework and part-time work made it too difficult for them to attend an extended series, and therefore they selected the condensed course. The rates for childbirth preparation courses were $235 at Holistic Center and $146 at Family Center. Several major insurance plans covered the cost of these courses, making them more affordable for participants holding such policies. Holistic Center also offered financial assistance for qualified applicants.

Childbirth education courses formed the core of offerings, to which classes in breastfeeding and newborn/infant care could be added. At each site, participants could purchase a "package" of classes at a slight discount, which included both breastfeeding classes (one or two sessions of two to three hours each) and infant care classes (two or three sessions of two to three hours each). Through these offerings, each site aimed to broaden its appeal to different parents, some of who wished to take the full array of classes while others wished to select only a particular course. Parents usually had to pay out of pocket for these courses (Breastfeeding/Infant Care courses were $60 each at Holistic Center, and $49/$65 at Family Center).

Researchers have noted that while participation in childbirth education classes has declined overall, participation remains high among white, older, wealthier, educated, and married women (Lu et al. 2003). Although I did not conduct a formal survey of childbirth course participant sociodemographic characteristics,[6] my observations during my participation in these courses reflect similar findings. In the courses I observed (including childbirth education series, infant care courses, and breastfeeding courses), the majority of participants were married (as evidenced by wedding bands), white couples in their late 20s and early 30s. I encountered one same-sex couple, Petra and Julia, who were married in a ceremony not recognized by the state. They were the only couple in my study who did not participate in the childbirth preparation course; they did not feel comfortable being the only same-sex couple amidst all heterosexual couples. Their experience reflects the heteronormative conventions of these courses (Reed 2005). I met only a few single mothers during my observations. Based on introductions at the beginning of class and in informal conversations during breaks, most participants held white-collar jobs and were well-educated. All of these trends reinforce the notion that more privileged groups are over-represented in these classes.

Part of the sociodemographic trends among participants could be explained by the composition of Green City since it reflects the geographic disparities in the region. Because Green City has a significantly more educated and wealthier population, these trends are apparent in the courses. Indeed, I noted the relatively high portion of foreign-born participants in these courses (from Europe, the Middle East, and a few from Asian and Latin American countries) compared with other studies of childbirth education conducted using nationally representative demographic samples (Lu et al. 2003). This trend reflects Green City's university's international reach, making this city exceptionally globally diverse in the state.

There were also, however, notable absences of certain groups based on Green City demographics. For instance, Asians, who constitute 12 percent of Green City's population (U.S. Census Bureau 2000), were under-represented. For some Asian couples, language barriers may have constituted a significant barrier, since it was often the men in couples arriving from Asia who worked at the local university while their wives might not have as much experience with English. In one class, I observed one such couple from Korea, where the husband translated for his wife. But it is also possible that there are different conventions that surround birth in various ethnic groups from Asia. In several Asian nations, pregnant women are expected to follow doctors' instructions and not have a plan of their own. In China and many areas of Korea, women face Cesarean section rates of 50–75 percent, essentially establishing surgical birth as a norm to which pregnant women not only submit but often welcome (Betran et al. 2007; Harvey and Buckley 2009; Lee, Khang, and Lee 2004; Lee et al. 2004). In these contexts, the need for childbirth education may not be perceived necessary since women and their families are simply expected to rely on the authoritative instructions of the obstetrician.

Another notable absence was the lack of African American participants in the courses that I observed.[7] Although Green City has a small black population of approximately 9 percent, over 30 percent of Neighbor City's population is black (U.S. Census Bureau 2000). Because Green City serves as the local hub of childbirth education, one would expect a larger number of black participants. Although blacks may be disproportionately affected by lack of access due to higher rates of poverty, I believe that another factor underlies this absence. Because childbirth education courses were started by and are run by educated white women, there may also be a sense that childbirth education courses are not inclusive and not directed to meet the needs of black families. Furthermore, there is a long tradition of white women and men being in authoritative positions over black women's reproduction that may also deter black expectant parents from participation (Roberts 1997). Similar arguments have been made by other researchers who have noted the underrepresentation of blacks in other studies (Lu et al. 2003).

In addition to these larger trends, I detected more subtle differences in the demographics of the two locations at which I conducted my observations. At the more mainstream childbirth education location I call Family Center, I observed a wider array of professions, some of which included blue collar workers (e.g., a truck driver), and a woman who expressed serious concern about being able to continue working once her baby was born due to job insecurity and the amount of time she had to take off.[8] In contrast, at Holistic Center the few blue-collar workers I met were men married to college-educated white-collar administrators. For instance, Gary was a welder, who was married to Lynn, a project manager. I did not hear any concerns about job security in the discussions during or after classes, although these concerns may have been simply kept private.

I also had a sense that participants at Holistic Center were slightly more educated, since many of them conducted research about childbirth prior to selecting their course and they had to do extra work to locate this resource in contrast to the larger and nationally recognized option of Family Center.

A major difference between the two sites was the larger proportion of women at Holistic Center who mentioned that they planned to take more extended time off or decided not to return to work after having their baby. In similar conversations, I also noted that several men planned to take lengthier leaves as well. In contrast, when an instructor in the breastfeeding course at Family Center asked participants about their plans for after their babies' birth, all women responded that they were planning to return to work. Furthermore, only a couple of men I met mentioned that they planned a more extended leave. Based on their jobs, couples planning for longer leaves and employment breaks did not seem to be significantly wealthier than other couples. Instead, it seemed likely that these families were prepared to live on a lower total income than those where both partners returned to work. The ideology of cutting back on work time in order to spend more time with children is aligned with the intensive model of parental engagement that "natural parenting" philosophies espouse (Bobel 2002).

Some of the sociodemographic differences I observed at each childbirth education site derive from the specific clientele of each organization. Attendees at Holistic Center were primarily clients of midwives and were referred to Holistic Center by their provider or through the same research into birth options with minimal medical intervention that led them to select midwives in the first place. They desired education that supported their birth plans as well as their strong commitment to breastfeeding. Because having a midwife and a deep interest in breastfeeding is not the cultural norm in the U.S., the families who could locate and take advantage of these community resources were likely to have distinguishing sociodemographic characteristics as well—probably most prominent in the area of educational attainment. In contrast, fewer of those at Family Center were interested in birth with minimal medical interventions. Similarly, not all decided to breastfeed their babies. Most were clients of obstetricians rather than midwives. Since they were more representative of mainstream cultural practices about birth, these clients likely reflected a wider range of sociodemographic characteristics than their counterparts at Holistic Center.

Despite distinguishing characteristics in the profiles of the two sets of clients, there was also some variability in who came to each course. There were clients who selected providers—both midwives and physicians—at Private Hospital in Green City but chose not to take that hospital's own courses, enrolling instead in either Holistic Center's or Family Center's courses. Jocelyn and Samuel, for example, chose a midwifery service at that hospital and courses at Family Center. Similarly, some clients at Holistic Center were cared for by physicians, and some clients at Family Center were cared for by midwives. For instance, Corinne selected a physician but chose to attend Holistic Center's courses because of her strong interest in "natural birth" and breastfeeding. Finally, the degree of interest in course offerings and commitment to each organization's philosophy was variable among participants. For example, Jocelyn and Samuel were strongly committed to natural birth but were enrolled in Family Center courses. Similarly, Johanna was open to the possibility of using anesthesia in labor but was strongly committed to breastfeeding, and she and her husband enrolled in courses at Holistic Center. Each organization's staff was aware of this diversity and wished to provide a respectful climate that offered learning opportunities for different clients.

The above contrasts in the availability of childbirth education by location and in the sociodemographic profile of the participants suggest that high quality childbirth education is a privileged good. Both organizations reflect a bias toward older, white, wealthier, more educated, heterosexual, married couples. Although books, television, and websites offer a wealth of information, many parents find it difficult to evaluate the credibility of this information. Those with fewer educational resources are at a particular disadvantage in being able to access materials such as scientific articles or expert discussion that evaluates childbearing practices. In addition to these outcomes, being able to locate and participate in extensive educational resources for childbirth and beyond reflect middle-class consumption practices. Consuming these high quality services not only helps to produce better outcomes in multiple aspects of childbearing (Lu et al. 2003) but also constitutes part of the rites of passage of becoming middle-class parents. Therefore, the process of selecting these courses and making the extensive commitment to participate in them reflects couples' efforts to become good parents for their baby.

The differences I have noted between the two childbirth education sites also point to more subtle dynamics of social class at work at the two sites that warrant greater attention. In the next section, I provide a more nuanced portrait not only of the specific knowledge parents can access about breastfeeding through childbirth education, but also of the different models of parenting these organizations offer in their courses.

## Learning to Breastfeed in Childbirth Education Courses

High quality childbirth education courses include courses not only on childbirth preparation but also on breastfeeding and newborn care. Breastfeeding education is situated within the larger context of the educational goal of these institutions, which retain a primary emphasis on childbirth. The legacy of the history of childbirth education, which emerged in the context of the natural childbirth movement, which challenged routine medical interventions in birth (see chapter 2), is apparent in the structure of the courses that devote six to seven weekly sessions to birth compared with one or two sessions to breastfeeding and newborn care each. Although breastfeeding is considered an important part of childbirth education, it receives considerably less attention compared with the enormous emphasis on preparing for childbirth.

Both physicians and hospital-based midwives recommend that pregnant women and their partners attend childbirth education courses. Many of these providers also recommend that those intending to breastfeed attend a breastfeeding course. Due to the history of breastfeeding in the U.S., breastfeeding beyond the first few months remains fairly limited. First-time mothers and their partners may never have seen a baby breastfeeding, and because birth takes place at the hospital and the next few weeks are most often spent at home, even fewer have first-hand experience with a breastfeeding newborn. Breastfeeding courses have been developed by childbirth education organizations in order to provide basic knowledge that enhances breastfeeding success as well as to support women in the process. As breastfeeding initiation rates have risen, breastfeeding courses have become a growing part of the business of childbirth education.

In Green City, three organizations provided the bulk of private options in breastfeeding education, of which I was able to observe two.[9] In addition, those receiving public health insurance assistance through Medicaid received breastfeeding education as well. Both of the above organizations provided high quality childbirth education that advocated for women and their partners to make informed decisions about childbirth and caring for their children. Despite the similarities between the two organizations and their support for breastfeeding, they had distinct approaches toward childbearing.

*Holistic Center*

Holistic Center was located on a side-street in a quiet, old residential neighborhood in Green City, near one of the local elementary schools. When visitors arrived during the summer months, Holistic Center was not easily visible while driving past the lush trees that lined the street. Walking up to the Center, I passed single-family homes on each side. The Center was located in a house that I could have easily mistaken for a family home until I saw the small signs on the door. The Center shared its space with a local lay midwifery practice. Since the end of my fieldwork, it has also developed a breastfeeding center and houses a massage therapy practice as well. During my study, the site also hosted an organization that provided doulas for those who could not afford them, which has since moved to a different location.

The front door opened into the classroom area where cushions, chairs, and couches were spread in a semi-circle prepared for the class that was about to begin. Slings for sale were hung on the wall, made in Guatemala by women with whom the home birth midwives worked during their summers. Bookshelves in the corner displayed a large number of books primarily devoted to "natural birth," breastfeeding, and caring for the newborn, as well as the whole family using non-medical resources, such as herbs, homeopathy, and massage. The rooms on the left housed the office of the director as well as the home birth midwifery practice, while the room in the back provided space for the doula service volunteers. This area included a supply cabinet for pregnancy tea packets and a table filled with snacks and drinks provided by doulas in training, who also observed these courses as part of their preparation. Plaster of Paris "belly casts" of pregnant women's bellies and breasts were displayed on the upper part of the wall. A small bathroom and kitchen completed this part of the space.

On a chilly winter evening, I attended one of the childbirth education courses offered here. Couples filed in and started filling the semi-circle of seats. Nearly all were white and in their late twenties to early thirties. Most had wedding rings on their ring fingers. The couples were casually dressed, with little to no make-up on women and hair that was minimally styled. Men primarily wore jeans and a sweater and women were similarly dressed in pregnancy pants and loose fitting clothing. Introductions revealed that many participants were interested in learning more about "natural childbirth," minimizing medical interventions, and avoiding a Cesarean section for their births. Dressed in a long, flowing skirt and a sweater, the instructor told participants that one of the primary aims of the course was "cultural deprogramming": to help unlearn what people have learned about childbirth and then learn a new way to think about the process.

The theme of challenging mainstream ideologies about childbearing reverberated in all the other sessions of the above course as well as in the breastfeeding and newborn care courses at Holistic Center. In the breastfeeding course, one of the aims was to discuss the cultural obstacles to breastfeeding and to help participants identify ways to overcome them. Similarly, in the newborn care course, participants were told that whereas they might encounter many "checklists" of how to prepare for having a baby, particularly in what to purchase, most of the recommended "gear" was unnecessary. Instead of accumulating the equipment, participants were told that the course would focus on interactions between mother, partners, and infants and the daily experiences of having a baby. All of these goals were manifest in different aspects of the courses, from the materials selected in class presentations to the objects that surrounded participants. Together, they offered an alternative path for parenting as well as for fashioning persons and families.

The course's structure replicated the history of the natural childbirth movement in its heavy focus on childbirth (seven weeks) and significantly less attention on caring for infants (two to three weeks). Furthermore, breastfeeding was addressed in a separate course from "newborn care," reflecting the history of breastfeeding in the United States where breastfeeding has become a potential aspect to infant care, rather than an assumed cultural norm. Issues about infant sleep and soothing babies were addressed primarily in the newborn care course, despite the interrelationship of breastfeeding with these topics. Indeed, the fragmentation of the three courses and their overemphasis on birth could make it challenging for parents to integrate what they learned in their actual experiences, which were physically and temporally contiguous.

At the same time, this organization systematically countered the fragmentation of themes in courses by incorporating breastfeeding into every course. It was assumed that those who wished to learn about minimizing medical interventions in childbirth or "natural" childbirth were also going to breastfeed their children. Breastfeeding was frequently mentioned in the childbirth preparation course, often as a default norm. When feeding was mentioned, the word "breastfeeding" was usually used. Having unrestricted skin-to-skin contact with the newborn and breastfeeding whenever the baby desired were cited as major benefits of having a birth with minimal to no medical interventions. This trope was reinforced when the final shots of videos and slideshows presented in class included a newborn baby latched on the breast of the mother or resting near the bare breasts of the mother. The visual display of naked bodies with breasts exposed and newborn babies near them or in the process of breastfeeding highlighted the primary role of breasts as feeding babies instead of their dominant cultural role as sexual objects.

The daily practice of breastfeeding was also incorporated into childbirth education through discussion as well as in the inclusion of a time-allocation activity in the final session of the childbirth preparation course, where couples were asked to individually map out their daily schedule after the birth of their babies.[10] This activity was designed to help participants visualize the time and labor of breastfeeding, and facilitate couples' planning for the radical reorientation of time and division of labor that they were about to face. Throughout the discussion, it was simply assumed that mothers would be breastfeeding, which was indeed the plan of all in the room. The only time I heard of women not breastfeeding was when I participated in a postpartum doula training at Holistic Center and heard of situations where, for various reasons, the mother was not able to breastfeed—after a difficult and/or surgical birth, for instance, or in the case of grave maternal or infant illness.

In the breastfeeding course, the instructor reinforced the connection between birth and breastfeeding. She mentioned the importance of selecting a provider that supports a "low tech birth," especially in light of rising Cesarean section rates both nationally and locally.[11] Furthermore, she cautioned that medications used in labor would likely impact the readiness of babies to breastfeed, reducing their alertness and desire to nurse. These points situated breastfeeding within the context of Holistic Center's overarching critique of biomedicalized childbirth practices.

The instructor incorporated a full discussion of co-sleeping (meant in the specific sense of bed sharing) into the newborn care course. She acknowledged that sleep was a highly controversial topic in the medical community, "probably the most controversial topic in the class," and in the parenting community as well. She explained that sleeping next to the baby was common in many cultures and did not necessarily lead to an increase in SIDS. She said, "I am not suggesting that you have to co-sleep—it may or may not be for you," but emphasized that research supported this practice and that there was more information about it in the packet of resources for the course.

The packet contained an article from *Mothering Magazine* in which anthropologist James McKenna (2002), a leading researcher of co-sleeping whose work I discussed earlier, authored a referenced summary of current research on co-sleeping that situates contemporary debates in an evolutionary biological context. The instructor also mentioned that "even" the American Academy of Pediatrics recently recommended that "it's important to at least have the baby in the room [with the parents]." This statement was another example of the critical approach this organization takes toward medical institutions, since the AAP was not simply used as an authoritative reference but instead was positioned in relation to anthropological research that challenged mainstream medical practices. Such statements assumed a sophisticated understanding of research evidence and its uses in biomedicine.

Material in the newborn care course similarly emphasized the primacy of breastfeeding by referring to breastfeeding as an activity in which mothers would participate rather than something that some mothers might decide to do. For example, when newborn potential health problems were discussed, the instructor spent considerable time explaining common misunderstandings that surround jaundice—a yellowing of the baby's skin and eyes due to the accumulation of bilirubin—and breastfeeding. The instructor made a strong argument that jaundice, rather than requiring supplementation with artificial milk substitutes, is an illness caused by "not enough" breastfeeding, that could be resolved with more intensive breastfeeding.[12]

The relationship between breastfeeding and infant sleep was also reinforced in later discussions. The instructor explicitly discussed the controversy surrounding co-sleeping and breastfeeding and referred back to McKenna's work featured in *Mothering Magazine* to suggest that co-sleeping while breastfeeding need not be harmful, and was, in fact, the biological norm for children. An article in the Newborn Care packet (Donohue-Carey 2002) referred to the work of biological anthropologist Katherine Dettwyler (1995), as well as McKenna's, to argue that breastfeeding and sharing a bed go hand in hand and are beneficial practices. Furthermore, the article challenged the Consumer Product Safety Commission's recommendation against co-sleeping (U.S. Consumer Product Safety Commission 1999). The packet also included an article from *Midwifery Magazine* (Quinn 2002) that used research conducted in Great Britain and New Zealand to argue that chemicals used to treat crib mattresses and bedding could, in the presence of a common fungus, be converted into toxic gases that caused Sudden Infant Death Syndrome. Adrianne and Doug, both scientists by profession, followed up on this research and used a special cover on the mattress of their Co-Sleeper (bassinet that attaches to the parental bed) in order to prevent the formation of this fungus and the escape of potentially harmful gases.

The materials parents were encouraged to purchase underlined the overarching parenting philosophy the organization promoted. After purchasing the services of a doula and picking up some pregnancy tea (a blend of nettles and raspberry leaves long used by midwives), parents purchased other products that signaled their interest in alternative approaches to parenthood. Some of these were available on site at Holistic Center, while parents could purchase additional items at other locations.

Slings featured at the top of the list, having recently become more mainstream due to their marketing and distribution in large chains, such as Target and Wal-Mart. This mainstreaming is largely due to the success of Dr. William Sears' books, the leading proponent of "attachment parenting" (see chapter 2), who has endorsed some of these products. Mothers were encouraged to make use of slings to carry their children and to support them during breastfeeding, the slings enabling them to keep their children close to their bodies and their breasts as sources of continually available nourishment and comfort while also freeing them to do other activities. Fathers were similarly told to carry their children close to their bodies in slings and similar carriers. Slings were mentioned in both the breastfeeding class as well as the newborn/infant care class where "sling or baby carrier" was listed as the third necessary item after "tiny nail clippers" and "low light or night light." Since participants were surrounded by slings hung on the walls of the room, these slings served not only as material reminders of this particular object's significance in parenting, but also became signifiers of the parenting philosophy promoted at Holistic Center.

The absence of certain objects and their replacement with alternative options similarly reinforced ideologies of parenting promoted at this site. For instance, in her discussion of necessary objects in preparation for the baby's arrival, the instructor did not mention purchasing a crib. The crib appeared as an "optional" item on the sheet entitled "Baby equipment—What's REALLY needed?" in the packet. In contrast, in nearly all such checklists in magazines, on-line publications, and parenting books, cribs appear as one of the first items parents need to buy for their baby. In omitting discussion of cribs and relegating them to an optional status, the instructor countered mainstream conventions and referred parents back to the discussion of controversies surrounding co-sleeping in the earlier portion of the course. Furthermore, directing participants to *Mothering Magazine* also connected them to resources advertised in that magazine for parents who chose not to have their children sleep in cribs. Interestingly, Co-Sleepers were not listed on the baby equipment sheet in the packet, although they were one of the important objects featured in *Mothering Magazine* advertisements and were also mentioned as possible options for sleeping close to one's child in the course itself. Dr. Sears has also endorsed Co-Sleepers as an object useful for parents practicing attachment parenting.[13] The omission of the Co-Sleeper from the list is likely due to Holistic Center's promotion of a minimalist philosophy that critiques the purchasing of potentially expensive and unnecessary equipment.[14]

Finally, the newborn care course devoted a large time slot to the discussion of cloth diapers. The instructor invited the owner of a local cloth-diapering store, who taught the class how to diaper a baby using stuffed animals and gave a presentation on the different kinds and varieties of cloth diapering options that are available. The packet featured an advertisement for cloth diapers as well as disposable diapers without chemicals considered harmful for the baby. Cloth diapers were promoted as both environmentally friendly as well as safer and at least as effective as disposable diapers. In addition, while the investment in cloth diapers could be initially quite high, depending on the style of the cloth diapers one uses (the more convenient styles that resemble disposable diapers and that are adjustable in sizing can be pricy at about $20 per diaper), the owner of the store emphasized that the total cost of cloth diapering is ultimately lower than that of disposable diapers. The presentation, practice session, and discussion took nearly an hour, reflecting the proportionally high level of care and attention paid to the issue of diapering and selecting the most appropriate materials for this task. The attention to diapering practices reflected Holistic Center's interest in reducing the use of potentially harmful materials on babies, which dovetailed with concerns about potentially harmful medical interventions. Purchasing reusable diapers fit into this Center's ideologies of reducing overall consumption of children's products. Furthermore, the instructor situated purchasing cloth diapers as an act of care for the child's body as well as for the environment.[15]

In contrast to the birth preparation course, which focused more on the selection of providers and negotiating the process of birth in a critical manner, the newborn care course shifted in emphasis to the discussion and purchasing of various materials in preparation for the baby. It was primarily in this class that parents could use objects that would be used to care for a baby and materially consolidate their parenting decisions. The socialization of the courses in which parents participated therefore not only conveyed information that actively shaped decisions about birth and caring for children, but also served as an introduction to a material culture associated with these decisions. These objects, carefully selected to surround the baby's body, in turn become signifiers of specific parental personas. I was witnessing the making of the "natural parent"—one who espouses birth with minimal interventions, extended breastfeeding, baby-carrying, co-sleeping, and cloth-diapering, among other characteristics. In this model, breastfeeding was situated amidst a series of other signs that consolidated around a specific persona of a breastfeeding parent.

*Family Center*

This significantly larger organization hosted courses at three different locations in Green City: one in a room within University Hospital's medical center, another at a community center, and the third located next to the main office of the organization within an office building occupied by a number of other organizations. Each of these locations was found in non-residential settings, with the medical center location clearly placing the course within the biomedical framework for childbirth. Upon entering the main building, I encountered an office with the director's area and the front office staff area where the bookshelf filled with resources for expectant parents was housed. The second room contained cushions and a few chairs spread around the room. This larger organization provided a large array of classes beyond childbirth preparation, breastfeeding, and infant care courses, including a new mother support class, a miscarriage support class, and playgroups. Accordingly, the closet housed a wide variety of teaching tools—posters with information about the stages of labor; diapers and stuffed animals and dolls that were used to practice breastfeeding positions, diapering, and bathing; and children's toys—categorized and labeled in large plastic bins that could be easily removed and replaced for each class.

The organization was directed by an energetic woman who had made a number of important changes to the organization since beginning her term as director. Among these was a greater emphasis on acquiring hands-on experience with childbirth for instructors, which was not previously required. The childbirth courses were taught by instructors trained and certified by the parent organization, and the breastfeeding course was taught by International Board Certified Lactation Consultants (IBCLC).

Breastfeeding was promoted within childbirth preparation, breastfeeding, and infant care courses in different ways, which helped to mitigate the fragmentation of course content among these courses to a certain degree. Nevertheless, Family Center's approach to breastfeeding significantly differed from that of Holistic Center. Importantly, Family Center presented breastfeeding as a "choice"; for instance, one instructor prefaced information about the benefits of breastfeeding with the statement "if you choose to do that." Instructors recommended taking the breastfeeding course if participants were intending to breastfeed. This discourse was intentionally and repeatedly used in order to be respectful of any participants who did not plan to breastfeed. Moreover, this approach suited the organization's emphasis on "informed choice" in all aspects of childbearing, wherein families were encouraged to use the information provided to make their own decisions. Furthermore, in the childbirth preparation course, breastfeeding was described as having many "benefits." The discourse of benefits replicates the rhetoric of earlier breastfeeding promotion efforts that I discussed in chapter 2. By presenting breastfeeding as a choice that conferred additional advantages, rather than the baseline for comparison, and by downplaying the potentially harmful effects of routine biomedical interventions in childbirth on breastfeeding, this framing also blunted the course's larger critique of institutional biomedical approaches to childbearing.

The breastfeeding course had a slightly different approach, since the instructors could assume that all enrolled participants wished to breastfeed. Nonetheless, the course content included a section on the "benefits" of breastfeeding. One instructor chose to briefly review the "benefits" while the other simply assumed that those in the course were already aware of these and went on to provide very specific information on the bodily skills that ensure successful breastfeeding.

In the infant care course, breastfeeding was only mentioned on a few occasions, once again as an option, not as a norm. The objects used in the course included several related to formula feeding, such as a baby bottle and infant formula. These objects were used as demonstration objects of common items used in the care of babies and the instructor picked up and discussed each item as she presented the course. The omission of breastfeeding as a topic and the presence of objects related to formula feeding suggested that the default way of caring for babies entailed formula feeding. Consequently, the infant care course could be perceived as a necessity, while the breastfeeding course as an additional option for those engaging in this less common practice.

The isolation of discussion of breastfeeding from sleep arrangements furthered the sense that support for breastfeeding within the organization was separated from the embodied experiences of breastfeeding. For instance, sleep arrangements were not mentioned in the childbirth preparation course, with the exception of when I was introduced at the beginning of class as a researcher interested in breastfeeding and sleep arrangements, including co-sleeping.[16] In the breastfeeding course, sleep was mentioned without reference to specific sleep arrangements. Instead, the instructor encouraged as much "skin-to-skin" contact as possible between mother and baby. She also told participants to keep the baby close to them at night. In describing the specific details of how to get a baby to learn breastfeeding well, she repeatedly emphasized unhindered contact between the bodies of mother and child from the first moments after birth through the learning process. The instructor also encouraged participants to pay close attention to the baby's early signs of hunger, rather than waiting for them to cry. Throughout the course, the instructor provided very detailed information about breastfeeding, with considerable time spent on the bodily positions for breastfeeding and ascertaining that the baby latched correctly to the breast and was transferring milk.

This highly focused approach toward the specific bodily skills for breastfeeding left little room for the daily experiences or cultural context of breastfeeding, but enabled participants to draw their own conclusions based on the information provided. If participants paid close attention to the instructor, they might have noted that such an approach to breastfeeding is facilitated by sleeping next to the baby either in a co-sleeper or in the same bed. Therefore, avoiding an explicit discussion of sleep arrangements might have opened possibilities for parents seeking their own paths in the context of the dominant cultural model of sleeping apart from one's baby without the instructor getting entangled in the controversy around bed sharing. The breastfeeding course's approach, however, was largely contradicted in the infant care course.

In the infant care course, the instructor simply assumed that all parents would set up a "nursery" in which there would be a crib and a changing table at the minimum, with a cursory mention of parents having bassinets in their rooms for the first few weeks. Detailed instructions were provided about crib safety, both in terms of structural safety to prevent falls and getting stuck and in minimizing any padding or other materials that might cause suffocation. Even the location of the crib was discussed in order to avoid getting entangled in the strings attached to blinds, for instance. Other possible sleep arrangements were not included, and the relationship of sleep and breastfeeding was simply not considered. The emphasis on sleeping in separate rooms and the omission of breastfeeding from the discussion of sleep arrangements once again reinforced the notion that breastfeeding and bodily proximity at night were non-standard practices.

In conversation with Family Center's director about this course, she noted that the curriculum was developed by a previous generation of instructors who had not necessarily breastfed or considered breastfeeding an important issue. The director was in the process of making revisions to this curriculum in order to shift the assumptions of the course to include breastfeeding. At the same time, she was cautious that the organization should not appear too pushy about the promotion of breastfeeding in order to respect parents' decisions and avoid alienating those who have chosen not to breastfeed. I was empathetic to this position in light of the increasing moral pressure on women to breastfeed in a cultural setting that offered little support for them (see chapter 2). At the same time, I wondered whether the organization could do more to transform cultural perceptions of breastfeeding.

The lack of systematic integration of breastfeeding with sleep was reinforced by the parent organization's informational packet,[17] which referred to cradles and bassinets as useful items and then had an entire page and a half devoted to crib safety. Under the heading "Crib and Proper Mattress" a bullet point stated, "Place your baby on his back in a crib with a firm, tight-fitting mattress," and later a sentence reinforced this point: "Put your baby to sleep on his back in a crib with a firm, flat mattress." This section omitted any possibility of sharing a bed with an infant. Under the later section "Keeping Your Baby Safe" and within the page on "Sudden Infant Death Syndrome" the packet stated,

> Bed sharing or co-sleeping with your infant may be hazardous under certain conditions. Care should be taken to observe the recommen-

dations outlined. Parents who bedshare with their infants should not smoke or use drugs or alcohol which may impair arousal. As an alternative, parents might consider placing the crib near the bed to promote ease of breastfeeding and contact.

This latter discussion hinted at the possibility that a parent might bring a baby to bed and indirectly implied that such an arrangement might promote "breastfeeding and contact." However, the reasoning behind such arrangements or their potential beneficial effect was omitted. Instead, even the potential benefits were only considered in the context of co-sleeping as a safety hazard that should be discouraged and replaced by a crib placed "near the bed." Since the packet originated from the parent organization of this childbirth education facility, it highlights the fundamental differences in different organizations' perceptions of how breastfeeding should be supported.

Despite the above differences, the two organizations also shared many important features of informational content in their courses as well as in the material objects they highlighted in parenting. For instance, the infant care course at Family Center emphasized the importance of baby-wearing both as a generally beneficial practice and as an excellent way of soothing babies. Although slings were not displayed in the classroom, the instructor's advocacy for this practice was clear. Similarly, she spent time identifying other resources for soothing babies, which included infant massage—a practice similarly mentioned at Holistic Center and listed in its packet of resources. The same instructor also recommended baby-care books by Dr. Sears. These overlaps were also notable in the birthing class, especially in both courses' emphasis on hiring a doula to attend childbirth. Finally, many of the practical aspects of how to initiate and sustain breastfeeding were quite similar because both organizations hoped to improve the care women received during childbirth and they wished to support breastfeeding.

In sum, the boundaries in the socialization of parents between the two organizations were permeable with significant overlapping areas. Nonetheless, different kinds of parental models emerged from each organization. At Holistic Center, despite a traditional curricular model that separated birth, breastfeeding, and infant care by course and emphasized birth among these three topics, breastfeeding was integrated into each course in relation to multiple topics. Furthermore, the daily experience of breastfeeding was considered in great detail, explicitly addressing and challenging cultural conceptions of breastfeeding, such as length of time of breastfeeding and sleep arrangements in relation to breastfeeding. In contrast, at

Family Center, breastfeeding remained mostly within the confines of the breastfeeding course, apart from its relationship with childbirth and sleep. Despite its attempts to advocate for breastfeeding, Family Center maintained the cultural norm of formula feeding, to which breastfeeding could be added as an option—an option whose traces were nearly erased in the infant care course.

## Consumption of Parenting Models

In the above sections I have argued that each of these courses constituted an important part of middle-class patterns of consumption in preparation for parenthood. Participants with somewhat different interests and characteristics gravitated toward each of the above sites, thereby selecting different consumer options for childbirth education. The two organizations then reinforced and shaped these interests toward their own specific models of childbearing/parenting. In this sense, each organization fulfilled the expectations of its participants. On the other hand, I also witnessed how participation in different childbirth education courses resulted in transformations in expectant parents' views as well as cases where participants found that their own plans and practices were misaligned with some aspects of the philosophies of the organization.

For instance, Angela and Oliver had initially planned to give birth at University Hospital, attended by midwives. However, upon listening to research about home birth presented at Holistic Center and looking into the safety of home birth compared to hospital birth on their own, they decided to switch to a local Certified Practicing Midwife (CPM) practice for their care. Their decision was particularly important in light of the controversy surrounding the safety of home birth in the U.S. While the U.K. supports women's access to home birth, the American College of Obstetricians and Gynecologists (ACOG) has remained staunchly against home birth on the grounds of safety (ACOG 2008; Craven 2010). Most recently, ACOG issued a statement about home birth that is more open to women making their own informed choices, but cautions that such a choice entails putting their babies at significantly greater risk (ACOG Committee on Obstetric Practice 2011).[18] Therefore, in switching to the care of home birth midwives, especially for their first birth, this couple broke with key medical recommendations. This change in providers, in turn, influenced their expectations for breastfeeding and sleep.

In home birth care, the midwife remains with the client for a few hours after birth, observing the new mother and baby and also providing breastfeeding support. Most often, this early breastfeeding takes place in the couple's bed and the midwife tucks in the mom and baby together and leaves them to rest.[19] Although Angela transferred to the hospital for a Cesarean section, upon their return to home, Angela and Oliver continued with their plans, aligning them with others who practiced "natural parenting" and its components of home birth or birth with minimal interventions, extended breastfeeding, and co-sleeping. They carried their baby in a sling, used cloth diapers, and researched routine medical interventions, such as immunizations.

Other participants had come to Holistic Center with an interest in having a "natural birth" but were uncertain whether they would use anesthetics in labor. Carol, for instance, attended Holistic Center's courses because her husband's cousin had recommended it. In the beginning part of her pregnancy, Carol received care from a physician, but due to a change in her insurance plan, needed to make a switch and had the opportunity to choose midwives at University Hospital. This switch was also supported by Holistic Center's advocacy for midwives. Carol had an interest in "natural birth," but did not want to make an explicit commitment to it. She wanted to leave room to use anesthetics if she wished to do so during labor. Nevertheless, Holistic Center's course reinforced her desire for an intervention-free birth, which she was able to accomplish with her husband's support. Prior to enrolling, Carol already developed the sense that she would like to breastfeed and stay close to her baby at night, which was also supported by her husband, Justin, and her doula. Holistic Center's curriculum once again reinforced these plans. Carol ultimately breastfed her son for over one year, and Carol and Justin slept next to him regularly for much of that first year. They also carried their son in a sling and also used cloth diapers. In each of the above two examples, participants became more aligned with Holistic Center's model of parenting than they had been prior to participating in the courses.

While Family Center's "informed choice" approach included advocacy for minimally interventionist birth and breastfeeding, this advocacy retained the sense that childbearing choices were ultimately of equal value in the long run. Furthermore, both the discourse of "benefits" and the material culture of the infant care course reinforced mainstream models of parenting in which breastfeeding only played a limited role. For instance, Kristen went into labor feeling informed and empowered after Family Center's courses and asked for an epidural during labor, with which she was very comfortable. She was very also committed to breastfeeding, and therefore made sure that she had ample opportunities to breastfeed after her daughter was born. Her husband was equally supportive of these efforts. She breastfed their baby "on demand" as well, but the couple did not carry her in a sling and they used disposable diapers. Their daughter slept next to Kristen for the first two months in a bassinet but then was moved to her own room. These arrangements were simply assumed as part of a normal and expected transition. Kristen's and Daniel's experience reflected mainstream ways of birthing and caring for children, except for their exceptional commitment to breastfeeding. While this commitment was supported by their childbirth education course, it was driven primarily by the couple's own previous knowledge and desires, and Family Center's courses reinforced but did not actively seek to shape the couple's birth plans, nighttime sleep arrangements, or the material culture of their parenting.

In a similar vein, Rachel wanted to keep her options open in birth and ultimately ended up having multiple anesthetics in labor. Rachel and Nathan were very committed to breastfeeding—a commitment that went far beyond that of most participants I encountered at Family Center. Their own experiences of breastfeeding ultimately prompted Rachel and Nathan to change their original separate sleep arrangements to sharing a bed with their baby as well as to breastfeeding far beyond one year. Unlike participants at Holistic Center, however, these arrangements did not arise in the context of ideas previously raised during childbirth education courses, and they lacked support from childbirth educators and from a community of other like-minded parents with whom they could share their experience. Similar to Kristen and Daniel, the material culture of caring for their baby was not altered—they used disposable diapers and a more conventional baby carrier instead of a sling, and the shift in their sleep arrangements did not result in the acceptance of other aspects of "natural parenting."

Jocelyn and Samuel represent an example of expectant parents who embraced "natural parenting" philosophies but selected Family Center. They did not wish for medical interventions in labor, selected a midwife at the second Green City hospital for their care, were thoroughly committed to breastfeeding, and were open to sleeping next to their baby when she was born. Although they differed from many other clients at Family Center, they felt informed and supported in their decisions there. They ultimately gave birth without anesthesia (albeit with other interventions), and slept close to their baby for most of the year, used cloth diapers, and carried her in a sling. While their decision to pursue a birth with minimal interventions was supported and enabled by Family Center, most of Jocelyn and Samuel's decisions that challenged mainstream parenting models originated from their own research and experience. Indeed, the pressures for intervention they experienced in their birth at Private Hospital steered them toward hiring a home birth midwife for their second birth, a philosophy strongly aligned with Holistic Center but omitted from Family Center. Once again, this transformation emerged from the couple's own strong desires instead of discussions at Family Center.

The differential ability of Holistic Center to shape an alternative model of parental personhood lay in the shared interest of participants toward "natural birth" and breastfeeding, which enabled Holistic Center to present a more cohesive model of parenthood to a receptive audience. Furthermore, Holistic Center encouraged participants to take their courses in their second trimester while the majority of Family Center's clients took the course in their third trimester. Beginning the courses in the second trimester offered greater opportunity to switch providers, locate doula services, and begin to purchase items in preparation for the baby's arrival. The early timing also enabled Holistic Center to lay groundwork for a different philosophy of parenting and increase the efficacy of its pedagogical goals; expectant parents had more time to absorb what they learned and to make decisions on the basis of their experiences.

Although Holistic Center offered a more unified model of "natural parenting," it is important to note that participants did not necessarily fully embrace every aspect of this model. Just as the examples I cited above from Family Center demonstrated considerable heterogeneity in childbearing approaches, Holistic Center's clients selectively incorporated different aspects of the model with which they were presented. For instance, Leslie and Alex desired a birth with minimal intervention. They hired a doula to support them in the process, but they were attended by a physician, and Leslie decided to ask for an epidural during labor. She felt comfortable with this decision. The use of anesthetics did not predict this couple's relationship to other aspects of parenting. Their baby remained on or close to his mother's body for the majority of his first few months, with his dad also participating in other attachment parenting decisions, such as bringing the baby into bed with them, a practice they continued for the duration of the study.

Similarly, Joy and Jonathan wished to have a birth without medications, and selected a certified nurse-midwife as well as a doula to support them during birth. However, Joy remained ambivalent about her ability to cope with the pain of labor. They were able to have a vaginal birth, but ultimately opted to accept Pitocin and an epidural. Despite these decisions that neither aligned with the primary goals of the Center, nor with their own initial desires, they followed many aspects of natural parenting ideologies, including "attachment parenting." For instance, although they did not share their bed with their baby, their son remained in their room very close to them for nearly the entire first year and was breastfed on demand throughout the day. They held their baby whenever possible and often carried him in a baby carrier. They also used cloth diapers in a similar fashion to many others in their Holistic Center group.

Finally, Bridget's experiences, described in detail in the following chapter, highlight the hierarchy of priorities in parenting approaches. For instance, although Bridget planned to use cloth diapers and breastfeed her baby for at least one year, when she faced breastfeeding difficulties, she quickly discarded her commitment to cloth diapers but persisted in breastfeeding. Thus, Bridget valued breastfeeding far more than she valued the use of cloth diapers, indicating that breastfeeding was a foundational and non-negotiable part of her construction of motherhood.

## Conclusion

In this chapter I drew on ethnographic observations of childbirth education, documenting middle-class couples' consumption practices in preparation for the birth of their babies. Avishai (2007), drawing on Linda Blum's earlier work (1999), has suggested that these practices fit into larger patterns of middle-class ideologies of motherhood in which breastfeeding is framed as a "project," which requires an enormous commitment of labor and resources in order to attain idealized notions of good mothers. Avishai argued that "by framing breast-feeding as a project, these middle-class mothers are able to access an otherwise potentially threatening, alien, or unintelligible embodied practice" (2007:136). Consistent with these insights, my participants used childbirth education courses as a pivotal resource for breastfeeding in a culture that promotes breastfeeding but provides little structural support for it. However, in an important departure from Avishai's discussion that focuses solely on mothers, in nearly all cases both members of couples participated in these courses, reflecting their shared commitment to breastfeeding.[20] In mobilizing their privileged ability to access high-quality childbirth education (and lactation services later on), these couples acquired important knowledge about how to successfully breastfeed their babies.

I have argued that, in the process of participating in breastfeeding education within the larger context of childbirth education, expectant parents not only consume knowledge but also consume different models of parental personhood. At Holistic Center, breastfeeding was enmeshed with a model of "natural parenting," while at Family Center, breastfeeding was an optional extension of more conventional parenting models. Although there were numerous distinctions between these two models, the boundaries between them were porous; parents undertaking the "project" of breastfeeding were attracted to the two childbirth education sites due to their different approach toward childbirth and parenting, yet they selectively embraced and were transformed by certain elements of parental personhood models. The ethnographic data reveal the complexity of particular couples' decisions, practices, and purchases, and resist stereotypical and reductionist media characterizations of parents into separate "camps."[21] The participants in my study, like most first-time middle-class parents in the U.S., forged their own unique paths based on their own histories and experiences that did not fully fit either model presented by the childbirth education organizations.

The role of breastfeeding within the two models of parenthood offered by the childbirth education organizations is particularly interesting. Despite the heavy emphasis on birth in both organizations, in explicitly weaving breastfeeding into discourses about childbirth as well as into conversations about caring for one's baby, Holistic Center consistently contextualized breastfeeding and highlighted the experience of birth, breastfeeding, and other aspects of caring for the baby as a unit. This approach highlighted the relational elements of different aspects of having a child, while also emphasizing the significance and lengthy duration of breastfeeding in the entire process of childbearing. In contrast, the links between breastfeeding and other domains of childbearing were downplayed at Family Center.

At the heart of these models of parenting is their relationship to capitalism. Holistic Center not only provided a cultural critique of capitalist models of childbearing (in which institutions of biomedicine play a crucial role), but of a capitalist way of life as a whole. Family

Center, in contrast, did not explicitly offer such a deep critique and worked largely within the accepted framework of capitalist ideologies (e.g., capitalist labor practices that make breastfeeding difficult were rarely mentioned or challenged except as something that is accommodated with breast pumps). Although the discourse of "informed choice" attempted to relocate decision-making authority and aimed to open new possibilities for educated consumers, the lack of social context for non-conventional choices made it quite difficult to attain these alternatives in actual parenting practice. In real life, choices are, of course, highly structured by cultural ideologies, socioeconomic circumstances, and institutional practices (Solinger 2001; Craven 2010).

On the other hand, while Holistic Center's broader critique is an important and valuable one, it failed to acknowledge that it, too, was a childbirth education (and a parental) model to be consumed, with specific recommendations for patterns of consumption, albeit ones that differed from mainstream conventions. These insights echo those of Chris Bobel (2002), who argues that critiques of consumerism such as those offered by Holistic Center are hypocritical in their lack of recognition that they rely on privilege. Bobel claims that this privilege among "natural mothers," who advocate for extended breastfeeding, homeschooling, anti-consumerism, and other similar goals, is asserted in both the knowledge and material privilege required to be able to participate in this alternative pattern of parenting. Bobel argues that while "natural mothers" successfully critique consumerist capitalism and the reliance on biomedical technologies (that are themselves intrinsically tied to capitalism), they ultimately reinforce their privilege in doing so.

Christa Craven's (2010) recent analysis of consumer choice rhetoric in home birth advocacy offers additional insights into these issues. Although Holistic Center explicitly critiqued aspects of capitalism, just as in the case of recent home birth advocacy movements, Holistic Center's approach relied on marketing this alternative set of consumer options. The ability of persons to access these consumer "choices" depends on their privilege, thereby furthering the stratification of reproduction.[22] Thus, it is important to note that critiques of capitalism are themselves situated within increasingly neoliberal capitalist regimes of "consumer choices."

The stratification entailed in "consumer choices" reinforces the need for further research into the social class differences among those who accesses these courses. While my study was limited in its capacity to illuminate these issues due to its small sample size as well as in the lack of access to detailed sociodemographic profiles of the clientele at Holistic and Family Centers, education appeared to be an important distinguishing factor among the largely middle-class participants at these sites. As Bobel (2002) also noted in her emphasis on knowledge in "natural motherhood," educational resources are key to parents' ability to seek out and purchase resources that provide alternatives for mediating the challenges presented by breastfeeding and sleep.

In addition to the perpetuation of socioeconomic inequalities, Bobel also found that the "natural mothering" ideology reinforced conventional gender roles, failing to overturn the intimate ties of capitalism and technology to patriarchy.[23] Women in her study disproportionately stayed at home, attended to labor-intensive domestic chores, managed their children's education, and marginalized the participation of men in parenting. My participants' ability to practice breastfeeding "on-demand" for several months, many beyond one year, similarly often relied on a male spouse's steady income and willingness to spend long hours at work in order to enable their partners to spend time with their babies during lengthy maternity leaves or while not being employed at all. Moreover, in evoking the "naturalness" of the childbearing options it promoted, Holistic Center deployed discourses about breastfeeding that have been used to confine women to traditional gender roles. Indeed, biological anthropology has been used in problematic ways to further such aims.[24]

At the same time, my decision to label Holistic Center's philosophy "natural parenting" instead of "natural mothering" reflects an important difference between Bobel's and my own study. Nearly always, it was couples, not simply mothers alone, who participated in these courses. By focusing on couples, I learned that the majority of spouses in my study actively participated in the breastfeeding process and in the entire process of childbearing/parenting and divided the labor entailed therein (see chapter 5). Thus, greater attention to mothers in the context of their relationships with their spouses, children, and others revealed a more complex portrait of participating families than that outlined by Bobel's study.

Finally, it is important to recall that although couples consumed different models of parenting and shaped their own parental personas in their own unique ways in the process, both patterns of consumption were important moral and sentimental acts.[25] The couples in my study partook in childbirth education because they wanted to be prepared for the arrival of their children, thereby constituting themselves as "good" middle-class parents who would provide the best possible care for them. Although Holistic Center more explicitly addressed the cultural barriers to breastfeeding, the embodied practice of breastfeeding nevertheless led to unanticipated dilemmas for most parents in both childbirth education courses, which I explore in the following chapters.

## Notes

1. Layne 1999; Avishai 2007; Bryant 2010; Bryant et al. 2007.
2. I borrow these terms from Rickie Solinger (2001).
3. Private Hospital had a prior working relationship with Family Center that ended shortly prior to my study when Community Hospital's network decided to institute and promote its own childbirth preparation courses.
4. For instance, expectant parents could also choose courses based on Robert Bradley's (2008) book "Husband-Coached Childbirth," which advocates no or minimal medical intervention in birth, or based on Pam England's and Robert Horowitz's (1998) *Birthing from Within*, which also advocates for minimal intervention but with more attention to scenarios when such intervention can be helpful. Both of these courses were offered through individual certified instructors rather than through a larger, center-like location, and neither were reimbursed by insurance plans.
5. These courses took place during one Saturday at Holistic Center or two consecutive Saturdays at Family Center, and consisted of six- to eight-hour sessions with breaks for lunch and snacks.
6. Such investigation would have been helpful but was not possible because of concerns over the privacy of those attendees who were part of my observations through fieldwork at the research sites but did not opt to become core participants of my research and the level of comfort for expectant parents in the courses.
7. During my observation period, I encountered one African American couple in a course that took place at the same time as the one that I was observing.
8. Although both Kristen and Daniel were laid off during the course of my study, their positions were both white collar, secure jobs when they took their childbirth education courses at Family Center. They were the most affected by the consequences of the financial crisis that was unfolding toward the end of my study.
9. I did not explore this program because of my focus on breastfeeding parents who had sufficient resources to carry out the recommended length of breastfeeding.
10. I discuss this activity in greater detail in chapter 5.

11. The Cesarean section rate in 2006 was 31.6 percent (MacDorman, Menacker, and Declercq 2008).
12. Treating newborns with infant formula supplementation continues to be a routine procedure at many hospitals despite evidence that it is not necessary and that the introduction of formula is disruptive to breastfeeding and potentially harmful for children (Gartner 1994).
13. See chapter 6 for more details on the significance of co-sleepers in nighttime breastfeeding practices.
14. See Bobel's (2002) discussion of natural motherhood.
15. See Wilk 2001 and Miller 1998 for a discussion of ethical consumption.
16. Perhaps aiming to reassure her audience, the instructor said, "It [co-sleeping] happens more than you think," but did not address breastfeeding and sleep further in the course. My sense was that although she intended to present my research as socially acceptable, since breastfeeding could not be assumed in this audience, she did not want to steer the discussion in this direction.
17. Citation information for the packet and the quotations from it are withheld in order to protect the confidentiality of the organization and its location.
18. This most recent statement, as well as the research upon which it is based, has generated enormous controversy among birth advocates. See, for instance, Declercq 2011.
19. See Davis-Floyd and Cheyney 2009.
20. See also chapter 5 on fathers' involvement in breastfeeding support.
21. While such polarization is apparent in the media, especially in the comment sections, I did not encounter these divisive patterns in my own ethnographic research.
22. These critiques also tie into anthropological discussions of "ethical consumption" trends outside reproduction, which similarly rely on knowledge and resources that enable the purchasing of goods in a socially responsible manner.
23. Previously discussed by Rothman (2000).
24. See Hausman's (2003) discussion, especially her chapter "Stone Age Mothering," pp. 121–154.
25. Daniel Miller (1998), in his study of shopping in North London, argued that shopping is an act of "lovemaking," a sacrifice through which shoppers' personhood and family relationships were constructed and reinforced.

*Chapter 4*

# Dispatches from the Moral Minefield of Breastfeeding

British sociologist Elizabeth Murphy (1999) first used the concept of the "moral minefield" to describe the complex cultural climate of infant feeding decisions in the contemporary U.K., wherein mothers use diverse strategies to justify their feeding plans in order to avoid being seen as morally deviant. Although Murphy's work documented multiple forms of moral judgment that surround both breastfeeding and formula feeding, she focused especially on how women who do not plan to breastfeed and those who switch from breastfeeding to formula feeding account for their decision. This focus was motivated by the emphasis in public health discourses in the U.K and elsewhere in the context of global initiatives to promote breastfeeding, as evidenced by the "breast is best" slogan as well as by health workers' infant feeding advice. In this chapter, I evoke Murphy's concept of a moral minefield to delve into the moral contradictions of breastfeeding in my own ethnographic setting. Although their exceptional commitment and resources enabled the mothers in my study to breastfeed, their embodied experiences revealed difficulties originating from the moral danger of potentially not being able to breastfeed, as well as from the moral hazards associated with the actual process of breastfeeding. My study documents the effects of this dual process of stigmatization (Goffman [1963] 1986) and the moral labor mothers undertake in order to mitigate them (Ryan, Bissell, and Alexander 2010; Stearns 2009).

Although spouses actively participated in many aspects of enabling the breastfeeding process, I found that mothers were disproportionately affected by the moral scrutiny to which breastfeeding is subjected. Because, in this cultural setting, children are breastfed nearly always by their biological mothers[1] and fathers are physiologically limited in their capability to lactate, mothers are the target of breastfeeding promotion efforts as well as most of the moralized discourses that surround breastfeeding. Consequently, the labor of managing breastfeeding stigma often becomes part of the larger set of gendered, embodied work that women undertake for the sake of breastfeeding (Stearns 2009). At the same time, throughout the chapter I remind the reader that in my study spouses provided crucial support for breastfeeding and often enabled them to continue to breastfeed amidst the challenges they experienced, thereby sharing and alleviating some of this labor.

Narrative accounts provide the primary source of evidence for exploring the effects and experiences of stigmatization associated with breastfeeding. Along with Ochs and Capps (1996), I view these narratives as inseparably tied to the construction of the self, "grounded in the phenomenological assumption that entities are given meaning through being experienced" (21). Narratives are self-fashioning devices par excellence through which narrators produce *"partial selves"* that "access only fragments of experience" (21). Thus, the conversations with me and sometimes with their spouses illuminate how mothers produce their own partial selves as they attempt to reconcile the moral contradictions in their breastfeeding experiences. Such conversations constitute an important part of the fashioning of gendered moral personhood[2] that conforms to cultural expectations of "good motherhood."

## The Moral Labor of Erasing Embodied Struggles

Many mothers anticipated the challenges of breastfeeding during pregnancy and aimed to prevent or mitigate them by taking breastfeeding classes. At the same time, during the childbirth education classes I attended, mothers also described their commitment to breastfeeding: they were prepared to compromise their sleep and feed their children as often as necessary in order to breastfeed. These expectations reinforced the sense that breastfeeding was a "project" that was to be carefully planned in order to produce desirable health benefits for children (Avishai 2007). This "project" came with a high bodily cost that needed to be endured in order to provide the best possible nutrition for one's child.

Although some challenges were anticipated, mothers were often surprised by the degree of difficulties they experienced with breastfeeding. Mothers nursed their babies in various states of exhaustion due to recovering from giving birth, sleep deprivation, and, for many, breastfeeding difficulties. Furthermore, over half of the mothers experienced pain as they worked to establish breastfeeding, struggling with engorgement, mastitis, cracked and bleeding nipples, and babies who could not breastfeed. These difficulties were often compounded or entirely caused by inadequate support for breastfeeding at the hospital and from the general lack of cultural knowledge about and support for breastfeeding. In a study of experiences of breastfeeding among a racially and socioeconomically diverse sample of women who gave birth in Toronto and in Boston, Kelleher (2006) similarly found that over half of her participants experienced pain or discomfort, and argued for greater scholarly attention to these negative embodied experiences. In contrast to some women in Kelleher's study who gave up breastfeeding because of these experiences, all mothers in my study persevered, relying on their spouses' and other family members' support as well as drawing on professional services. This finding confirms both the exceptional commitment of my participants to breastfeeding, and the resources they were able to mobilize to fulfill their desire to breastfeed.

Although pain and embodied struggles emerged as a major theme in many of my conversations, chronicling these experiences proved challenging. I found that mothers repeatedly downplayed or erased their negative experiences in order to realign their experiences with a positive image of breastfeeding that highlighted the ultimate value of breastfeeding. While ideologies of sacrifice are part of discourses of "good motherhood," mothers' negative experiences disrupted idealized images of mothers who joyfully breastfeed despite encountering obstacles. Mothers' marked reluctance to discuss negative embodied experiences drew attention to the social unacceptability of this issue and the contradictions in moral tropes surrounding breastfeeding.

When I first sat down to talk with Petra shortly after the birth of her son, she told me that in terms of breastfeeding, "I had no problems, *I almost feel guilty about how easy it was*" [emphasis mine].[3] Petra, a tall, fair, lively woman nearing her mid-thirties, always welcomed me with warmth and a smile, and carried an enthusiasm toward life that was infectious. Thus, it took me some time to understand the contradictions in her accounts. As I reflected on our conversation, however, it became clear to me that Petra's experience was far from "easy." In fact, Petra had an abrupt ending to her pregnancy because of signs of preeclampsia[4] and an induction before her due date. Despite the emotional upheaval of an unexpected hospitalization and painful contractions caused by the artificial induction hormone, Pitocin, Petra delivered their son, Anders, without anesthesia with her partner, Julia's, support and began to breastfeed him.

From the beginning of her pregnancy, Petra was absolutely determined to breastfeed. After her baby's birth, her son latched on to her breast without any difficulty. As her transitional milk[5] came in, however, Petra's breasts became painfully engorged and she also noticed that Anders was becoming jaundiced.[6] She was encouraged to feed him more but found it challenging to do so because he was "too sleepy to eat." When she brought Anders in to the pediatrician, she discovered that her son had lost 10 percent of his body weight and feeding him became an urgent concern.

Petra was determined not to give Anders formula and was trying everything to persuade him to breastfeed. She said, "That's when I panicked, everything was there, all you have to do is to stay awake." Petra knew that one way to wake a sleepy baby was to strip off his clothes and wipe him with a wet washcloth. Petra's mother and her sister, who were both visiting, inadvertently heightened Petra's worries by expressing their concern about Anders' weight loss but also discouraging Petra from using the washcloth to wake him. With Julia's ongoing and unfailing support, Petra ultimately persisted and Anders began to gain weight. Petra's initial statement of having had an easy time with breastfeeding needs to be evaluated in the context of the intensity of the experiences of childbirth and the breastfeeding difficulties she shared with me. Petra worked hard to downplay these difficult parts of her experience, even when her own description of her experiences directly contradicted her characterization of the ease of breastfeeding.

Petra similarly downplayed her exhaustion from nighttime breastfeeding in our first conversations, only hinting at it briefly in a brief comment that she was "doing fine, except for the sleep-deprivation," a state that she seemed to expect as part of the natural course of events.[7] Even as I learned more about Petra's growing exhaustion over the course of the study, and the various arrangements she and Julia devised to address this while also continuing to breastfeed, Petra maintained a relentlessly positive view of her breastfeeding experiences. Our conversations suggested that these contradictions and selective erasures in Petra's narratives emerged partly from comparisons with friends who were unable to breastfeed due to medical conditions. Petra was grateful for her ability to breastfeed and felt that her difficulties were insignificant and did not warrant attention when compared to the challenges her friends endured. These comparisons, however, also buttressed ideologies that breastfeeding mothers should be joyful about their ability to breastfeed regardless of the difficulties they encounter. Petra, therefore, performed "moral work" in her narratives in order to align herself with these social expectations (Ryan, Bissell, and Alexander 2010).

## The Moral Hazards of "Failing" to Breastfeed

Some of my participants, like Petra's friends, faced the distinct possibility that they would not be able to breastfeed. Bridget's experience below demonstrates the pain and moral anguish some mothers endure in order to avoid the grave moral risks of "failing" to breastfeed their children. When Bridget and I first met during her childbirth education course at Holistic Center, I learned that she was enthusiastically preparing for the birth of her and Roland's first child. In her late twenties, with medium-long brown hair that she often wore in a ponytail, Bridget projected a sense of purpose and energy. Seven weeks after the birth of her daughter, Angelina, Bridget looked at ease with her transition to motherhood and breastfed Angelina on and off during our long conversation at a local café. As we sat together on that sunny, but still cold late winter day, I had little reason to suspect that the journey to this day had been far from simple. Indeed, Bridget joyfully recounted the details of her labor, during which she felt fully supported by her husband and doula, and which ultimately culminated in a birth with virtually no medical interventions with the midwives of University Hospital in attendance.[8]

Bridget told me that right after her birth, Angelina was not interested in breastfeeding, and the midwives let her rest so she could breastfeed when she was ready. When Angelina did begin to breastfeed, however, she did not stay attached to the breast for very long. The staff at the hospital noticed that Angelina was having difficulty and the nurses helped with the latch, and the breastfeeding process seemed to be working at the time. In accordance with the experiences of many others, however, upon returning home from the hospital the situation deteriorated. Angelina had such strong but ineffective suction that Bridget was getting "compression stripes" on her breasts and her nipples began bleeding.

The pain prompted Bridget to return to the hospital's labor and delivery service where she was seen by a lactation consultant who also concluded that Angelina was not latching on correctly. The nurses offered Bridget a finger-feeding system to take home that would allow her to rest her breasts.[9] This system entailed Bridget expressing her milk using an electric pump as many times during the day and night as possible, and then feeding the baby the pumped breastmilk using the finger-feeder. In between finger-feeding sessions, Bridget also "tried to breastfeed and it hurt so badly" that she could only breastfeed for ten minutes at a time. She felt that Angelina was "not getting enough, so she's crying," and these sessions would inevitably end in a frustrated and upset mom and baby.

Feeding Angelina with the finger-feeder partially relieved the situation because it enabled Bridget's husband to feed the baby and for the first time Bridget "felt that it was not all about me." Roland took on the complex and time-consuming finger-feeding process, while Bridget's mother, who was staying with the couple, made sure that Bridget got up to pump regularly during the night and stayed up to wash all the pump parts to prepare them for the next pumping session. Although Bridget was grateful for Roland's and her mother's help, she also "had a lot of mixed emotions [... and felt like] I wasn't mothering her [Angelina] because I wasn't feeding her." Despite Bridget's recognition that Angelina's inability to breastfeed could not be attributed to any external factor, she labeled herself as an inadequate mother because breastfeeding involved her body.

Enduring a heavy emotional and physical toll, Bridget—with the support and encouragement of her family—continued to seek help to address the breastfeeding problems. She sought help from a private lactation consultant recommended by nurses at the hospital, who referred them to a craniosacral therapist. Craniosacral therapists (CSTs) provide alternative medical care by performing subtle manipulations of the bones of the skull that have led to improving breastfeeding problems for certain babies (Vallone 2012). The practitioner made adjustments but was also surprised by how Angelina appeared to seek the breast but could not latch on and continue feeding normally. The CST practitioner sought additional advice from her mentors and colleagues and encouraged Bridget to return for an additional visit.

The situation reached crisis proportions when Roland had to return to work two weeks after the birth of their daughter. Bridget's mother was no longer staying at their home, although she continued to provide support. During the day, Bridget was alone with Angelina and with the challenges of feeding her. Already exhausted from giving birth and the continuing trials of the past two weeks, getting through the day seemed an insurmountable challenge. Angelina "needed to be held" at all times, otherwise she would begin to cry immediately, and Bridget continued to be unable to breastfeed her. In addition, Angelina would not accept a bottle, which meant having to rely on the finger feeder. Bridget spent her time either engaged in the long process of finger feeding or pumping her breasts. Pumping was nearly impossible, however, because Angelina was upset by being put down or not being held close. Bridget described how she was caught in a cycle of "pumping while she [Angelina] is laying on my lap screaming." Bridget was also worried about the rapidly diminishing supply of breastmilk because she could not pump enough to keep up. Although she never wanted her daughter to have any artificial milk substitutes, Bridget "finally gave her formula." Bridget still attempted to breastfeed "but [Angelina] would scream at the breast, this high-pitched scream. I'm thinking it's me. She is really upset because she can't feed." Bridget blamed herself because of her inability to provide nourishment and comfort through breastfeeding for her daughter. This acute self-blame and despair became part of a constellation of symptoms that led Bridget to seek therapeutic help for postpartum depression.

For Bridget, as for Petra, losing sleep was simply to be endured in the process of trying to breastfeed her daughter. In fact, she did not mention sleep in our conversation until I explicitly asked her about it. Yet, when Bridget did address these issues it became clear to me that both fatigue and sleep arrangements compounded the severity of the situation. Bridget told me that in the first few weeks after birth she wanted to make sure that Roland would have enough sleep due to his long commute and thus removed herself and Angelina to the couch at first and then to the guest bedroom. This made Bridget feel more isolated from her husband and contributed to a sense of acute despair. Roland's repeated encouragement led her to return to the couple's bed along with the baby, which helped relieve this sense of isolation. Although Angelina slept well next to her parents, Bridget's sleep was greatly disrupted by the nighttime pumping sessions she undertook in order to maintain her milk supply. In our conversation, Bridget mentioned the exhaustion from having to wake up to pump her breasts at night and then carrying on with a virtually unending cycle of pumping, attempting to breastfeed, and soothing her daughter. Thus, while Bridget's concern of not being able to breastfeed Angelina overshadowed her experience of exhaustion in her account, the extreme fatigue she experienced was a significant factor in producing the severe situation that led to her postpartum depression.

Bridget's mother intervened and insisted on teaching Angelina to use a bottle. Along with continued help from the cranial sacral practitioner and the lactation consultant, the breastfeeding problems slowly began to improve. Using a bottle freed up time for Bridget during the day and Roland during the night. Bridget's work with her therapist, who supported her through her postpartum depression, also began to bear fruit. Still, it took Bridget about five to six weeks to be able to breastfeed Angelina. Even then, she experienced some initial pain and had to assist Angelina by holding her breast while the baby fed. Only certain positions worked for breastfeeding, such as the "football" hold, which entails holding the baby against the mother's side under her arm. The football hold requires positioning pillows to support the baby's body and is often not a particularly comfortable position for mothers, since they cannot use the back of the chair or sofa for support. By the time of our conversation, Bridget mastered the football hold and nursed Angelina with relative ease while also continuing to talk with me. In the meantime, lying in bed and nursing, a position Bridget felt was most restful during the night, remained out of reach. Nonetheless, Bridget ultimately managed to breastfeed and by the time of our first postpartum conversation she told me that her daughter was "one hundred percent" breastfed. Bridget's description emphasized individual achievement (or failure) and de-emphasized the social factors that made breastfeeding challenging.

Toward the end of our conversation I asked Bridget to reflect on why she persevered and kept working on breastfeeding despite all the difficulties she encountered. Bridget replied, "I wanted to quit so many times, but I couldn't make myself." Bridget recalled that in conversations with her therapist, Bridget identified her inability to breastfeed her daughter as a major contribution to the depression. She often felt that if she could just figure breastfeeding out, her depression would resolve. Even the therapist, who was a strong supporter of breastfeeding, questioned her about her decisions.

Bridget continued: "I don't know how long I would have gone before calling it quits." Yet, Bridget noted, "I didn't feel like I had any other choice." I asked Bridget what she meant by that, and she said that although she felt that way about breastfeeding, she changed her mind on many other aspects of parenting. For instance, while Bridget spent a great deal of time researching cloth diapers and planned to use them for her daughter, when she encountered the breastfeeding difficulties, "cloth diapers went out the window." Similarly, Bridget noted that she had planned to carry her baby in a sling, yet Angelina would scream when she was put either in a sling or in a front-pack carrier. Bridget's family purchased a stroller a few weeks after Angelina was born, since they did not have it prior to the birth. Although Bridget easily discarded the aspects of material culture that she had planned on using in her parenting,[10] her desire to breastfeed never wavered.

Upon further reflection, Bridget shared with me that she was "really worried about what [Roland] would think [if she] quit." Roland learned about breastfeeding primarily in the breastfeeding class they took together at Holistic Center. He was very supportive of breastfeeding and felt strongly that infant formula was not the best way to feed a baby. Both he and Bridget shared the sentiment that they did not want their daughter to have formula. Bridget said she "felt that I made this commitment to him to do this." In this sense then, breastfeeding was not only a relational practice that involved the mother and child, but also a "commitment" that entailed Bridget's relationship with her husband.

Throughout this process Bridget's husband was extremely supportive of Bridget and shared the care of their daughter as much as he could (see chapter 5). Bridget noted that her sense of failure did not derive from Roland; in fact, "he never said anything, never 'You are doing it wrong.' He's been nothing but proud of me." Despite his support and reassurance, Bridget couldn't shake the sense that although "Her not feeding was both of our problem, it was really my problem. Hard to explain, because it comes from my body." Thus, Bridget located their daughter's inability to transfer breastmilk from Bridget's breasts in a failure of her own body, and then linked this bodily "failure" to her sense of "failure" as a mother.

Bridget's narrative demonstrates that, for her, the potential hazards of not breastfeeding were grave. Bridget's difficulties of breastfeeding led her to self-blame and guilt despite her supportive husband and mother. Bridget felt that she did not adequately mother because of her inability to feed her baby, and this sense was compounded by her misgivings about formula. She was exhausted from pumping, attempting to breastfeed and finger-feeding around the clock, frustrated and in pain, yet she did not give up on breastfeeding. The moral blame of "failing" to breastfeed in Bridget's case did not originate from specific interactions with others; instead Bridget internalized the cultural pressure to breastfeed and turned the blame on herself. Bridget's ordeal confirms the stigmatization of mothers who do not breastfeed (Murphy 1999). My data also indicate, however, that the cultural imagination of an idealized version of breastfeeding and the moral hazards of not being able to breastfeed also lead to the stigmatization of mothers facing breastfeeding difficulties. In Bridget's case, even the continuing attempts to resolve these difficulties and her provision of expressed breast milk for her baby did not shield her from the toxic influence of mother(self)-blame.

## Encountering Moral Judgment during Breastfeeding

Corinne's initial experience of breastfeeding was also filled with pain and exhaustion (see chapter 5 for a detailed description). A librarian in her early thirties with bright blue eyes and brown hair in a bob haircut, Corinne had a wry sense of humor that she used often when reflecting on her harrowing experience. Corinne nursed through cracked and bleeding nipples while also spending nights holding her son, Finn, upright on the couch because he would not sleep without her and could not sleep in any other position during the first few weeks.[11] Corinne, like many other mothers in my study, anticipated that breastfeeding would be difficult and did not dwell on these experiences in our conversations. Similar to Petra and Bridget, it was only after I directed my questions toward these experiences that she provided more detailed descriptions of this extremely challenging beginning to breastfeeding.

As we got to know each other better over time, however, Corinne became more willing to share her negative experiences with breastfeeding. Through these conversations it became apparent that Corinne's difficulties in the first few months were greatly compounded by the moral judgment of various, ostensibly "supportive" relatives who questioned her approach to breastfeeding. While Corinne's sister and her sister-in-law breastfed their own children and were advocates of breastfeeding, they subjected Corinne's breastfeeding to intense scrutiny. Corinne's and Jacob's baby fed frequently and spent several hours at the breast in the evenings. The visiting nurse and the baby's pediatrician assured the couple that he was gaining weight, and both of these health care providers as well as Corinne's doula explained that this pattern of feeding, called "cluster feeding," was completely normal. Corinne's relatives, however, continued to question her approach to breastfeeding: "In between talking to them [the health care providers and doula], I talked to relatives who said, 'This is not normal, you are not producing milk, the baby is starving.'"[12]

Corinne described that the image of the starving baby was so "scary," that she constantly questioned her own breastfeeding: "It was weird. All the professionals—doula, nurses, doctor, said everything is fine, he is growing. And it should have been enough but it really upset me. Is something wrong with my milk production?" Both Corinne's sister and her sister-in-law felt that cluster feeding was a sign that Corinne was not producing sufficient breastmilk and that the baby was starving. Corinne's sister, who breastfed her own son for two years and was also a La Leche League leader, said, "I don't know if your milk really came in." Thus, even without physical evidence of inadequate weight gain, Corinne's body was perceived as not being able to provide an adequate milk supply, and ultimately she was blamed for subjecting her baby to starvation.

These fears about not having enough milk recall Bridget's similar worries and Petra's urgency in waking the baby to feed him. Although Corinne's relatives were advocates of breastfeeding, their worries about the embodied process of breastfeeding revealed underlying anxieties and danger associated with breastfeeding. Bernice Hausman (2003:33–68) argued that images of malnourished breastfed babies in the media reflect ongoing cultural skepticism about breastfeeding, the legacy of the many decades within which infant formula feeding became the normative standard against which breastfeeding is measured. Hausman has developed these concepts further in her second book, and suggests that despite medical perceptions of breastfeeding as important to reducing risks of illness, breastfeeding is also simultaneously conceived as a risky practice, full of potentially dangerous infectious agents and toxic materials (Hausman 2011). Despite their understanding of breastfeeding as the preferred and superior feeding method, by accusing Corinne of "starving" her baby, Corinne's relatives' unknowingly replicated this skepticism and undermined Corinne's breastfeeding confidence.

The relatives' solution to the so-called breastfeeding "problem" was similarly contradictory. They felt that Corinne needed to feed *less* often, yet provide *more* breastmilk for her "starving" baby. Corinne's account of her relatives' comments revealed that cluster feeding was not only problematic in their eyes because it implied a hungry baby, but that Corinne's and her baby's pattern of breastfeeding disturbed other social expectations:

> Corinne: Like both of our families are disturbed that he doesn't use a pacifier. They think he wouldn't cluster feed if he used a pacifier.
> Author: Why? What is so bothersome about cluster feeding?

Corinne: They think I'm getting into a bad habit, that I'm spoiling him.[13]

Consequently, this breastfeeding pattern not only violated social expectations for the use of the pacifier (itself a substitute for suckling at the breast), but also indicated Corinne's unwillingness to conform to ideologies of children's personhood that emphasize self-reliance. According to these ideologies, which echo Watson's behavioralist approach from the earlier part of the twentieth century, parents must carefully regulate and limit their response to children in order to avoid over-dependence and "spoiling" them.

Corinne explained that her sister-in-law and her husband's parents felt that "we need[ed] to be having meals with hours in between rather than snacking on the breasts all evening."[14] But Corinne identified the profound contradiction between breastfeeding advice given in classes and in books and her relatives' view: "But what I don't understand is feed on demand, seems to me, like, if he wants to snack, what am I supposed to do? He demands it."[15] Corinne, therefore, was stuck between the contradictory obligations to feed her child and to limit his breastfeeding. She also noted that the same relatives "are all snackers" and that "people allow adults to eat at different times" while they want to regulate babies' eating habits.[16] Thus, cluster feeding was a touchstone of breastfeeding criticism because it presented a number of moral concerns about Corinne's ability to adequately nourish her child as well as to regulate her child's feeding behavior in order to produce a desirable (non-spoiled and well-regulated) person.

In Corinne's encounter with the stigmatization of breastfeeding within her own kin network, Corinne was blamed for using her body to engage in socially unacceptable and potentially dangerous patterns of breastfeeding. Although Bridget did not encounter this stigma through personal interaction, she internalized the same tropes when she located blame for not being able to successfully breastfeed her daughter in her own "failed" body. Ironically, Corinne's baby grew in length and put on weight so quickly that his measurements outpaced nearly all other babies in his age group. Corinne later laughed as she told me, "He stopped wanting to cluster feed, and also the family would have a hard time making the argument that he is not growing or not eating enough, so I think this argument is put to rest."[17] The visual evidence of her thriving son then not only proved Corinne's breastfeeding success but also removed any further moral concerns surrounding her approach to breastfeeding.

## The Compounding Effects of Sleep in the "Moral Minefield" of Breastfeeding

Sleep was thoroughly enmeshed in the moral landscape of breastfeeding in a variety of ways, from concerns over infant sleep practices while nursing to debates about sleep locations. As I spent time with participants, I became increasingly aware that sleep deprivation was simply part and parcel of the many sacrifices couples believed they needed to make in order to breastfeed their babies. In this sense, breastfeeding was a form of providing nourishment that required nearly heroic work.

First, using breastfeeding to fall asleep was a highly problematic practice. Mothers who breastfed their babies to sleep were discouraged from doing so by their pediatricians as well as relatives and many friends. For instance, Corinne said, "[The] pediatrician told me that I should start to disassociate the breast from sleeping. She said if he looks sleepy, don't offer the breast. I said, well, OK, I can do that but it's gonna be hard. I can't really disassociate the two, it's the only trick I have. How am I gonna get by? I just don't want to do that. I've got nothing then."[18] Corinne assumed that, in line with her other beliefs about breastfeeding, this strategy was "one of those things, if it's more difficult it must be better."[19] She ultimately decided, however, not to follow her pediatrician's advice, taking the risk of potential moral judgment from the doctor or others in her family.

Carol, her thin frame and youthful presence belying that she was in her early thirties, had already mastered breastfeeding after a difficult start, when at two months postpartum she decided to attend a group for new mothers sponsored by Private Hospital in order to see if she could make some good connections among the mothers and learn a few things that might be helpful in taking care of her very lively son, Jeremiah. During the course of the group, which turned out to be more of an instructional class, Carol was told that children must be awake when being put down to sleep, rather than being breastfed to sleep. The group leader, a nurse, repeatedly told the mothers who attended the group that putting them down this way would help their babies acquire "self-soothing"[20] skills. The brochure Carol was given in the group reinforced these messages. While we chatted in Carol's living room with Jeremiah bouncing along in Carol's lap, Carol read out to me some of her favorite sentences from the brochure in a sarcastic tone: "Make sure your child has plenty of opportunities to fall asleep on his own" and *"Never* let the child sleep next to you [Carol's emphasis]."[21] Although Carol dismissed these ideas, she was careful not to reveal her own family's bed sharing practices in the group. Furthermore, Carol carefully researched and discussed with other (supportive) mothers her initial decision to keep her baby in bed to ensure her baby's safety.

In both of these cases, mothers were expected to follow medical advice in order to produce children who possess desirable qualities of self-regulation and self-reliance. Their failure to follow such advice, in turn, signaled their moral failure to produce this culturally normative person. Corinne managed the stigma associated with the disclosure of not having complied with medical advice by suggesting that such advice was too difficult. Carol used a different strategy of secrecy, a common technique for managing stigma that is not apparent, since disclosing the "secret" would lead to moral judgment that discredits the character of the stigmatized person (Goffman [1963] 1986).

Although the moral peril of not following a physician's advice was significant in the above cases, defying medical guidelines on bringing a baby into bed in order to facilitate breastfeeding led to much more serious moral dilemmas. As Jocelyn's and Samuel's experience demonstrates, bringing babies into the couple's bed was equated by some with potentially killing one's baby. Jocelyn, an administrator in her early thirties at Green City's University, and Samuel, a purchaser for a local delicatessen in his late thirties, had planned an unmedicated "natural" birth and prepared by attending Family Center's courses, hiring a doula, and selecting their care with certified nurse-midwives at Private Hospital. The three of us were sitting together in the couple's cozy living room as Jocelyn nursed their daughter, Deirdre, and they described the details of Deirdre's birth. Despite their preparation, Jocelyn had an emotionally trying birth experience with an unsupportive nurse-midwife at Private Hospital. After managing to give birth vaginally without anesthesia despite being pushed into using Pitocin, the couple faced a new problem. Jocelyn stated,

> I had a rough time at first. Well, partially it was like realizing that she wasn't gonna sleep if she isn't next to somebody and then realizing that well she wants to sleep in the bed and at the hospital we had this doctor come in and just like do the horror stories of like "babies die when they sleep in beds" [using a deep, serious voice]. It was really horrible.[22]

Although Jocelyn was still smiling when she said these words, the expression in her bright blue eyes darkened along the way. It became clear that this exchange at the hospital had a deep effect on Jocelyn and made it very difficult for her to cope when she found that her daughter would not sleep on her own.

Prior to birth, Jocelyn and Samuel were open to bringing their daughter into their bed but also set up a bassinet next to their bed. Now, with their daughter unable to sleep in the bassinet, Jocelyn was at a loss: "Yeah, I had a rough time. She was not going to sleep in her bassinet, she just wasn't ... as most kids don't. And, I mean, why would she? [Jocelyn laughs and then we all laugh.] She's been right next to me inside." Her daughter's need to sleep next to her made sense to Jocelyn, but this left her with the only option of bringing Deirdre into bed with them, which frightened Jocelyn after talking with the pediatrician at the hospital. Samuel and Jocelyn, both highly informed parents who examined biomedical advice carefully, spent a great deal of time researching the pediatric literature about the risks of bed sharing. They quickly found out about the controversy in the pediatric community dividing the AAP's breastfeeding experts and the SIDS experts (see chapter 2). They concluded, along with the AAP's Section on Breastfeeding, that bed sharing was safe if the mother was breastfeeding and if bed sharing is carried out in a safe manner. Reading, however, could not allay Jocelyn's fears. Jocelyn felt that the pediatrician might have reinforced fears of bed sharing that were instilled by her mother. She explained:

> Jocelyn: I was thinking back, my mother never sort of came out with don't sleep with the baby—she said I slept with your older brother and it *scared* [Jocelyn's emphasis] me because I was just afraid that I was gonna roll over him. So she never said don't do it but she put all these things in my head enough so I was a little bit freaked out [by the pediatrician] and on top of just not sleeping at all and nursing ...
> Author: That's really hard, that's not a good time to think about ... [overlap]
> Samuel: [...] killing your baby [laughs]

In this account Jocelyn's mother used her own experience to caution Jocelyn about the potential dangers of sharing her bed with her daughter. In the exhaustion after giving birth, the pediatrician's much more direct warning compounded the moral hazards Jocelyn's mother introduced earlier. Samuel co-constructed the narrative account and used the verb "killing," to specify the implication of the pediatrician's statement and thereby identified the enormous moral hazards of bringing their baby into their bed in order to facilitate breastfeeding.

In response to the above dilemmas, Jocelyn and Samuel slept in shifts so that they could maximize Jocelyn's sleeping time while also enabling Deirdre to breastfeed. But Jocelyn, even with having lots of room for herself and her daughter, could not sleep. Over the course of the next few weeks they worked out a system where Deirdre spent part of her time in the bassinet and part of the night with Jocelyn in the bed. While Jocelyn initially said that she could not go to sleep because of the noises that their daughter made, Samuel clearly felt that Jocelyn could not sleep because she was worried about rolling over on their daughter: "She is not as worried about moving over the baby and I think that's what worried her [earlier on]." My own sense was that while the noises probably did keep Jocelyn awake, her worry about rolling over played an important part in sensitizing her to a heightened awareness as well.

Even with the new system, Jocelyn continued to worry about her husband potentially rolling over on their daughter, and Samuel simply left when Jocelyn was ready to have their daughter in bed with them. Jocelyn was clearly torn by her own experience:

> Jocelyn: The rational part of my brain says Samuel has never rolled over me—why would he ever roll over on [our daughter] [laughs] but that's just ... I'm not gonna be able to sleep through it.
> Samuel: Yeah, she won't sleep period with me in there.
> Jocelyn: Because I've read stuff and I know, I know it's OK, and I know that if we do it safely it's just as safe as any other safe thing.

Jocelyn's intellectual knowledge could not alleviate her embodied experience of not being able to sleep.

The situation left Jocelyn in a double bind. Initially, Jocelyn was confronted with the paradox of having a baby who could not sleep away from her body, but bringing her to bed meant willfully ignoring her mother's caution and defying a pediatrician's advice. As Samuel pointed out, while bed sharing facilitated easy breastfeeding and longer sleep periods for Deirdre, the decision to bring Deirdre to bed also implied that Jocelyn potentially endangered Deirdre's life. Furthermore, although Jocelyn determined that sharing a bed would be safe and beneficial for her daughter, she was unable to overcome her insomnia caused by bed sharing. Jocelyn's embodied response to bed sharing shows the powerful internalized effects of moral danger, which originated from her mother and the hospital pediatrician. While Jocelyn's inability to bed share resolved the potential danger of killing Deirdre, because Jocelyn understood bed sharing with breastfeeding to be beneficial, separate sleep arrangements also produced a sense of guilt and failure.

Jocelyn's experience demonstrates that in this "moral minefield" there are no "winners." Despite Jocelyn's success in breastfeeding Deirdre, the sleep arrangements—all of which were developed in relation to breastfeeding—meant that she felt morally compromised as a mother. Jocelyn's feelings of failure and guilt were compounded by displacing her husband, despite his complete support and willingness to leave the bed. These sentiments echoed Bridget's concerns about disrupting Roland's sleep by bringing Angelina into their shared bed. Finally, the severity of the situation also derived from sleep-deprivation, since Jocelyn felt "delirious" from frequent nursing and from her inability to sleep either next to or away from her daughter. Once again, the moral hazards surrounding breastfeeding produced an acute period of struggle.

Other participants' experiences reinforced the sense that family sleep arrangements, which were developed in relation to breastfeeding, led to similar moral dilemmas. Rachel and Nathan, a couple in their late twenties, made the switch from keeping their daughter, Maya, in the bassinet next to their bed, except for nursing, to sharing a bed with her a week or so after her birth.[23] Rachel felt conflicted about the shift for two reasons. First, she initially researched sleep recommendations and determined that separate sleep was safer, partly influenced by her professional training as a nurse. Rachel recognized that sleeping next to Maya presented a potentially serious safety risk.

Rachel, unlike Jocelyn, was able to overcome her worries and quickly adjusted to the new bodily practice of sharing a bed with Maya and breastfeeding her during the night. Rachel found this arrangement "so much easier" and discovered that she could sleep through some feedings because "sometimes she just latches on" without fully awakening Rachel. She was not worried about her husband either, although Nathan worried about himself potentially rolling over on their daughter in the early days.[24] Reflecting on this transition Rachel jokingly said: "I feel like she is safe. She hasn't stopped breathing yet [laughs]." Despite the marked differences between Jocelyn's and Rachel's experiences, Rachel's laughter revealed a similarity in their narratives. Jocelyn and Samuel both laughed when they described the pediatrician's gory depiction of babies dying in beds and at similarly tense moments where the possibility of death arose. I suggest that humor and laughter were narrative tools to cope with the gravity of the implication of potential lethal harm to their babies. Furthermore, Rachel's insertion of "yet" in the end of the sentence demonstrates that the possibility of danger is still present—her daughter could stop breathing in her sleep at any time. Despite the embodied ease with which Rachel adjusted to sharing a bed with her daughter, the specter of death continued to be on her mind.

The moral problems associated with bringing her daughter to bed to facilitate breastfeeding were compounded by Rachel's training as a nurse. Part of her guilt derived from the contradiction between her own practice and the instructions she provided. At first Rachel's training made her question the safety of her own decision to share a bed with her daughter. But once she resolved that she was not going to endanger Maya by sleeping next to her, there was still an element of discomfort: "I feel like a jerk sort of because I'm this nurse who tells people 'always in the bassinet on their back' and then I'm sleeping with my baby." Rachel's guilt was assuaged by her conversations with other moms, when she discovered that they often lied about sleep arrangements to their pediatricians: "Well it's funny when you talk to other moms, too, 'cause they'll be like, 'Oh yeah, I slept with all my kids,' you know. And I'm like, OK. ... Everybody is telling their pediatricians that their baby sleeps in the crib on their back but they are totally in your bed." Rachel realized that this was probably one of the most common "secrets" mothers keep from their children's doctors, thereby minimizing the potential effects of stigmatization. In the process of investigating sleep practices, she learned that her mother and sister also slept with their babies.

Rachel herself did not have to lie to her pediatrician because, although the pediatrician recommended separate sleep, she also accepted Rachel's and Nathan's decision to share a bed with their daughter (this was their second pediatrician after they made a switch from a practice that they did not feel adequately supported breastfeeding). In fact, the pediatrician seemed aware that the daily realities of breastfeeding often entailed bed sharing. For instance, on their two-month pediatric check-up, Rachel recalled the following conversation:

[Pediatrician:] So where are you all sleeping?
[Rachel:] Well, there is a bassinet next to our bed.
[Pediatrician:] How often is she really in that?
[Rachel:] Well, not so much.

This kind of acknowledgement of bed sharing did not constitute outright support, but eased the moral burden of sleep arrangements prompted by breastfeeding. Several participants switched to pediatricians during the course of the study whom they felt were more supportive of breastfeeding and thereby also of sharing a bed to facilitate breastfeeding.

Aside from avoiding this topic with pediatricians, some participants also hid their bed sharing from colleagues and friends who were not supportive of this practice. Leslie, a lawyer in her early thirties at Green City's university, recalled,

> I think it is, they make it sound so alarming like you are doing a bad thing, even when you are talking to other people, they assume he is sleeping in his own room, 'Oh, how many times you have to get up to feed him? And then you have to calm him down and do all these things.' Well, that's not really what's going on. I just didn't tell the people at work, [it is] almost like a generational thing. Before we had him I mentioned co-sleeping[25] as one of the options we might try and they were just like 'get that baby out of your bed.' They have very different ideas, so OK, I'll just not bring it up.[26]

Leslie attributed her colleagues' negative reaction to bed sharing to a generational difference, suggesting that younger people may be less alarmed by this practice. Nonetheless, these negative moral judgments from senior colleagues prompted Leslie to conceal her family's sleep arrangements. These colleagues were similarly surprised by Leslie's continued breastfeeding months after her son was born, reflecting that such "long-term" breastfeeding remains unusual in mainstream practice as well as their lack of understanding of the connection between breastfeeding as the driver of family sleep arrangements.

All of the above evidence suggests that bed sharing remains a stigmatized practice in the U.S., which can be equated to placing one's baby in mortal danger at worst, and limiting their ability to become self-sufficient at best. Bed sharing to facilitate breastfeeding, a practice that ostensibly attests to mothers' commitment to the health of their babies, is not sufficient to redeem bed sharing. Shweder and colleagues (1995) identified three key moral norms in U.S. middle-class sleep arrangements: the value of autonomy for children, the importance of the "sacred couple" that highlights the necessity of married couples to sleep together, and incest avoidance. In their comparative study of Indian parents and white middle-class parents from Hyde Park, IL, the authors found that, for the Hyde Park parents, incest avoidance was the most important value, followed by the value of maintaining a separate sleep space for the married couple, and finally by the value of autonomy. In a similar vein, McKenna and McDade (2005) argued that the extreme negative attention in the medical literature on bed sharing reflects deep cultural taboos about sexuality and incest as well as concerns about independence, rather than rigorous discussions of scientific evidence.

Viewing my findings through this lens, it is apparent that sharing a bed with children in the context of breastfeeding presents enormous challenges to these values. Although parents in my study rarely mentioned anxieties expressed by others about sexuality in relation to bed sharing, this clearly was an underlying issue that might be also implied in Leslie's colleagues' reaction. The efforts to disassociate sleep from breastfeeding by pediatricians more explicitly addressed the issue of breastfeeding/bed sharing inhibiting the development of independence, reflecting concerns about children's acquisition of culturally normative characteristics of personhood and about parents' moral responsibility to facilitate this process.

Since bed sharing is a significantly less common practice in the U.S. than sleep arrangements that separate couples from children, it remains to be seen if the current increase in bed sharing in relation to breastfeeding manages to reduce its stigmatized status. The *New York Times* has devoted several articles to the topic of co-sleeping in relation to breastfeeding, some of which focused precisely on the "secret" nature of this practice. These articles similarly suggested that while some couples were able to reveal their "secret" to supportive friends or family members, others experienced considerable negative reaction to their sleep arrangements that discouraged them from sharing their experience with others (Harmon 2005; Parker-Pope 2007). Furthermore, Kendall-Tackett and colleagues (2010) reported that parents who bring their babies into bed are much less likely to report this practice to health care providers than other sleep arrangements, due to the negative feedback they receive. Thus, bed sharing practices are likely to be underreported since their concealment continues to offer parents (especially mothers) some protection from the consequences of stigmatization. Yet, as we have seen from the ethnographic examples, the management of this stigma still involves labor and has embodied costs.

The stigma attached to sleep practices is further complicated within the community of breastfeeding parents, where the practice of not sleeping next to one's child, and especially using sleep training to achieve separate sleep, could also be stigmatized. Many participants expressed that they felt guilty considering or pursuing separate sleep from the baby and/or sleep-training. For instance, recall that Jocelyn felt bad about having to move her baby into a bassinet for part of the night in order to be able to sleep close to her without sharing a bed. In a similar vein, as I describe in chapter 7, when Johanna began to feel more comfortable with bed sharing, she could not physically manage it without bodily pain. Later, she also shared that she felt "guilty" about telling me about her sleep-training because it had involved "crying it out" or letting the baby cry itself to sleep unattended, a strategy that is often criticized by supporters of long-term breastfeeding. These statements showed that, despite their non-mainstream status, parenting ideologies that fully embrace breastfeeding—in mandating the specific form of breastfeeding practices—could be morally oppressive, similar to those that dictate the establishment of autonomy for children despite the challenges that this poses for some breastfeeding parents. Thus, regardless of their specific form, sleeping arrangements devised to facilitate breastfeeding plunged breastfeeding mothers into further moral quagmires.

## Conclusion

Mothers' narratives in this chapter point to profoundly conflicted cultural ideologies about breastfeeding. On the one hand, breastfeeding was considered a desirable moral good whose attainment was supposed to produce joy for mothers. Its valorized status, however, directly contradicted mothers' painful and exhausting experiences of breastfeeding and forced mothers to selectively downplay and erase their negative experiences. Breastfeeding difficulties were interpreted by Bridget as a sign of maternal failure. At the same time, the daily practice of breastfeeding violated moral norms surrounding mothers' and children's personhoods. Corinne's and Carol's ability to provide adequate nourishment for their children and to produce children who conform to expectations of self-regulation and autonomy came under intense scrutiny through monitoring specific feeding practices and sleep arrangements. Finally, mothers' personhood as supreme providers of care was most profoundly challenged by their potential failure to keep their children alive in the context of bed sharing, as in Jocelyn's account. At the same time, medically "safe" sleep arrangements could also lead to questions about the adequacy of mothers' caregiving, as in the case of Jocelyn and Johanna. The enormous moral hazards associated with on-the-ground experiences of breastfeeding attest to multiple sources of stigmatization. Ironically, this insight suggests that neither those who "fail" to breastfeed, nor those who "succeed" to do so can escape stigma and its embodied consequences.

Previous scholarship on breastfeeding and morality has primarily focused on the experiences and strategies of mothers who decided not to breastfeed.[27] Murphy's research of women who decided not to breastfeed in the U.K. showed that women were not simply ignorant of public health advice; instead they drew on their own understandings (e.g., formula is as effective as breastmilk, breastfeeding is inappropriate, etc.) to make rational decisions about infant feeding in a particular cultural context. Blum's (1999) research similarly highlighted how working class white women and African American women make decisions about feeding their babies in structural and cultural conditions that make it virtually impossible for them to do so. African American women explicitly questioned the exclusionary nature of breastfeeding and decided not to breastfeed as a form of resistance to the dominant white middle-class ideologies of motherhood.

Significantly less attention has been devoted to the moral praxis of women who are committed to breastfeeding, although the body of research that signals the complex relationship of breastfeeding women to their own embodied breastfeeding experiences points in this direction.[28] Although Faircloth (2009, 2010a, 2010b) does not situate her work primarily in the framework of moral contradictions, her ethnographic study of full-term breastfeeding mothers in London and Paris illustrates the morally contradictory position breastfeeding mothers occupy when they engage in the medically-recommended practice of breastfeeding, yet do so for lengths of time that extend beyond cultural norms. Faircloth employs Goffman's construct of identity-work to discuss how mothers construct themselves in relation to these contradictions and deploy the medical concept of risk to defend themselves against marginalization.

Ryan and colleagues (2010) explicitly situate their discussion within the framework of "moral work being undertaken within the act of breastfeeding and related practices that may be neither risky nor deviant nor resistant" (2010:952). The authors carry out their analysis using Foucault's concept of "technologies of the self" and "ethics" as a "relationship to oneself" (2010:952) to discuss how mothers perform moral labor to address and resolve, through narrative practices, the moral contradictions they encounter in their breastfeeding. Drawing on video interviews with a diverse sample of U.K. women, they suggest that the moral work women undertook in their narratives was constitutive of their subjectivity. [29]

I suggest that considering the role of stigmatization in the context of infant feeding practices provides an alternative to the above approaches. My ethnographic findings indicate, on the one hand, that the moral frameworks that valorize breastfeeding not only stigmatize those who do not breastfeed, but also those who struggle with breastfeeding because of the danger of "failure." On the other hand, most aspects of the actual practice of breastfeeding are also directly stigmatized, because they violate moral expectations for mothers' and children's personhood and their kin relations. Although privilege can facilitate the attainment of "successful breastfeeding," thereby avoiding the moral charge of "deviance," it does not offer an escape out of moral dilemmas presented by breastfeeding. I believe that the relational, embodied negotiation of stigma enables us to capture the complexities in breastfeeding mothers' and their families' moral experiences.[30] Longitudinal ethnographic methodology is particularly well-suited to examine the social dynamics of moral experience over time, including the role these experiences play in the making of kinship, personhood, and capitalism. In this framework, my ethnographic material provides evidence of the gendered effects of the stigmatization of breastfeeding and its embodied effects. In the next chapter I turn to men's contributions to breastfeeding that play an important role in mitigating the effects of this stigmatization.

## Notes

1. With the exception of rare cases of cross-nursing and professional wet-nursing (Bartlett and Shaw 2010).
2. See Zigon 2008.
3. Fieldnotes, March 2, 2007.
4. Preeclampsia, signaled by elevated blood pressure during pregnancy and protein in the urine, is a condition that carries significant risks of death for both mother and her fetus. Depending on the stage of the pregnancy and the severity of the condition, preeclampsia is addressed with bed-rest, medication and/or medical induction of labor in order to hasten the birth (Cunnigham et al. 2009)

5. Transitional milk refers to the milk that is produced a few days after birth (usually two to five days) after colostrum and before the production of fully mature milk.
6. Newborn jaundice is caused by the accumulation of bilirubin in the body that can be addressed by providing additional breastmilk or infant formula, which facilitates the breaking down and removal of the substance (Gartner 1994). Additional treatment, usually phototherapy, may be necessary in acute cases (Maisels and McDonagh 2008).
7. Fieldnotes, April 14, 2007.
8. Fieldnotes, March 28 2007.
9. The finger-feeding system enables the infant to suckle breastmilk or infant formula from a tube attached to an adult's finger. Suckling on a finger resembles the suckling motion from the breast, helping infants strengthen their suck in hopes of eventually transitioning them to nursing at the breast (Oddy and Glenn 2003). This system requires a fairly complex set-up and clean-up after the feeding, and each feeding session takes considerable time, often lasting one hour to an hour and a half.
10. See the previous chapter for a detailed discussion of the association of material culture with different parenting philosophies.
11. Fieldnotes, March 13, 2007.
12. Ibid.
13. Ibid.
14. Ibid.
15. Ibid.
16. Ibid.
17. Fieldnotes, April 30, 2007.
18. Ibid.
19. Ibid.
20. Fieldnotes, July 24, 2007.
21. Ibid.
22. Fieldnotes, September 23, 2007, for this entire account.
23. Fieldnotes, February 13, 2007, for this entire account.
24. See chapter 5.
25. Leslie meant the specific practice of bed-sharing here.
26. Fieldnotes, March 20, 2007.
27. See Blum 1999; Murphy 1999, 2000, 2003, 2004.
28. C. Stearns 1999, 2009, 2010; Kelleher 2006; Shaw 2004; McBride-Henry and Shaw 2010.
29. Ryan and colleagues' approach resembles Zigon's (2011b) discussion of the ethical process of working on the self to construct a moral person, although Zigon's theoretical approach (2008) engages a richer construct of morality and personhood.
30. Yang et al. 2007; Kleinman and Hall-Clifford 2009.

*Chapter 5*

# BREASTFEEDING AS MEN'S "KIN WORK"

In a controversial *Atlantic Monthly* article titled "The Case Against Breastfeeding," journalist Hanna Rosin (2009) compared breastfeeding to "this generation's vacuum cleaner—an instrument of misery that mostly just keeps women down." Rosin argued that breastfeeding mothers' exclusive involvement in breastfeeding leads to a fundamental rearrangement of the division of labor that results in greater freedom and power for fathers and a restricted domestic role for mothers. Rosin's investigation of the medical literature prompted her to conclude that the minimal benefits of breastfeeding in an industrial society simply do not warrant undertaking this gendered labor of breastfeeding.

Rosin's critique calls attention to breastfeeding promotion efforts that fail to address the lack of structural support for breastfeeding, uncritically enshrine women's domestic roles, and compound the moral burden for those women who cannot or choose not to breastfeed. While these perspectives merit attention, ethnographic evidence can offer a wider array of perspectives that can take us beyond dichotomous views of breastfeeding as either a tool for women's liberation or oppression. Moreover, ethnography can broaden the scope of analysis beyond mothers to their relationships with others that shape their breastfeeding practices and experiences. Marcia Inhorn and colleagues' recent edited volume, *Reconceiving the Second Sex: Men, Masculinity, and Reproduction* (Inhorn et al. 2009), argues for the importance of careful, ethnographically grounded studies of how men construct and perform masculinity and participate in reproduction.[1] In this vein, my study documents men's vital support for breastfeeding among a group of middle-class families in the U.S. and provides unique insight into breastfeeding as a kin-, person-, and class-making process.[2]

The focus on men in this chapter offers several important analytical insights. First, my ethnography provides an interesting example of the reversal of the gender relations described in di Leonardo's (1987) classic study of "kin work" among Italian American families in California. In di Leonardo's study, women were central to sustaining inter-household kin relations, a previously unrecognized category of gendered labor di Leonardo termed "kin work," so much so that these relationships often diminished in the women's absence. I argue that spouses in my study carried out similarly essential "kin work," without which many mothers would have found it impossible to continue to breastfeed. This "kin work" required the commitment of substantial resources and labor and played an important role in building kin relations and fathers' personhoods.

Second, drawing upon the insights provided by Inhorn's (2003) study of infertility in Egypt, I suggest that breastfeeding in the U.S., similar to producing children after experiencing infertility in Egypt, is a special site where kin bonds between spouses are renegotiated and social class is reproduced. Infertility in Egypt is a highly stigmatized condition characterized by systematic discrimination and expensive, but often painful and ineffective, treatments. In a similar vein, in the previous chapter I have argued that breastfeeding (as well as not breastfeeding) is subject to continued stigmatization, producing serious embodied consequences for mothers. The inability to comply with cultural expectations in both cases is considered morally problematic, particularly for women whose bodies are considered the sites of reproductive "failure." Furthermore, finding a way to produce children or to breastfeed requires considerable financial, educational, familial, and emotional resources in societies that lack broad structural support for these processes. Just as in Egypt, where learning about, locating and purchasing high quality fertility diagnostics and treatments is difficult and expensive, obtaining sufficient knowledge, medical support, and equipment to breastfeed can be fraught with challenges in the U.S., albeit in a less extreme form.

In both Inhorn's study and my own, the enduring support of spouses mitigated the effects of stigmatization. Because obtaining infertility treatments and the resources necessary to sustain breastfeeding beyond a few weeks are elite goods in these two societies, securing spousal support in the production of children among previously infertile couples in Egypt and in breastfeeding in the U.S. become signs of and, ultimately, sites for the reproduction of social class. This chapter, along with Inhorn's work, illustrates that men make critical contributions to reproduction and simultaneously participate in the construction of kinship, personhood, and social class.

## Fathers, Work, and the Politics of Breastfeeding in the United States

Historian Jacqueline Wolf (2001) has argued that the development of companionate marriage is one of the pivotal influences that have shaped the shift away from breastfeeding to artificial milk substitutes in the end of the nineteenth century and the beginning of the twentieth century (see chapter 2). In her study of breastfeeding in Chicago, Wolf used letters and other written materials from wealthy couples that documented their romantic affections and longing for another as well as how such relationships superseded those with their children. Wealthy mothers often hired live-in domestic servants, "nurse-maids," to care for their children from birth, who also breastfed the baby. Later on, medical recommendations that echoed capitalist regimes of efficiency and self-regulation reinforced the necessity of the nighttime separation of couples and children as well as the feeding of children according to strict schedules with the scientifically engineered infant formulas (Apple 1987). In these idealized models of parenting that presumed middle-class status, fathers provided the income for the family while their wives ran an efficient household that included the socialization of children according to similarly efficient models. Wolf's account highlights the importance of the rise of companionate marriage in the separation of mothers and babies and ultimately in the replacement of breastfeeding altogether.

Yet, marriage was also at the heart of grass roots movements that promoted its return. Julia Ward (2000) documents that the seven founders of the La Leche League were married to men who were very supportive of breastfeeding, some of whom held medical degrees that leant them credibility and moral authority in the women's promotional efforts. Without these men, the League's mother-to-mother support may not have resulted in a sufficiently powerful movement to begin to alter physicians' views of breastfeeding. Furthermore, it was the League that also enshrined a model of breastfeeding based on Catholic ideals for companionate marriage in which husbands supported breastfeeding and shared the division of labor in the home in order to enable its continued practice (Ward 2000; Tomori 2005). Nevertheless, these marital ideals continued to assume gendered roles for men as the providers of a family income and women as the primary caregivers of children. Furthermore, the League continued to presume the presence of a loving and supportive father, largely ignoring the experiences of women raising children on their own, with a same-sex partner, or in any other configuration (Hausman 2003; Weiner 1994). The League has only more recently shifted its rhetoric to be more inclusive of women employed full-time outside the home (Weiner 1994; Hausman 2003; Ward 2000).

The lack of support for breastfeeding women in the labor force is particularly notable in light of the dramatic increase of employed women since the middle of the twentieth century. Little has been accomplished to alter family leave and employment practices that make breastfeeding difficult, if not impossible, for the majority of U.S. women (Galtry 2000; Galtry and Callister 2005; Calnen 2007; Blum 1999). As a poignant illustration of this point, during the summer of 2009 the Ohio Supreme Court upheld a decision in support of the firing of a woman from her job at Totes/Isomer for taking fifteen-minute breaks from her work to express breastmilk for her five-month old child. Furthermore, the Ohio Supreme Court ruled that breastfeeding discrimination was separate from gender discrimination and did not comment on the language of the previous decision, which claimed: "Pregnant [women] who give birth and choose not to breastfeed or pump their breasts do not continue to lactate for five months. ... Allen's condition of lactating was not a condition relating to pregnancy but rather a condition related to breastfeeding" (Shellenbarger 2009; Harding 2009). By severing the relationship of pregnancy, birth, and breastfeeding, the Court placed the burden of sustaining breastfeeding on the working mother, removing any responsibility of the employer. This move also reinforced moralizing discourses surrounding breastfeeding that highlight individual responsibility instead of viewing breastfeeding in the larger context of the many obstacles that hinder women's ability to breastfeed.[3]

It is no surprise then that educated, wealthier women are breastfeeding at disproportionately higher rates and for significantly lengthier periods of time. These women have secure middle- and upper-middle-class status with sufficient income from two partners, more generous leave policies, and the educational resources necessary to be able to breastfeed. Since sustaining many months of breastfeeding is challenging even for these women, however, some decide to take a more extended break from employment in order to enable them to continue to breastfeed and provide an intensively engaged model of parenting of which breastfeeding is a part.[4] Although these decisions enable women to negotiate the demands of childrearing, they also have important negative consequences for their earning potential and career trajectories (Moe and Shandy 2010). Furthermore, research on women who left the labor force to raise children indicates that such decisions can also lead to the entrenchment of traditional gender roles that naturalize women's role of childrearing and men's role as income-providers (Bobel 2002; Hays 1996). Following Hochschild's (1989) classic argument about the "second shift" working women take on when they return home, Hays (1996) has argued that new intensive parenting ideologies that include breastfeeding constitute a new "second shift" for women. These are precisely the concerns that led Rosin (2009) and others to their critique of breastfeeding.

As a feminist anthropologist troubled by reductive perspectives on breastfeeding, I was interested in learning more about how middle-class U.S. families who are considered more likely to breastfeed their children negotiate the challenges of breastfeeding. In contrast to Rosin's research, however, my own ethnography revealed that among highly educated middle-class participants, both members of the couple were intimately involved in the entire breastfeeding process and the labor entailed therein. Situating my discussion of breastfeeding in the context of kinship enabled me to broaden the scope of my analysis beyond mothers to examine the role of men's "kin work" in the construction of kin ties that bind spouses and children together.

## Kinship, "Kin Work," and Breastfeeding

While prior ethnographic research outside the U.S. has shown that acts of nurturance, including breastfeeding, are primary ways in which kin ties, including enduring sentimental bonds, are created,[5] these ethnographies leave unexplored how men might also participate in the construction of kinship through their involvement in breastfeeding. In particular, my ethnographic data on the daily practices through which spouses enabled and supported breastfeeding demanded an integrated analysis of kinship, breastfeeding, sentiment, and work. Micaela di Leonardo (1987), reflecting on her ethnography of Italian American families in California, argued that women participated in "three types of work: housework and child care, work in the labor market, and the work of kinship" (1987:442). She suggested that the work of kinship was a highly gendered form of labor that constructed and sustained kin relations across multiple households. In the absence of an adult woman, this kind of work often dwindled or simply ceased to exist. By describing spousal involvement in breastfeeding as "kin work," I draw upon di Leonardo's concept quite loosely, without the above demarcation of three labor categories. While di Leonardo's categories were helpful in drawing attention to the previously neglected domain of the maintenance of inter-household kin relations, my own ethnographic data indicates that spouses were involved in all of the above elements of labor in establishing and maintaining breastfeeding. Therefore, conceptualizing these spousal activities as "kin work" draws attention to the network of kin relations entailed in making breastfeeding possible while also serving to remind readers of the interconnected nature of work and affective ties.

In pursuing this analytical direction, I build most clearly on Sallie Han's ethnographic research on pregnancy undertaken in a similar ethnographic setting to my own, which has yielded many productive insights. For instance, Han (2009) described how the embodied practice of "belly talk," which entails talking, reading, and singing to the fetus and touching the mother's pregnant belly, becomes an important part of constituting kinship and producing fatherhood. In my own study, men's deep involvement in making breastfeeding possible reinforced affective ties with their spouses, forged new ties to their children, and thereby also produced their personhoods as fathers.

This material-affective process provides groundwork for thinking through the multidimensional involvement of fathers in breastfeeding in my own work and seeks to develop new, ethnographically rich perspectives on an important dimension of kinship in the United States, while simultaneously expanding discourses on the politics of motherhood to a wider network of social relations.

## Men as Pivotal Sources of Breastfeeding Support

Although couples in my study were not aware of the complex interrelationship of marriage, gender, and work in the history of breastfeeding in the U.S., they had to contend with its legacies in their daily practices. Participants in my study were aware even prior to giving birth that breastfeeding could be challenging, and they mobilized extensive resources in order to accomplish their goal to breastfeed. During the course of my study, spouses actively supported breastfeeding in the following key areas: participation in childbirth education, provision of support in birth and the immediate postpartum period, construction of new divisions of labor, nighttime support, and breastfeeding advocacy in later months. These areas reflect the emphasis on these realms in my data as well as the design of the study that investigated nighttime arrangements in great depth. The diversity of these five realms of support and their continuity in time demonstrates that spouses can play pivotal, yet inadequately documented, roles throughout the entire pregnancy/birth process/postpartum period that enable and support breastfeeding.

### *Childbirth Education as a Site for the Socialization of Men's Support for Breastfeeding*

Drawing on interviews and ethnographic observations with middle-class fathers,[6] Richard Reed (2005) argues that just as taking these classes constitutes part of a rite of passage that transforms pregnant women into mothers (Davis-Floyd 2004), through participating in these courses men also begin their transformation into fathers. Reed claims that in this sense childbirth education is a form of couvade, a set of ritual preparations that men undertake that parallel and engage with their spouses' pregnancies. Through these classes men learn their roles as the primary source of support for their partners during childbirth as well as facilitators between medical care providers and their laboring spouses. Furthermore, Reed suggests that birthing classes constitute important ritualized interactions through which men can fulfill new ideals of involved, emotionally engaged fatherhood. For Reed then, childbirth education classes play a role in both person- and kin-making processes; men begin to acquire their new personhood as "fathers" and in the process they construct their kinship with their children-to-be and re-affirm their relationship with their spouses. Sallie Han's more sustained and wide-ranging research on pregnancy situates childbirth education classes as part of a larger set of practices that enable men to actively partake in the pregnancy (2009a, 2009b, 2006).

In accordance with Reed's and Han's research, for men in my study participation in childbirth education courses was an important step in preparing for the baby's arrival and for supporting their spouses in birth, breastfeeding, and other caretaking activities for their children. At both childbirth education locations where I conducted fieldwork, spouses were encouraged to attend classes together. As I described in chapter 3, expectant parents made a significant time commitment to participate in these classes, which often stretched from the second trimester of pregnancy to the middle or end of the third trimester.

The class sessions primarily emphasized spouses' active role in facilitating the birth process—for instance, in the creation of a birth plan. The aim to minimize medical interventions, often featured as a central component of these plans, was partly motivated by the desire to avoid the potentially adverse effects of pharmaceuticals or procedures used in labor, or complications whose treatment necessitates the separation of mothers and babies, all of which can reduce babies' ability to breastfeed. Men also participated in breastfeeding classes with their partners. In these sessions, they learned about the importance of breastfeeding as well as about specific ways in which successful breastfeeding can be established and sustained. Although the largest portion of the classes focused on birth itself, instructors made clear that the process of birth had implications for breastfeeding. By inviting spouses to participate in these sessions, each field site's instructors emphasized that spousal support is essential throughout the entire childbirth/breastfeeding process. In turn, men's participation in these classes signaled that they would play an active role in supporting their spouses and caring for the baby once he/she was born.

In his ethnographic observations, Reed (2005) found that men were being socialized into gendered models about their role in childbirth. They were expected to act as defenders and protectors of the birth process, while also recognizing the authority of medical personnel. The role of birth advocate was particularly significant in the courses that advocated for childbirth with minimal medical interventions and went against mainstream childbirth practices. At the same time, Reed also found that men also served as birthing companions—sources of emotional support for their spouses. My own research in Green City replicates these findings and extends them to breastfeeding.

At both of the childbirth education sites where I conducted research, expectant fathers were encouraged to advocate for their partners during childbirth, especially in times when laboring women encountered difficulties. There was at least as much emphasis, however, on men's roles as primary sources of support for their partners during labor, indicating that men were also being socialized into more traditionally feminine roles of caretaker. Furthermore, making sustained eye contact, holding their spouse close and verbally asserting their love for their partners were encouraged at both sites, as acts that helped laboring women regain a sense of groundedness during the hardest parts of labor. These acts reinforced ideologies of partnerhood that emphasize close emotional connection.

These approaches were also extended to breastfeeding. Men were encouraged to learn about breastfeeding in order to advocate for it, should such advocacy be necessary in the postpartum period. For instance, if the couple decided that the child should not receive any supplemental feedings besides breastmilk, fathers were entrusted to make sure that this plan was followed. These encouragements reinforced men's role as protectors of the breastfeeding process. This role was then complemented by the companionate approach to breastfeeding promoted at these childbirth education sites that encouraged men to support breastfeeding by reducing mothers' workload and providing encouragement for mothers as they worked to establish breastfeeding.

Although both organizations encouraged men's involvement in supporting breastfeeding, there was considerably more emphasis on men's role in breastfeeding at Holistic Center, which treated spouses as a decision-making unit that together could enact an alternative model of childbirth and parenting. Accordingly, there was also more discussion of the challenges that breastfeeding babies could pose in re-establishing sexual relations between spouses, including having a breastfeeding baby who demanded constant bodily contact with his/her mother and the potential challenges of having a baby sleeping in the parental bed. Men were encouraged to be understanding of the physical exhaustion and bodily challenges of breastfeeding for women, to engage in open communication with their partners, and to reconnect with their partners emotionally during this new phase of their relationship. While the topic of sexuality was touched upon, and the physical demands of breastfeeding in relation to sexuality were also mentioned at Family Center, these issues were addressed in less specific ways with far less emphasis on breastfeeding.

Holistic Center also addressed the bodily labor entailed in breastfeeding in very concrete terms. Their childbirth sessions concluded with an activity that asked expectant parents to estimate the time each of them would spend on different aspects of life in the first few weeks postpartum using a pie chart. When the instructor filled in a larger model pie chart to show the average time one would spend on the tasks related to caring for the baby, a stunned silence usually filled the room. I witnessed several such moments during my participation in these courses. In particular, participants were often taken aback when shown that breastfeeding took approximately six hours each day. In several cases, attendees commented on how different their own and their spouses' charts looked because most spouses knew that they would return to work shortly after the babies' birth, while new mothers would stay at home to care for their baby during their maternity leaves or for even longer periods of time, and would spend the majority of their time breastfeeding the baby in the first weeks after birth. This recognition of the demands of breastfeeding prompted several men to express their support in the class for helping with household activities to support their spouses to breastfeed their babies, which was then reinforced by the instructor's comments.

These educational activities strengthened spousal bonds and prepared spouses for an active, supportive role in the birthing and breastfeeding processes. Childbirth education courses played an important role in eliciting and socializing spouses into providing support to enable breastfeeding for their partners through acting as protectors of the process and as emotionally engaged companions. This support was not only pivotal in reinforcing kin relations with their partners, but simultaneously served as a building block for developing the persona of the caring and committed father.

### *Enacting Breastfeeding Support in the Birth Process and Immediate Postpartum Period*

During the birth process and immediate postpartum period, men largely fulfilled the roles for which they prepared during childbirth education courses. They supported mothers during the birth process in multiple ways, including encouraging the mother's intentions to minimize medical interventions and/or helping them come to terms with the need to accept these interventions, such as the augmentation of labor with the synthetic hormone Pitocin, epidural anesthesia, and surgical birth via Cesarean section. Once the baby arrived, spouses played a particularly important role in seeking lactation support and advocating for breastfeeding.

New mothers were tired from the birth process, often having endured long and painful labors and/or surgical birth, which made breastfeeding especially challenging. Mothers who underwent Cesarean sections were sometimes separated from their babies for several hours in order for neonatology specialists to follow up with the child in order to rule out possible infections or because the babies had lower vital signs than those set by medical standards. In these cases men helped to ensure that both mothers and children were attended to and facilitated their reunion. For instance, after their planned home birth ended with a Cesarean section, Oliver spent several hours shuttling between his wife, Angela, and their son, Max, who was undergoing testing on a different floor of the hospital.[7] Oliver told me that he felt quite torn between attending to his wife, who had just undergone major surgery, and his newborn son. Therefore, Oliver provided support for both Angela and Max, in turns, but his primary objective was to ensure that Max was returned to Angela as soon as possible so that she could breastfeed him. His attention to this greatly speeded up the pace of completing the tests necessary so that Max could be released and returned to Angela. Once there, Oliver also helped her position Max so that he could breastfeed without touching Angela's incision, a delicate balancing act that involved multiple pairs of arms. Thus, Oliver was pivotal in facilitating this early period of breastfeeding (as well as breastfeeding later on).

Lactation support at the hospital was not always consistent or readily available, making new mothers wait or receive contradictory information from different medical personnel. When mothers experienced breastfeeding difficulties, spouses advocated on the mothers' behalf in order to receive more comprehensive support. In one such case, although Leslie's and Alex's baby, Connor, was born via an uncomplicated vaginal birth with epidural anesthesia at University Hospital, they faced some unanticipated obstacles to breastfeeding. Leslie and her husband, Alex, were already exhausted from the birth process and from the interruptions caused by routine hospital procedures in the postpartum period, which included checking vital signs, heel pricks for Connor, and other medical check-ups. When Leslie and I met a couple of weeks after she gave birth, her voice was still filled with annoyance as she described her distraught reaction to a resident's orders for a special kind of light therapy to treat jaundice due to slightly elevated levels of bilirubin in the baby's blood.[8] The nurses who conveyed the order recommended taking Connor to the nursery for the night while being treated with phototherapy[9] so that the couple could "get a good night's sleep."

The parents both agreed that they did not want to be separated from their baby and offered to stay with him, holding Connor under the two different kinds of light blankets throughout the night. One important reason for staying with Connor was to be able to breastfeed him whenever he desired. Leslie and Alex took turns sleeping and holding Connor and asked for further clarification on the plan from the resident on duty. The resident physician's explanation suggested that he was treating a different kind of jaundice based on maternal-child blood type incompatibility, which both Leslie and Alex recognized to be an incorrect diagnosis based on their knowledge of Leslie's and Connor's blood types. Alex explicitly questioned the resident's explanation, thereby challenging the authoritative position of the physician. Although Alex's concerns were initially dismissed by the resident, Alex's advocacy and the couple's continued insistence on a better explanation the next day from a different physician resulted in the correction of the treatment plan and in their continued ability to stay with their baby. Since the establishment of breastfeeding is greatly facilitated by the proximity of mother and child, Alex's advocacy most certainly contributed to the success of the breastfeeding process.

Fathers also played a crucial role in helping mothers overcome breastfeeding difficulties, many of which only emerged once they returned home. For instance, during Bridget's ordeal of trying to breastfeed her daughter that I described in the previous chapter, her husband took over feeding Angelina expressed breastmilk with the finger-feeder during the nighttime. This was a very time-consuming process, which resulted in minimal sleep for Roland in the first few weeks. The couple used the finger-feeder in order to help Angelina develop and maintain the suckling motion used in breastfeeding. Furthermore, the finger-feeder delivered expressed breastmilk, whose expression facilitated the maintenance of Bridget's milk supply and Angelina's connection to breastfeeding. Roland carried out these feedings without complaint, affirming his support for his wife by enabling her to get rest while also facilitating the establishment of the breastfeeding process. Moreover, Roland provided unfailing emotional support for Bridget during her struggles, helping to alleviate the effects of the stigma associated with breastfeeding difficulties and potential discontinuation of breastfeeding. This theme of men's importance in overcoming particularly stressful times was echoed by other couples.

Thus, fathers played a pivotal role in supporting breastfeeding throughout the birth process and subsequent immediate postpartum period. Through defending/protecting the birth/breastfeeding process, and providing emotional and instrumental support that facilitated breastfeeding, they enacted the paternal personhoods that they began to craft during childbirth education courses. Through these processes of kin work they actively constructed kin ties with their wives and children and forged an emotionally engaged model of fatherhood.

### Breastfeeding and the Renegotiation of the Division of Labor

The minimal provisions built into the U.S. employment system for supporting the intensive caretaking involved in rearing children presented an especially difficult challenge for breastfeeding families. Indeed, due to the significance of maintaining regular contact between the mothers and their babies and/or having access to breaks for expressing breastmilk for the baby, breastfeeding played a pivotal role in the configuration of couples' work arrangements after their babies' births. Several spouses supported their wives by taking advantage of workplace policies that enabled extended unpaid family leaves or flexible work arrangements from home. Some of these arrangements were made to reduce the burden on mothers in the early postpartum weeks when the establishment of breastfeeding was the central activity in which the new mothers and babies were engaged, while in other cases spouses became primary caregivers for a period when the mothers returned to full-time employment.

Joshua and Kate, whose breastfeeding and sleep dilemmas opened the book, worked together to divide the labor of caring for Anna and the household as equitably as possible. Joshua took extended unpaid family leave, available as part of his employment benefits, to support Kate and to spend time with their baby. Joshua took on the bulk of housework as well as many other baby-care tasks so that Kate could focus on securely establishing breastfeeding, recovering from giving birth, and getting some rest. During our meetings, Joshua clearly focused on the details of how he could make it easier for Kate to manage the demands of breastfeeding. For instance, I watched as Joshua diapered Anna and helped Kate get situated in an armchair in the living room for breastfeeding in the early days, when positioning the baby was still pivotal to being able to latch her on.[10] Joshua prepared a glass of water for Kate right next to her chair, in anticipation that she would get thirsty while nursing Anna. Indeed, Kate was getting thirsty within a minute and was grateful to find a glass already within her reach. These were among the many seemingly small but important acts of care that I observed during our meetings, which greatly facilitated Kate's breastfeeding process.

Breastfeeding was seamlessly integrated into the everyday activities of the family. After taking the maximum amount of leave from her work as a teacher, Kate later decided to take a more extended leave so that she could spend more time with Anna (who breastfed far beyond the basic biomedical recommendation of one year) and to continue with her master's degree part-time. Thus, Joshua ultimately became the sole breadwinner for the family for at least some time. In this and other similar cases, fathers undertook a variety of employment arrangements that facilitated the establishment of the breastfeeding relationship and later enabled its continued maintenance.

Similar to Kate and Joshua, Leslie and Alex meticulously planned for their baby's arrival, relying on a sequence of Leslie's paid and unpaid maternity leave from her work for five months as a lawyer, followed by six weeks when Alex cared for Connor during the day and worked from home in the evenings. Leslie's retired mother provided the final stretch of support until the parents felt that their child could enter childcare full-time at about eight to nine months old. Once Leslie returned to her job, she used an electric pump to express breastmilk at her office as well as at home, so that her husband or mother could feed Connor her milk during the day. In this case, Alex's weeks as a primary caregiver were a part of a larger set of arrangements that enabled the couple to delay placing Connor in childcare, to minimize the time that Leslie spent away from him, and to reduce the stress caused by needing to leave Connor during her work.

Despite these efforts, Leslie became increasingly dissatisfied with full-time employment. The inability to breastfeed her son during the day and the burden of pumping greatly contributed to her desire to alter work arrangements. At eight months postpartum, Leslie proposed a plan to her supervisor that would enable her to complete all her responsibilities in a part-time format that could be easily accommodated into the office structure. When her supervisor rejected this proposal, Leslie eventually decided to leave her job nine months after Connor's birth.

Throughout this situation, Alex was supportive of Leslie's breastfeeding and employment arrangements. When Leslie was working, he enabled her to breastfeed by supporting pumping and breastfeeding at home during the day and night, and feeding their son the pumped breastmilk during the day. In fact, when I spent part of one of these days with Alex and their baby, Alex told me that he usually took Connor on a walk and "then we do the breastfeeding, I mean the bottle-feeding [laughs] breastmilk feeding."[11] Alex's linguistic slip demonstrated how, through feeding Connor breastmilk, Alex himself had become thoroughly integrated into the couple's overall breastfeeding process. Indeed, after we went for a nice walk in the neighborhood that helped Connor take a nap, Alex took out some of the breastmilk Leslie had expressed and stored in the fridge and got it ready by pouring it into a bottle with a nipple for Connor. He was careful only to take a few ounces at a time, and handled the storage bag delicately, so as not to waste any of the milk that Leslie had worked so hard to save for Connor. Alex also gained more insight into the process of breastfeeding itself. For instance, Alex told me that he learned that while Connor enjoyed drinking breastmilk from a bottle, Alex saw that this was not the same as the process of breastfeeding, which provided comforts beyond food. Alex told me that when he was first learning how to care for Connor throughout the course of the day without Leslie being there to nurse him, he worried that he could not soothe Connor without breastfeeding. By the time of our meeting, however, he developed more confidence and his own repertoire of how to best help Connor when he was upset, incorporating "breastfeeding" via the refrigerated milk and bottles into this process.

Later, when Leslie's part-time arrangement for employment became unattainable, Alex supported Leslie's decision to leave her job and became the family breadwinner. In this and similar cases, spousal employment became pivotal, since the entire family now depended on the income and the employer-provided benefits of the spouse. Thus, both taking time off from work and participating in paid employment outside the home[12] for long hours are often very important yet potentially overlooked ways in which some spouses enable and support mothers' efforts to continue breastfeeding.

In other families, spouses shared primary caretaking due to part-time work arrangements, and one father, Samuel, became the primary caregiver of their child. These families developed such work arrangements mainly because the mothers held employment that provided the primary income of the family and/or health care benefits upon which they depended and because they could not negotiate longer leaves or reduction in hours. These arrangements resulted in physical separation of mothers and their children, necessitating the implementation of regular times during which the mother used an electric pump to express breastmilk, which then could be fed to the child by the spouse or another person.

For instance, after her eight-week maternity leave, Jocelyn returned to work full-time while Samuel became the primary caregiver of their daughter, Deirdre. Samuel fed Deirdre with Jocelyn's expressed breastmilk and cared for her during the day, and completed some of his work at home while Deirdre napped or at times when Jocelyn was home. Furthermore, Samuel took on the bulk of household work with baby in tow and during the times when his wife was nursing or pumping. Samuel, a food connoisseur and excellent cook, enjoyed preparing meals while Deirdre played or slept nearby. He also did much of the cleaning and laundry while carrying her in a baby carrier strapped to his body. Samuel often finished dinner preparations while Jocelyn nursed Deirdre after her return from work.

This arrangement was complicated by a visit to the pediatrician a few months postpartum, when the couple learned that Deirdre was not gaining weight at an adequate pace, indicating that the electric pump could not adequately stimulate Jocelyn's milk production. Despite increasing the number of pumping sessions at home and at work, Jocelyn's milk supply continued to dwindle.[13] In order to facilitate breastfeeding, Samuel drove to his wife's work every day, often twice, so that Deirdre would have adequate opportunities to breastfeed, providing her with a greater supply of milk than what Jocelyn could provide by pumping alone. I was able to meet with the couple on one such occasion[14] and observed how smoothly Samuel handled this process, updating Jocelyn about Deirdre's day as Jocelyn breastfed on a couch at her office. Samuel also made sure that Jocelyn had a chance to eat and brought her some lunch, thereby helping to complete the circle of care and nourishment. Both Jocelyn and Deirdre benefited greatly from this arrangement, since the visits relieved pressure on Jocelyn to pump (something she did not enjoy) and enabled mother and daughter to reconnect through breastfeeding in the middle of the day, while the frequent contact with her baby ensured that Jocelyn would continue to produce sufficient breastmilk. Thus, this case represents a reversal of traditional gendered patterns of employment and household labor but with important accommodations that facilitated the ongoing sustenance of breastfeeding.

Rachel and Nathan found themselves in a similar situation because their daughter, Maya, would not drink from a bottle the breastmilk Rachel expressed. Despite Nathan's repeated efforts, each feeding session ended with Maya hysterically crying, having only swallowed drops of breastmilk. Rachel worked twelve-hour shifts at University Hospital and their family depended on both her income and her benefits. Nathan worked part time while also completing his bachelor's degree at Green City's university. Nathan was quite panicked when he first realized that he could not feed Maya from the bottle and questioned his fathering abilities, but then he and

Rachel worked out an arrangement that worked for all involved.[15] Since their daughter could not go without breastmilk for the duration of these lengthy shifts, Nathan drove to the hospital at least once during each shift in order to enable their daughter to breastfeed. Thus, despite employment arrangements that resulted in physical separation of the mother and child, spouses caring for the baby during the mothers' work actively participated in supporting and maintaining breastfeeding by feeding the baby expressed breastmilk as well as by transporting the baby to the mother when the alternative feeding system failed.

Regardless of their employment arrangements, a primary way in which spouses enabled breastfeeding was through completing household chores. Cooking, doing dishes, cleaning the house, and doing laundry were some of the most common tasks that often shifted fully to spouses in addition to their previous household work and usual paid employment responsibilities. Yet fathers were also engaged in caring for their babies when they returned to work, enabling mothers to get a break from them. Leslie, for instance, commented that even though she was worried about how she was going to manage during her maternity leave with Alex returning to work a week after their baby was born, "My husband is just so good when he comes back—he took over bill paying, cleaning up the kitchen, making dinner, all the household stuff. All I did was rest and take care of him. But he is also involved, I can just give him the baby and take a shower."[16] Thus, Alex simultaneously took on household labor and caretaking tasks, both of which facilitated Leslie's breastfeeding. This new division of labor often became particularly important for mothers who returned to work soon after giving birth. Overburdened by the physical aftereffects of childbirth, the labor involved in breastfeeding and expressing milk at home and at work, the separation from their babies, and/or by the organization of childcare in addition to the usual stresses of work itself, mothers found their spouses' willingness to take on the bulk of housework proved essential to their ability to maintain breastfeeding.

In sum, when men became the primary breadwinners, they reproduced more traditional models of paternal personhood. This traditional role supported a new(-old) phenomenon of some American mothers breastfeeding their children for many months. At the same time, the above examples also show men's willingness to participate in more complex employment arrangements that included taking longer leaves or even the reversal of primary employment. Supporting the ongoing maintenance of breastfeeding was an important consideration in these arrangements as well. Furthermore, even the most traditional labor arrangements included new takes on the division of labor that supported and facilitated breastfeeding. In contrast to Hays's (1996) argument about the "second shift" constituted by intensive parenting, due to their prenatal preparation and their engagement with their partners, men were aware of the labor entailed in breastfeeding and made a great deal of effort to alleviate its burdens. Thus, men demonstrated considerable creativity in their negotiation of employment, household labor, and caretaking tasks, reworking many elements of conventional models of paternal personhood in the process. These efforts, in turn, constituted a central part of the daily enactment of kinship.

*Nighttime Support*

Many couples found the negotiation of nighttime practices the most labor-intensive aspect of supporting breastfeeding.[17] Men played an important role in developing and facilitating sleep arrangements that facilitated nighttime breastfeeding, which often resulted in profound upheavals of spatial and temporal orders. Discussions among couples also shaped their stance toward biomedical guidelines about solitary sleep and their own assessment of the safety of their sleep practices. Regardless of whether the men perceived sharing their bed with their babies as problematic, if mothers found this arrangement helpful, they were willing to play a supportive role so that the mothers could breastfeed and get some sleep.

Men took on a wide variety of roles during the night that helped their wives breastfeed or reduced their wives' time awake. For instance, during the difficult period after their daughter's birth described in chapter 4, Samuel and Jocelyn slept in shifts in order to enable Jocelyn to rest. When Jocelyn brought their daughter to bed, Samuel willingly left the bed in order to help allay her fears about Samuel rolling over on the baby. Later on, Samuel often took care of Deirdre during the night when she simply needed soothing and/or would provide pumped milk for her so that Jocelyn could sleep longer and be adequately alert for the next workday. Joshua similarly took on shifts of soothing their baby when Kate needed rest. Finally, Daniel took over some nighttime feedings using a bottle in order to reduce fatigue for his wife, who was working full-time. Daniel, as other men in my study, simply did this along with any other work in the household in a matter-of-fact way, as part of the normal routine of care. He made sure that he attended to what to put in the bottle, too, since Kristen was struggling to maintain her milk supply. Thus,

Daniel always double checked ahead of time with Kristen so that he knew whether to use breastmilk, formula, or a certain combination thereof, according to Kristen's needs. In these examples, and in the many others' in my study, spouses' acts of nighttime caretaking reduced the burden of breastfeeding and extended sleeping time for their wives. For these men, this work was not special or sacrificial; they simply did what needed to be done. These fathers actively worked against a paternal persona that does not entail sharing the labor of caring for children.

Fathers also actively participated in negotiations of specific sleep arrangements. For instance, their willingness to participate in bed sharing was essential in cases where mothers felt that they could not manage breastfeeding otherwise. Just as some mothers had difficulties with sleeping next to their babies, some fathers were also concerned about their babies' safety, which made it difficult for them to feel comfortable sleeping next to their babies. Nathan, for instance, was initially worried about potentially rolling over their baby and spent several nights sleeping on the edge of their bed, with his arm hanging over the side. After a few days, however, he began to adjust to sharing their bed and came to enjoy sleeping next to their daughter. Nathan and Rachel continued to share their bed with their daughter for the rest of her first year and beyond. When Nathan reflected on their decision to bed-share, he made it clear that these sleep arrangements were constructed collaboratively and were prompted by the couple's joint desire to facilitate breastfeeding: "Our process is centered on breastfeeding, and the fact that we are co-sleeping is driven by the fact that we are breastfeeding."[18]

Bed sharing often resulted in the rearrangement of the surface of the bed to reduce the risk of suffocation—such as removal of duvet covers, pillows, and other objects so that nothing could cover the face of the infant. Furthermore, bringing the baby into the bed also entailed the spatial rearrangement of couples' bodies. In some cases the baby slept between the spouses, while in others the baby slept on the side of the mother, both of which arrangements required adjustments on behalf of fathers and mothers, with a significant reduction in sleep space. Carol and Justin, for instance, worked on adjusting their son's nighttime position as he began to squeeze Justin into ever-smaller areas of the bed. Justin attached a bed rail in order to enable Carol to place Jeremiah closer to the outer edge of the bed for part of the night. This arrangement helped increase both of their sleeping space to a degree. Finally, during bed sharing both spouses needed to acclimate to the sleep patterns of the infant that included new sounds as well as awakenings during the night. In some cases, as in Samuel's example above, fathers left the bed and slept elsewhere so that mother and baby could sleep and breastfeed comfortably and safely together. Thus, the support of breastfeeding involved significant changes in many spouses' sleep patterns and locations.

For fathers who slept next to their children and wives, incorporating the child into the parental bed also constituted a set of important embodied practices the produced powerful affective bonds that brought the three sleepers together into a family unit. Leslie, for instance, mentioned that if Alex went to bed sooner than herself, he would take Connor to bed with him and she would find them snuggled up against each other when she entered the bedroom. Both Alex and Leslie enjoyed the closeness of their son and looked forward to sleeping in the same bed together. Even though Alex would have liked to be able to spend more time alone with his wife, he felt that he "had moved past that."[19] He believed that sleeping together in the same bed would help their family set the foundations for being emotionally connected with their son that would have lasting effects even many years down the road. Thus, sleeping in the same bed simultaneously facilitated breastfeeding and united the couple with their child.

Not all changes during the night were welcomed by new fathers or mothers. For example, some men acknowledged that having the baby in the middle of the bed and frequent night-nursing presented new obstacles to spousal relations. Fathers mentioned the challenges of having bodily contact with their partners as well as the opportunity to spend time together, even when the baby did not share the bed but was present in the same room, as most participants started out with the baby sharing the parental bedroom in at least the first few weeks. Thus, the baby's awakenings, which were primarily seen as driven by the desire to breastfeed, often resulted in the rearrangement of sexual relations. Yet, many couples found inventive ways to work around these issues, with nearly all bed-sharing couples laying down with their babies as they went to sleep earlier in the evening and then moving to another space to spend time together. Spouses' ability to support their partners' breastfeeding and productively contribute to new arrangements once again played an important role in the successful continuation of breastfeeding.

In some cases, spouses supported long-term goals for breastfeeding by helping to revise nighttime arrangements and implementing changes the couple had discussed. For instance, during a period when Carol's and Justin's son, Jeremiah, woke frequently at night,

Justin, despite his long day-time work hours in the auto-industry, took on a period of time during the night when he went in to soothe Jeremiah instead of Carol nursing him. This arrangement was pivotal in the couple's plan to enable Carol to get some rest and begin to wean their son from night-nursing, while also maintaining the continuation of breastfeeding during the daytime.

Similarly, as I describe in chapter 7, Carl assisted Johanna in developing and implementing a series of sleep-training plans in order to reduce Johanna's fatigue from nighttime breastfeeding. The first couple of nights of the implementation of a plan to eliminate nighttime feedings were emotionally difficult for both parents because their baby, Haden, cried for several hours. Johanna felt very torn about her decision and questioned it throughout the process but found comfort in her husband's support, who sat with her and listened to Haden's cries to make sure that he was going to be fine. Johanna felt that this change in nighttime practices ultimately helped her continue to breastfeed Haden during the day as she desired. In this case then, Carl's support played an important role in enabling continued breastfeeding on Johanna's terms, thereby extending the total duration of breastfeeding.

Spouses, therefore, performed several different kinds of labor during the night that supported breastfeeding. They engaged in the embodied labor of disrupting their own sleep in order to perform care-taking tasks that minimized the burden on their breastfeeding spouses, and they accommodated a variety of different sleep arrangements. Moreover, they supplied emotional support and active engagement in the process to develop and implement a sustainable sleep arrangement for tired breastfeeding mothers and for the whole family. All of these acts reinforced a model of highly engaged paternal persona and reinforced the affective ties between spouses.

### Breastfeeding Advocacy beyond the Hospital

Although this chapter has emphasized dimensions of spousal support in kin relations, relatives could also undermine breastfeeding. For instance, as I described in the previous chapter, Corinne's sister, sister-in-law, and parents-in-law all unwittingly undercut Corinne's confidence in breastfeeding and contributed to significant difficulties. In such cases, some spouses took on the role of defending their partners' breastfeeding. In a poignant example, Nathan encountered unexpected challenges to breastfeeding at an Easter holiday dinner with Rachel's family.[20] Since Rachel had to work, having recently returned from maternity leave, Nathan took Maya to the dinner, along with several bottles of expressed breastmilk that Rachel had pumped earlier. During the event, Nathan was asked to play with a cousin for a few minutes, so he handed Maya to Rachel's brother-in-law and stepped out of the room. Upon his return to the room, Nathan found Maya with a bottle of formula that belonged to another child and that the brother-in-law had given her. Rachel's family was well aware that Rachel was exclusively breastfeeding Maya and that, during Rachel's work, Nathan would feed Maya only Rachel's milk. In fact, they made light of the expression of shock on Nathan's face. Nathan was appalled by his brother-in-law's blatant disregard for their breastfeeding plans and left the gathering with Maya. Nathan's departure from the event was particularly significant since it added another element of already existing tension between the couple and Rachel's family. When Rachel first told me this story, she expressed that she appreciated Nathan's strong commitment to supporting breastfeeding and her desire to breastfeed. The couple's unified stance in protecting the breastfeeding relationship not only subverted Rachel's family's effort to sabotage breastfeeding but also reaffirmed the primacy of Rachel's and Nathan's relationship and their shared commitment to their daughter, which constituted the foundations of their family.

Echoing Nathan's experience at the Easter dinner, other men also engaged in conversations with family and friends that affirmed their commitment to breastfeeding. In these instances men again reasserted their persona as a defender and advocate for the breastfeeding process.

### The Limits of Breastfeeding Support

Despite their shared support for breastfeeding, couples and spouses within each couple negotiated unique ways of making breastfeeding possible. Couples' actions were clearly bound by structural inequities that made it much more difficult for women to remain employed, even if they desired to do so. These inequities reinforced American cultural ideologies of women's primarily domestic roles. Furthermore, men in my study varied in their contributions to supporting breastfeeding. For instance, some mothers pointed out that at first their spouses were not aware of how difficult it would be for the mothers to complete housework while staying home with the baby, who often nursed frequently throughout the day. Yet, each of these situations was followed by discussions that resulted in new divisions of household labor that better accommodated the needs of the mother. Since breastfeeding was valued by participants per the selection criteria for the study, it is also possible that couples were less willing to share information that could be interpreted as hindering breastfeeding. Finally, since I met with mothers more regularly in most cases, my study design may have limited my ability to learn about spouses' ambivalence about breastfeeding or about their concerns about sensitive areas such as sexuality and breastfeeding. Despite these limitations, my findings repeatedly reinforced the significance of men's acts of caring and support for breastfeeding.

## Conclusion

The previously neglected realm of men's "kin work," documented in these pages, demonstrates that, in the U.S., middle-class men's contributions to the breastfeeding relationship can help overcome the lack of structural and cultural support as well as mitigate the moral challenges generated by breastfeeding's embodied praxis. Just as men's support was crucial in overcoming and coping with infertility in Inhorn's study (2003), men's "kin work" in my study provided pivotal support that enabled their wives to successfully breastfeed their children. Additionally, these findings offer new opportunities for the analysis of gender, kinship, and labor practices. First, the acts of caring and support men provided highlight the significance of the relational elements of reproduction and the importance of developing more complex perspectives of men (Inhorn et al. 2009). Far from escaping the demands of parenthood, men in my study emerged as complex figures who strove to be engaged fathers and supportive spouses as they navigated many different obligations of demanding jobs and household tasks. Second, couples' incorporation of breastfeeding into their daily lives by rearranging the division of labor within and outside the household and by reinforcing the affective ties of their relationships provides insight into the construction of kinship and fatherhood in contemporary middle-class U.S. families.[21]

In a study of middle- and working-class men from Northern California, Nicholas Townsend (2002:2) argued that "having children, being married, holding a steady job, and owning a home" are part of a "package deal" of closely interrelated cultural norms. Townsend found that men struggle to resolve contradictory desires within this scheme to be emotionally close to their families while also supplying the material foundations seen as necessary for their family's existence. Certain elements of my findings, particularly fathers' support for their wives' desire to cut back on paid employment, as well as willingness to become primary breadwinners after the birth of their children, reinforced these culturally valorized aspects of being a father. At the same time, my participants were younger and more educated than those of Townsend's study and were more willing to take advantage of family leave policies and flexible work arrangements as well as to share the labor of housework and childcare, often despite extensive work obligations. These men's participation in the lengthy childbirth education classes signaled their future involvement and their provision of support for breastfeeding throughout the entire birthing process and postpartum months.

In a similar vein, building on Reed's (2005) work, men's support for breastfeeding both reinforced and renegotiated gendered expectations for their role as fathers. On the one hand, becoming the defenders and protectors of the birth/breastfeeding process reasserted traditional paternal roles of the protectors of the family. At the same time, fathers' ongoing emotional support in the face of difficulties and their pragmatic support for alleviating the burden of breastfeeding for their partners suggested the simultaneous creation of a different model of "involved" and emotionally engaged fatherhood (Gerson 1993).[22] Inhorn's work shows that the emotional ties between spouses cannot be overlooked in studies of reproduction, regardless of setting, but must be investigated in the specific forms they take in each ethnographic case. Moreover, my findings, along with Han's (2009) research on belly talk, point to the importance of embodied praxis in the construction of affective relational ties. In my own findings, fathers' embodied care for their partners and children as well as sharing sleep with them are the loci of constructing such emotional ties.

Each of the above gendered expectations for men has moral dimensions. Fathers' support for breastfeeding in my study was a part of constructing their own gendered moral personhood that simultaneously participated in the relational construction of mothers' complementary gendered personhood. By enabling their spouses to breastfeed, fathers mitigated the impact of stigma on their wives in multiple ways. First, through their active labor and emotional support they helped mothers avoid the moral danger of not breastfeeding or "failing" to breastfeed their babies. Second, their participation in negotiating sleep arrangements ensured a supportive environment for mothers to navigate the embodied challenges resulting from contradictory sociocultural expectations for infant sleep and feeding practices. Finally, their direct advocacy for breastfeeding explicitly challenged the taken-for-granted set of norms that make breastfeeding problematic in everyday life.

Unfortunately, the model of fatherhood articulated in the above pages continues to be an ideal situated within the constraints of social class. Men's ability to support breastfeeding relies on their access to knowledge about breastfeeding as well as material resources that supply the income, benefits, and overall economic security for the family. Due to the enormous commitments of these resources, the sheer ability to sustain breastfeeding reinforces norms for fatherhood and spousal partnership that are nearly always attainable only to the middle and upper-middle classes. Spousal support for breastfeeding therefore not only produces fathers' personhood and kin ties, but also participates in the reproduction of social class. In the final two chapters, I turn to a closer examination of families' negotiation of the spatial and temporal aspects of nighttime breastfeeding and sleep, and its implications for personhood, kinship, and capitalism.

## Notes

Material for this chapter has appeared in Tomori 2009.

1. See Dudgeon and Inhorn's (2009) article in that volume for an overview of anthropological approaches to men in reproduction.
2. In this chapter I restrict my analysis to male spouses in order to address feminist concerns about men's involvement in breastfeeding. Julia, the only woman spouse in my study, was similarly involved as the men I discuss. In fact, Petra felt that because they were both women, they understood each other's needs in a more profound way and therefore Julia was better able to support Petra during breastfeeding than most men. While Petra and Julia worked toward an equitable division of labor and shared involvement with their child, the men in my study had similar desires and acted in quite similar ways, reflecting shared ideologies of parenthood among middle-class Americans. At the same time, each heterosexual couple negotiated these arrangements in different ways, some of which replicated more traditional models of division of labor than others. Research that compares same-sex and heterosexual couples is needed to develop greater insight into the division of labor in relation to breastfeeding and infant sleep.
3. The Patient Protection and Affordable Care Act contains an important provision for ensuring adequate breaks for expressing breastmilk at work in Section 4207 (United States Breastfeeding Committee 2011), but no systematic changes to parental leave or on-site childcare.
4. See Moe and Shandy 2010; Kukla 2005; Bobel 2002; Hays 1996.

5. See, for instance, Carsten 1995; Lambert 2000. Breastfeeding is a documented part of this process in several different cultural settings (Dettwyler 1988; Khatib-Chahidi 1992; Wright, Bauer, and Clark 1993; Zeitlyn and Rowshan 1997; Lambert 2000; Parkes 2001; Cassidy and El-Tom 2010). Janet Carsten has explored these links in great depth in her Malaysian ethnography (1995, 1997, 2004). In her book *Performing Kinship*, Krista Van Vleet has argued that while considerable work has focused on undermining assumptions of "deep-seated connection of feeling" within families, "Few anthropologists ... have explored just how the affective aspects of relatedness emerge between people in the process of their interactions" (2008:9).
6. Reed did not conduct a systematic ethnography in a community. Rather, he drew on his friends, acquaintances, and later a group of men who participated in childbirth education courses, presumably near the author's home near Trinity University in Texas (he did not specify his research site).
7. Fieldnotes, October 2, 2007.
8. Fieldnotes, January 11, 2007.
9. Phototherapy for treating newborn jaundice is used when bilirubin levels are elevated to a degree where breastfeeding or formula feeding cannot adequately resolve the buildup of the substance. The therapy involves placing the infant under special lights either built into a blanket that can be wrapped around the child or placed above a hospital bassinet (Maisels and McDonagh 2008)
10. Fieldnotes, February 23, 2007.
11. Fieldnotes, June 11, 2007.
12. These hours were often supplemented by additional work hours completed at home, sometimes during the night.
13. See Dykes 2005; Stearns 2010; Lepore 2009; Bartle 2010 on the ways in which lactation becomes focused on breastmilk production and is infused with capitalist machine metaphors.
14. Fieldnotes, February 4, 2008.
15. Fieldnotes, June 14 and 24, 2007.
16. Fieldnotes, March 20, 2007.
17. Considerable recent sociological research suggests that nighttime caretaking is gendered, with women disproportionately taking on the "fourth shift," and that this pattern extends far beyond infancy (see, for instance Burgard (2011); Williams, Meadows, and Arber (2010); Venn et al. (2008). Since my study is ethnographic and is not drawn from a representative sample, I cannot quantitatively compare the division of nighttime labor and relate it other factors. In the context of the existing literature, my data suggests that couples' behavior in this regard may also differ from others (they already clearly differ in their long-term breastfeeding behavior), with men mitigating the embodied burdens of nighttime breastfeeding. Nevertheless, there are gendered inequities in my study as well that merit further consideration. The variation in

breastfeeding and sleep practices both at any given time point and over the course of the year (see chapters 6 and 7) suggests opportunities for fruitful collaboration between large-scale quantitative sociological research and ethnographic anthropological research in this area. This research would be greatly enhanced by biological anthropological work on the physiological dimensions of solitary and shared sleep practices in relation to breastfeeding, and close attention to the spatial dimensions of nighttime sleep arrangements.
18. Fieldnotes, June 24, 2007.
19. Fieldnotes, June 11, 2007.
20. Fieldnotes, June 14 and 24, 2007
21. Carsten 2004; Franklin and McKinnon 2001.
22. According to some social historians, this kind of fatherhood has deep roots in middle-class ideologies of fatherhood that date back at least to the nineteenth century (Johansen 2001).

*Chapter 6*

# BREASTFEEDING BABIES IN THE NEST
## PRODUCING CHILDREN, KINSHIP, AND MORAL IMAGINATION IN THE HOUSE

A rich body of anthropological research addresses how the house, its occupants, and the relations among them co-produce one another through the material qualities of the house and the activities and movements that take place within its spaces.[1] This chapter explores how nighttime breastfeeding and related sleep arrangements offered similarly important sites for the mutual production of persons, kinship, and houses in Green City. In seeking houses suitable for raising children, and especially in the process of constructing new spaces for their babies during pregnancy, expectant parents actively located and produced their children's personhood in and through the house. Separate parental and child bedrooms within the house instantiated middle-class moral ideals for family relations that produce children—children who are simultaneously separate and "independent" from the bodies of parents and connected through the objects that surround them. Although such spatial sedimentations of cultural ideologies structure specific kinds of persons and gendered family relations, the spatial practices of nighttime breastfeeding pushed participants to challenge, renegotiate, and materially transform these morally laden ideologies.[2]

The cultural image of the house as a "nest," drawn from Gaston Bachelard's classic study of space ([1958] 1994), possesses rich affective qualities that evoke past memories and future dreams,[3] and serves as a site for the actualization of middle-class moral norms in the present and the future.[4] In my study, the child's bedroom within the house became an especially charged site wherein the past, present, and future were joined through heirlooms and specially crafted objects from relatives that were imagined to surround the future slumbering body of a much-desired child. Situating the experiences of nighttime breastfeeding in the metaphor of the "nest" serves as a reminder that these intimate processes that take place in the house are at the heart of much larger constructions of space, time, and morality that bind together multiple generations in the process of reproduction.

## Domestic Spaces and Household Economies: A "Nest" for Raising a Family

The purchasing of a home in which to raise a family was of primary significance for study participants. The house thereby become an anchor in space (and time) for the creation of a family and was imbued with enormous significance as families prepared for the arrival of their children. For most families, the selection of a specific location for a house was made on the basis of a complex calculus of proximity to work and a network of family and friends, as well as the economics of being able to be in a desirable location rich with resources for couples and future children. Over two-thirds of my participants had a rich network of connections to this region and state, with relatives of at least one member of the couple living fairly close by. The remaining families, as expected in this affluent university town, moved to this area because of their work and studies.

Study participants could be divided into two categories—three families lived in towns closer to a nearby large industrial city, while the remaining fifteen families resided in Green City itself or in the city right next to it. The average cost of housing in Green City was much higher than in many other neighboring areas, although there was considerable variation among neighborhoods.[5] The higher cost of housing also reflected a greater abundance of local resources, such as in the case of childbirth education courses as well as maternity care providers mentioned in previous chapters.

The three couples who commuted to their childbirth education courses from outside the Green City/Neighbor City area resided in towns that differed considerably from Green City.[6] Lynn and Gary lived close to a major airport in a small, tree-lined neighborhood near a large highway.[7] Although they lived close to both sides of the family, they wished for a larger home. Furthermore, because Gary had children from a previous marriage and the children resided in Green City during the week, they spent considerable time traveling back and forth to Green City. Paula and Matthew lived in another nearby town whose residents primarily relied on work at nearby industries.[8] They chose a neighborhood right across from a park and an elementary school. Yet, they also contemplated moving to a bigger home and/or to a wealthier town. Paula had some concerns about the size of the space for multiple children as well as for the neighborhood itself as nearby industries began to leave the area or scale down their operations in response to the economic downturn. Although both of these families seriously contemplated moving, they had not yet moved at the end of the study period.[9] Finally, Kristen and Daniel lived on a property that had been in Kristen's family for over a hundred years and her mother as well as many other relatives remained close by.[10] They enjoyed this proximity, and were situated close enough to be able to commute to their work and to other resources they sought, such as the childbirth courses and the hospital they selected for childbirth in Green City. Kristen and Daniel's house was located closest to Green City in a small town surrounded by an area that used to be farmland but is now dotted with developments.

Those living in or around Green City emphasized Green City's many positive characteristics, especially for raising a family. Green City is renowned for its excellent schools, cultural resources, and large number of parks. Of the fifteen families who resided in or very near Green City, three lived in Neighbor City, where the average cost of housing was lower. The visual characteristics of these neighborhoods were very similar to those found in Green City, with tree-lined streets and sidewalks. Although several participants had lengthy commutes to their work, usually at least one spouse worked closer to home. Nonetheless, those living in and very close to Green City preferred their location compared to other areas they could have chosen. Several couples also mentioned the importance of living in a good school district. Those residing within Green City paid attention to the geography of the public school system that begins with small neighborhood elementary schools that feed into increasingly larger middle schools and high schools.[11] Thus, finding a "good" location could be quite specific, because of the significance of having a good neighborhood elementary school as well as the presence of other families with children and nearby parks and playgrounds. Such concerns also underlie some of the segmentation of Green City along lines of age into neighborhoods that have a larger or smaller proportion of young children.

Although Green City was a desirable location for most participants, some families anticipated moves in the future either to new areas of the country or within the city. Johanna and Carl, who initially moved to Green City for Carl's work, were planning their impending move due to Carl's new job as they awaited the birth of their baby, and purchased a house in a southern state. Rachel and Nathan, who lived in Neighbor City, had planned to move closer to Nathan's family on the West Coast after Nathan completed his studies in Green City, and they made the move after the study's conclusion. Finally, Joy and Jonathan and Jocelyn and Samuel moved to more spacious homes in neighborhoods that they considered better during the course of the study.[12] In planning each move, finding a suitable home for raising children was an important consideration.

In addition to the specific location of the home in a "nice neighborhood" and its condition as well as aesthetic qualities, participants paid close attention to the space within the home, measured in square feet. In our discussions it was clear that couples considered the number and size of bedrooms in the house as they imagined their future children. In turn, participants also shared their worries about not having adequate space in their homes to accommodate the children they planned to have. As mentioned above, two families moved to larger homes during the period of the study, both in part so that they could better accommodate their first child as well as other future children.[13] Others shared these concerns and planned similarly motivated moves or alterations to expand usable space within the house in the future.[14]

The ability to purchase a single-family home, and to be able to do so in a safe and attractive neighborhood, is of primary concern to most Americans and has been so since the Fordian era when the purchasing of single-family homes was first subsidized by the government (Townsend 2002). In the history of the United States, the stand-alone family home has become a key identifying characteristic of being middle class and a path toward achieving middle-class status. The economic burden of a home in a desirable location with what families consider adequate space within, however, requires sufficient earnings and access to lines of credit to purchase and maintain it. The inability to purchase suitable homes in desirable areas due to socioeconomic differences and discrimination is a key driver of segregation by race and class (Charles 2003; Lands 2009). Therefore, sustaining the middle-class household not only supported individual families, but also reproduced systems of labor, property, and social relations that are replete with inequality.[15]

The economic burden of home ownership also has gendered implications. A primary reason for purchasing a home is to provide a domestic space for raising a family, which paradoxically makes other middle-class ideals of intensive caretaking for children difficult.[16] Increasingly, two incomes are required to pay for mortgages as well as for the associated expenses to maintain a middle-class lifestyle (Moe and Shandy 2010). These expenses put considerable pressure on parents after the birth of their children as they also attempted to meet the demands of this intensive parenting. These pressures, in turn, resulted in the increased gendering of daytime spaces, as mothers took time off from employment to care for their children while fathers worked long hours at work mostly outside the home. Furthermore, for many families these arrangements become more consolidated with the birth of their second children, demonstrating the gendered difficulties of raising children and securing longer leaves and/or reduced-hour employment. Although there were important variations among participants, this rearrangement of spatial relations prompted couples to wrestle with implications for the division of labor.[17] Despite these gendered oppositions, my analysis must also attend to continuities.[18] Although it is tempting to imagine men and women in separate, contrasting spaces, families reconnected each evening and night, as well as on weekends and days off from work. Their connections within the domestic spaces as well as their outings together sustained the cohesion of the family and warrant additional analytical attention.[19] Many families actively worked against these spatial separations by renegotiating their division of domestic labor as well as employment practices. Nevertheless, even these efforts to restructure gender relations remained constrained within the system of inequities engendered by the political economic relations of class, race, and global capitalism. Although in the remainder of this chapter I shift the focus to the interior of the house, and the embodied practices within it, I do so with these inequalities in mind.

## Preparing the House for the Baby's Arrival

As families prepared for the arrival of their babies, their activities imbued their houses with heightened symbolic significance. These preparations were now the actualization of dreams of "having a family" materialized in the house itself. Although some of the activities involved "child-proofing" the home—making a less dangerous environment for babies and toddlers—most parents focused their attention on the baby's future room.

## The Baby's Room

In nearly all the households I observed, parents created a separate room or at least a separate space outside the parental bedroom for their babies prior to their births, which became the center of preparations within the house.[20] Some families who lacked a dedicated bedroom for the baby in their homes transformed spaces that adjoined the parental bedroom and were spatially separate from it, but did not have a separate door. These rooms/spaces were usually called the "baby's room" or the "nursery".[21] The assumption that babies require this separate space is incorporated into the architecture of many homes with smaller bedrooms that could be used as children's rooms, usually situated near a "master" bedroom that is intended for the parents. These architectural norms originated in the late nineteenth and early twentieth century (Abbott 1992; Stearns, Rowland, and Giarnella 1996), reflect similar changes in England (Crook 2008), and have since spread to many other areas of the world.

In light of the overwhelming emphasis on preparing a separate sleep space prior to the birth of the baby, Natalie's departure from this model offers insight into the significance of such labor. In our first meeting over lunch during her pregnancy, Natalie explained that her husband Carsten's family was unhappy with her because she did not set up the baby's room ahead of time.[22] Her lack of investment in this room shocked Carsten's family who took it for granted that Natalie would devote great attention to beautifying the space and filling it with the necessary objects that surround a middle-class American baby. Instead, Natalie continued with her normal routine of dedicating her energies to her studies. My conversations with Natalie, who grew up in Eastern Europe, indicate that she was not raised with a similar cultural emphasis on the "baby's room," and therefore she felt that it was perfectly fine to prepare the baby's space after his birth. To her in-laws, as I will argue below, Natalie's reluctance to create this space did not simply signal her lack of interest in home decoration but a potential inadequacy of maternal commitment to the baby, whose room was a culturally significant site for the consolidation of his personhood.

Although my study began in childbirth preparation classes and I did not always witness the process of creating the children's spaces, some couples mentioned their work on these spaces even before I visited their homes, and nearly all couples discussed these spaces and showed them to me when we met at their homes. During these first visits I was usually given "tours" of these spaces. In several cases I had the sense that the parents had given several similar "tours" to relatives and friends, since their presentation was well-rehearsed and they occasionally mentioned others who had visited and viewed these spaces before me. As parents presented these spaces to me, their demeanor revealed the sense of pride they took in their work as well as their excitement and anticipation before their babies' birth. Participating in several of these "tours" prompted me to reflect on the powerful role of domestic spaces in shaping expectations for the children's future sleep. Despite the fact that no family in the study planned to have the baby sleep in the baby's room immediately after birth, most couples worked hard to ensure that the room was ready for the baby's arrival.

As I visited these rooms, I noted the significance of careful planning and manual labor in creating these spaces. Several families had turned a space they had previously used for other purposes into the baby's room. For instance, Joy and Jonathan converted a guest bedroom they mostly used for storage into the baby's room. They thus had to empty the room of its previous contents and then repaint, furnish, and decorate it in accordance with an aesthetic that the couple had developed together. Since both Joy and Jonathan worked full time outside the home, this work took up quite a bit of their evenings and weekends. Thus the creation of the baby's room was an important locus where couples worked together to prepare for their babies' arrival. Based on her ethnography with expectant couples in the Midwest (U.S.), Han (2009) has similarly argued that the construction of nurseries were special sites of men's "kin work," where they could build their own relatedness to their children through performing the often heavy labor entailed in these projects.

The most prominent objects parents placed in their babies' rooms were cribs and changing tables where dirty diapers would be removed. Most of these cribs were quite large, attractive, and solidly built for long-term use (see Figure 6.1). Some could be converted to daybeds without rails and even child beds with part of the crib forming the headboard in future years. Parents often spent several hundred dollars on the purchase of an attractive, solid wood crib with a matching changing table. In addition, rooms usually had a large armchair or rocking chair for nursing, soothing, and reading to the baby. The rooms usually had containers for storing additional diapering and clothing supplies, as well as shelves for books and toys.

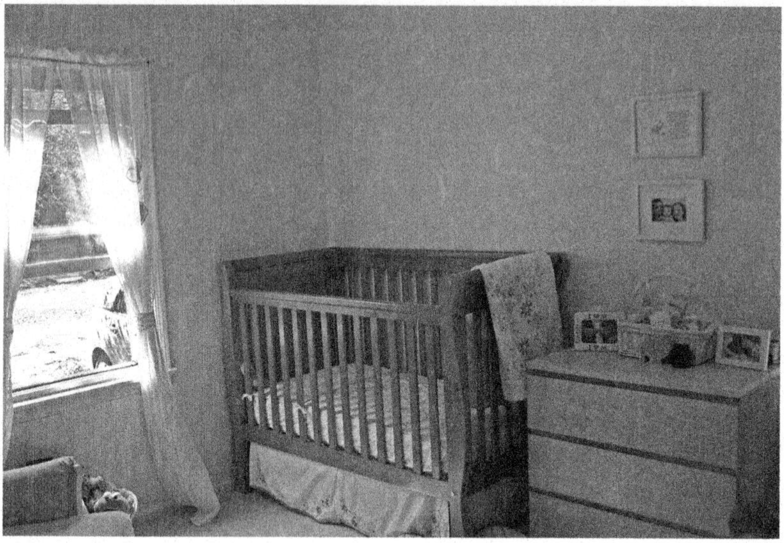

**Figure 6.1.** Rachel's and Nathan's nursery with their crib for Maya. Photo courtesy of Rachel.

The walls and the decorations were assembled to "coordinate" with one another—often in accordance with a particular color theme and embellished with common U.S. childhood motifs, such as baby animals, the alphabet, or other similar elements. Han (2009) has argued that these decorations also serve as person-making devices, for example through baby animals standing in for the future baby.

Most families had done the painting and stenciling, placement of decorative borders, and so on themselves. Furthermore, handmade objects featured prominently in these spaces. For instance, the crib might feature blankets hand sewn by a female relative, as in Petra's and Julia's nursery. Erik had built a unique bookshelf of tree branches that supported the shelves that the two of them had already filled with books in anticipation of their baby's arrival. Erik's wife, Camilla, along with several others, also knit clothing for the baby, and this was laid in her room. Corinne, a librarian with a passion for reading, spent many hours selecting books she looked forward to reading to their baby. The room thus became a powerful signifier of the baby's impending arrival and his/her emerging personhood. Although I did not specifically investigate participants' notions of fetal personhood from the beginning of their pregnancy, in my discussions with participants and families in childbirth education courses, as well as when I had the opportunity to repeat home visits, I could glean a gradual material consolidation of the baby's personhood and kin relations in the rooms and objects that were carefully selected and made to fill it. This gradual emergence of personhood was extensively documented in Han's study (2009, 2009, 2013).

Scholars of material culture have documented the person-making significance of creating, furnishing, and decorating children's rooms. Alison Clarke (2004), for instance, writes that such spaces "ideologically ... have become a key means of valorizing the otherwise ostensibly mundane and utilitarian aspects of caring. ... [T]he conjuring up of the nursery ... is a key means of imagining the physical presence of an infant-to-be and its objects" (2004:61). Similarly, Linda Layne's work on miscarriage and infant death demonstrates how these objects become involved in the process of grieving and in acknowledging the reality of personhood for the lost infant (Layne 2000). Thus, middle-class infants become "real" persons through the objects with which they are surrounded. Indeed, the danger of creating this space and filling it ahead of the baby's birth was not lost on expectant parents. Petra shared with me that after she gazed upon the nursery after a shopping trip, she asked Julia whether they were doing too much: "What if something happens and we don't bring a baby home?"[23] For Petra, filling the room with new purchases was a recognizable person-making process—and the emotional weight of the material goods that shaped that person-in-the-making was sometimes too much to bear.

Such conceptions of space are, as we have seen in chapter 2, historically specific. At the same time that parents and children were separated in sleep, bedrooms also increasingly became associated with interiority and subject-formation (Crook 2008). Indeed, Bachelard's ([1958] 1994) writings on the phenomenology of the house are an eloquent exploration of the consequences of this cultural-historical transformation. In his descriptions, the house emerges as a protective enclosure, a site wherein children's subjectivity emerges and to which adults return in their daydreams, often filled with nostalgia and longing. Bachelard pays close attention to small, enclosed spaces within the house that children experience in solitude, including the attic and the bed chamber, which seem particularly potent sites for sensual experiences and their reworkings in memories. Although Bachelard mentions that children who have had frightening experiences in a house, such as during wartime, do not imagine the house as a place of safety, his analysis does not focus on these issues in great detail. Thus, Bachelard reinforces the image of the house, and enclosures within, as particularly important sites for the formation of a safe and protected subjectivity. Just as finding a suitable family home can be viewed through the image of a nest, parents' dedication to children's bedrooms can be seen as creating a protected space within the interior of the house where children can safely grow. Indeed, Han's (2009) participants used the image of the nest in their descriptions of their nurseries.

In sum, the emphasis on intimate personal involvement through planning, purchasing, and creating these spaces shaped personhood within a network of significant social relations—the baby was most prominently woven into relations with his or her parents, but also with other relatives and friends whose objects and work were featured in the room. Although these relations were prominently featured in these spaces, the emphasis on a separate space for children also materialized individualistic ideologies of personhood. Thus, the entire space of the baby's room was involved in the creation of a particular kind of middle-class American personhood—one that is nested in the webs of kin relations through carefully selected objects, but where the child is imagined as an individual in a "space of her own," separate from the bodies of her parents.

### The Parental Bedroom

In contrast to the baby's room, the parental bedroom underwent significantly fewer changes in preparation for the baby's arrival. Prior to the birth of their babies, all couples in the study slept together in one bedroom. The ideal space for couples at night remained this shared bedroom, despite exceptions in cases where spouses experienced insomnia, worked late, or traveled. In middle-class U.S. homes, bedrooms are assumed to be used primarily during the night, and master bedrooms are culturally linked to the occupant couple's sexuality (Shweder, Jensen, and Goldstein 1995). As a daytime visitor invited to cross the threshold of the family's home, I was already granted access to a "private," familial space where persons outside of kin relations occupied only a temporary space. Unlike other visitors, however, I was interested in the family's specific sleep arrangements, which often took me into couples' bedrooms.

When I was visiting participants at their houses, I was acutely aware of the demarcation of the bedroom within the home as a private space. Most of our conversations took place in the living room of the house, and with the passage of time, in kitchens and dining rooms. While parents happily showed me the fine details of their babies' rooms even on a first visit, and we had relaxed conversations elsewhere in the home, I usually had to ask to see the setup of their own bedroom in order to better understand specific and often evolving sleep arrangements. I did not always feel comfortable asking to see the bedroom and only asked when I felt that our relationship was secure enough to do so. I was grateful for the few parents, who, upon seeing the look of confusion on my face as I attempted to understand the details of their latest sleep configuration, offered to show me their bedrooms and help me visualize how they slept. For instance, when Alex and I discussed their sleep arrangement, which at the time sometimes involved laying Connor down to sleep in his own room in a crib and then moving him to the couple's bedroom, he realized that I was confused about the location of their son's room in relation to their own as well as about the height of their bed. Alex then invited me into their bedroom and provided a detailed description of their sleeping arrangement that cleared up my confusion and enabled me to better situate my conversations with both Alex and Leslie. These visual observations of select households' bedrooms and verbal descriptions and discussions thereof guided my learning.

When I was invited into the bedroom, several families apologized for the state of the room—its messiness—and some families walked ahead of me and tidied the covers on the bed so that I would not see an unmade or "imperfectly" made bed. The importance of the tidiness of the bedroom reflected another emphasis on the orderliness—both material and moral—of the house and its occupants. The association of bedrooms and especially beds as sites for sexual activity was an unstated but important factor in drawing this boundary. As time went on, however, most families became increasingly comfortable with my presence, and I was invited back to the bedroom to observe any changes, discuss plans for the space in the future, or to talk while a mother was breastfeeding a resting baby. The increasing level of comfort with my presence in the bedroom mirrored the growing closeness of our relationship.

Despite the significant association of conjugal, and especially procreative, sexuality within the marital bedroom of the house, Bachelard ([1958] 1994) does not explore this subject in his extensive and sensuous descriptions of the house. Indeed, although sexuality is implicit in the production of children, it presents a number of difficulties for the image of the home. Although procreative sexuality is culturally appropriate within the confines of the bedroom, fears of "dangerous" sexuality abide at the margins. First, the normative nature of conjugal sex in the bedroom exists in contrast to the socially inappropriate sexuality outside the home—for instance, provided by prostitutes in the "street" (Baldwin 2002). Second, sexuality is spatially sequestered within the interior of a room within the house, away from the eyes of children (Shweder, Jensen, and Goldstein 1995). In Victorian England, the historical separation of parents' and children's bedrooms was partly driven by transformation in marital relationships and middle-class concerns about inappropriate sexuality in working class homes due to the intermingling of bodies (Crook 2008). Survivors of parental sexual abuse also remind us that, despite architectural divisions, boundaries between children and potentially dangerous parental sexuality are permeable. For these children, the image of safety and protection of one's own room was violated, and the bedroom often became the locus of terrifying memories (Halley 2007). Breastfeeding adds another layer of complication to this already charged terrain since it involves bodily contact between a baby's mouth and the mother's breast—a highly sexualized part of the body in the U.S.[24] Breastfeeding could also incite societal fears of incest between parents and children (Smale 2001).

Although concerns about children's relationship to parental sexuality were rarely brought up by my participants, the history of bedrooms and their associations with potent sexuality remains an important unstated—and perhaps even unconscious—factor in concerns over sharing beds and bedrooms with children. In Schweder and colleagues' (1995) comparative exercise of sorting hypothetical fathers, mothers, and children into a limited number of bedrooms, the avoidance of incest and the preservation of the couple emerged most significant for the U.S. participants. Within my research, the lack of attention to altering the parental bedroom prior to the baby's birth, as well as the purchase of equipment for the parental bedroom that accommodated only very little babies, confirm this cultural imperative to separate parents and babies during the night and offers further evidence to the significance of sexuality in shaping these decisions. The presence of young babies in the parental bedroom, likely due to their assumed lack of awareness, did not seem to present as great a problem as older children did.

Since families planned to keep their babies close to them for the first few weeks, particularly to facilitate nighttime breastfeeding, they purchased additional equipment to include in the parents' bedroom to accommodate newborn babies' presence. Families made primarily two plans for where the baby was going to sleep during this early period: a free-standing bassinet or an attachable bassinet such as a Co-Sleeper, each of which is described below. These pieces of equipment were supposed to facilitate the initial period of intensive breastfeeding by enabling children to stay in their parents' bedroom. In their design, these temporary beds embodied mainstream conventions of a brief period of nighttime bodily proximity, while also maintaining norms of separate sleep surfaces for parents and children.

The first group of parents (eight couples) purchased a bassinet or received a bassinet from an important relative or friend. Bassinets are small baskets made of wood or plastic, with padding and decorative cloth surrounding the baby's sleep area, that stand on a raised platform so that they are easily accessible to parents without much bending. Bassinets are suitable only for infants from about one to three months, since they quickly outgrow them and can also fall out of them as they acquire increased mobility. Bassinets sold in stores often evoke nostalgia of the past with designs that imitate woven baskets and with decorations that resemble those women would have made by hand in the past. More modern designs, such as the one given to Elise and Adam at their baby shower, may be equipped with electronic musical options and lights that can be used to entertain the baby. That specific bassinet had a canopy that shielded the baby from light as well as offered a surface for a built in mobile that hung down from the top. Buttons for the electronic entertainment options, including light vibrations, were provided at the top of the canopy. This bassinet could be moved using the casters on the bottom of the legs of the platform or by detaching the basket from the platform. Similar bassinets can be purchased for approximately $100.

The aesthetic qualities of the bassinets were important for both store-purchased and heirloom bassinets. In Petra's family, the bassinet was passed around to the next person in the family who was expecting a baby. Petra's mother made blankets, each with different colors and bows for each new baby, and came to install the decorations on the bassinet prior to the birth of the baby, in addition to staying with each of her daughters after they had given birth to help with the new baby. Thus, for this family, the bassinet was another site of significant decorations and adornment with familial labor or objects that were made by previous generations.

Joy and Jonathan decided against the bassinet and selected a Pack 'n Play instead, a plastic bed with mesh sides that most resembles a portable form of a crib (see Figure 6.2). Portable play yards such as Pack 'n Plays are similarly priced to bassinets and they resemble them in that they are also freestanding objects. Unlike bassinets, however, they can be folded up and used as travel beds for children. Furthermore, they provide a considerably larger protected surface

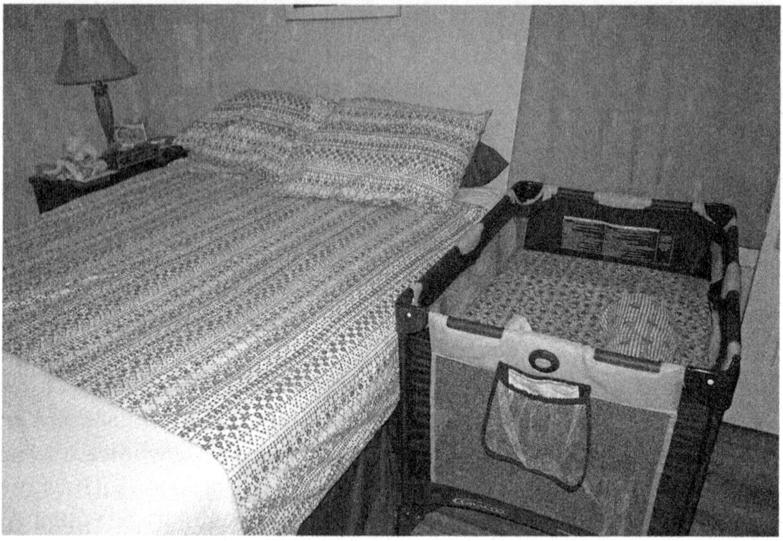

**Figure 6.2.** Pack 'n Play. This portable play yard is set up right next to the parents' bed, in the same configuration that Petra and Julia used in their bedroom. Photo courtesy of Jessica Smith Rolston.

area for sleeping as well as for playing in the later months than bassinets do, making them suitable for sleeping for a much longer period of time. The mesh enclosure on the sides enables babies to see the world around them, but prevents them from crawling out of the area—something many parents find useful in the later months to help keep their babies away from danger while they step out of the room (e.g., when they go to the bathroom). This versatility was one of the main reasons why this couple selected a portable play yard for their sleep plans. The play yards vary in design and additional features, such as a play area or an attachment of a smaller basket for newborns across the top of the main bed, complete with mobiles, etc.

A second group of parents (another eight couples) purchased Co-Sleepers, bassinets that attach to the parental bed so that the baby can be within arm's reach of her mother, but sleeping on a separate surface from her parents. Co-Sleepers differ from standard bassinets in three key ways: 1) they are attached to the parental bed itself, while the standard bassinet remains separate from the parental bed; 2) they are the same height as the parental bed, while free-standing bassinet height does not necessarily coordinate with that of the bed; 3) one side of the Co-Sleeper is open so that it provides easy access to a parent reaching over from the bed, while both sides of standard bassinets are closed to protect the infant from falling out of it. Attachable bassinets are a relatively recent arrival in the large market of baby goods and have gained ground among parents who are planning to breastfeed. They are marketed to this population of parents who would like to stay close to their babies to facilitate breastfeeding but who do not wish to sleep in the same bed with their babies.

Purchasing an attachable bassinet was more common in the group of parents who attended the childbirth education classes that were geared more toward "natural childbirth" at Holistic Center, where Co-Sleepers were explicitly mentioned (see chapter 3). This finding is not surprising in light of the fact that parents whose childbirth plans vary from that of a heavily biomedicalized and medicated childbirth are also often those parents who plan to breastfeed their children beyond the usual few months and who wish to stay close to them at night. Dr. Sears, the primary physician advocate of attachment parenting, has endorsed the use of Co-Sleepers, and his recommendation has certainly contributed to the growth in sales of these products, which usually cost approximately $200.

Only four couples seriously considered sleeping in the same bed with their babies. Elise and Adam initially worried about having to potentially make changes to their bed in order to accommodate the infant, but then later decided to have their son, Luke, sleep in the bassinet that was given to them at their baby shower (described above). The unanticipated arrival of the gift of the bassinet became incorporated into the negotiations of this couple's sleeping plans; the bassinet provided a new and potentially convenient space for the baby's sleep. Jocelyn and Samuel were open to having their baby in the bed with them, but also purchased a bassinet to supply a separate space for the baby at night. In a similar way, Adrianne and Doug purchased a Co-Sleeper as their primary plan, but included the possibility of bringing their baby into their bed for short periods. Finally, Angela and Oliver modified their own bed by setting up a Snuggle Nest—a special mat that has a raised edge for the purpose of protecting the baby from rolling over, thereby creating a partially separate sleeping space within the parental bed (see Figure 6.3). This object aims to bring a sense of safety and protection—a truly Bachelardian nest—to the surface of the parental bed itself, something that no other equipment for the baby attempted. Angela and Oliver made the fullest commitment to bed sharing within the study, although they also purchased a crib that they later used as a separate surface that was immediately attached to their bed. This couple's level of planning for more sustained bed sharing aligned

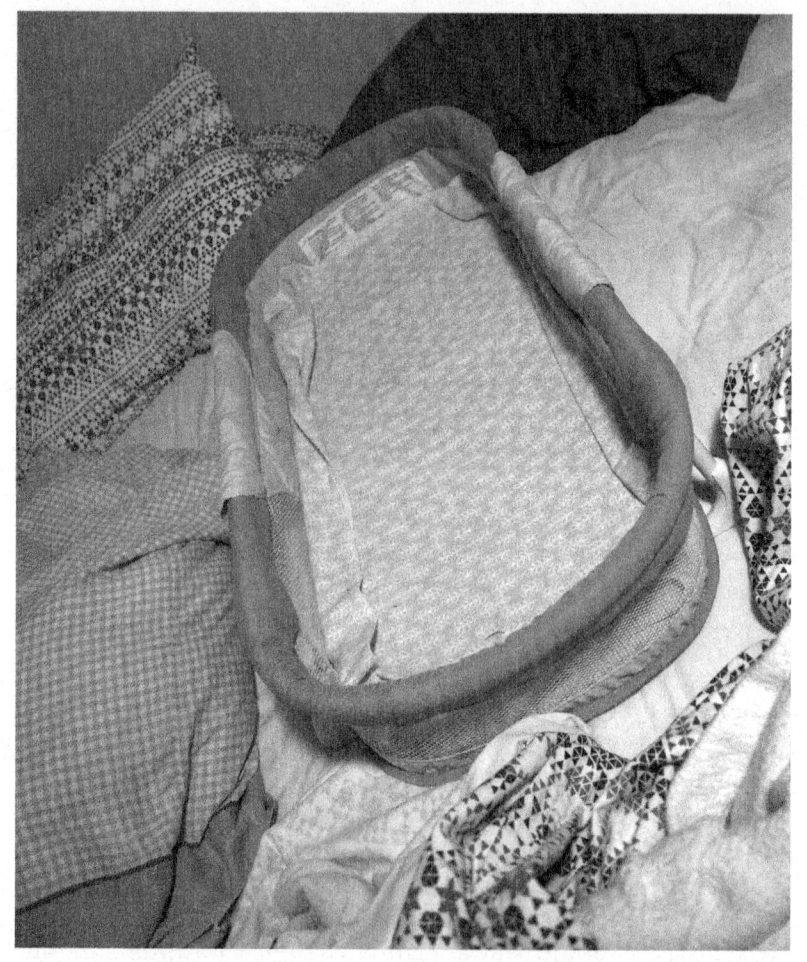

**Figure 6.3.** Snuggle Nest. This mat with raised sides is placed in the middle of the parents' bed, as Angela and Oliver had also done. Photo courtesy of Jessica Smith Rolston.

with their philosophy of birth (home birth), as well as other dimensions of their "natural parenting" approach.

Most parents directed their efforts toward building, furnishing, and decorating the baby's future room instead of modifying their own bedrooms, reflecting the significance of the consolidation of their children's personhood in this separate space as well as concerns about morally inappropriate shared sleep arrangements. In accordance, comparatively little attention was spent on modifying parental beds and bedrooms that were only to be shared for a short period of time after birth. Instead, parents incorporated few new items into their bedrooms, such as bassinets, Pack 'n Plays, and Co-Sleepers, which signaled the necessity of a degree of spatial separation of parents and babies' bodies even within the bedroom and emphasized the temporal limitations on sharing the parental bedroom. The material resources required to create and maintain such spaces as well as the moral orders associated with them reproduced social class distinctions—these objects and spaces were accoutrements of a middle-class baby. Confronted with the realities of breastfeeding babies, however, most parents found that their carefully designed sleeping plans required significant adjustments.

## The Return to Home

### *The Beginning: Upheavals to Previous Spatial Orders*

Parents were quite relieved to be back in their own house after the exhaustion from the effort and excitement of birth itself as well as the stream of interruptions by staff at the hospital. Upon returning home, however, new spatial challenges awaited them that further hindered their ability to rest.[25] At the hospital, Corinne had been in such awe of her son, Finn, that she was unable to sleep the night after she had given birth. While her husband, Jacob, and Finn both slept, she could not. When she returned home, everything started out just right. Their doula stopped in to check on the family, and things were going well. But right after the doula left, Finn started crying, and would not stop. Corinne described this as the baby not "feeling like" sleeping, and although both she and her husband tried everything they could, Finn would not settle down: "That first night was really rough. No one slept, then the next day we were all really tired, and I held him and he fell asleep in my arms." In the meantime, Corinne and Finn were learning how to breastfeed. Finn was only soothed at the breast, so Corinne and Finn spent most of the day breastfeeding.[26] As Corinne struggled to figure out how to breastfeed, she ended up with severely injured nipples—cracked and bleeding from trauma likely caused by Finn latching on in an incorrect way.

After breastfeeding her son nearly constantly the day after they returned home, Corinne figured, "Well, he will sleep if he is held and so I, you know, determined that that was the way that he was gonna sleep. He didn't like it if I lied down." Deciding to do "whatever you [the baby] want," Corinne "propped [herself] up on the couch and held him" while her husband returned to their bed. And this is how

Corinne slept every night for the next two and a half weeks: holding her baby at her breast on the couch, with her feet propped up on the coffee table. In describing this experience Corinne recounted, "I really wanted to lie down. I really felt like I wasn't even circulating right. It was one of the hardest things to go through, never lying down." Thus, Corinne's and Jacob's plans were radically altered. Instead of the baby slumbering peacefully in the Co-Sleeper while his parents slept, with Corinne nursing the baby every few hours, here they were with an inconsolable baby who only slept in Corinne's arms, preferably upright, and was soothed only when she put him to her increasingly traumatized breasts.[27]

Corinne's transitional milk (that follows colostrum) came in within a few days, but the situation failed to improve for several more weeks (until Finn learned to sleep lying down) due to ostensibly supportive relatives who questioned Corinne's ability to produce sufficient milk for the baby (see chapter 4). Although Corinne resisted these suggestions, the doubts seeped into her own thoughts, amplified by the exhaustion and pain she was already feeling. These worries about her child raised by Corinne's relatives, combined with her already exhausted and vulnerable state, made the first couple of weeks nearly unbearable.

States of complete upheaval and extreme sleep deprivation and exhaustion in the first weeks following the birth were common among participants. Most parents entered a similar liminal period where their lives were radically rearranged under extreme conditions. Mothers' experiences were particularly shaped by frequent breast trauma mostly caused by difficulties with latching their babies on and positioning them for breastfeeding. At night, most parents initially acted according to their prior plans and placed their babies for sleep in a separate container next to their beds. Few parents, however, were able to figure out how to get their babies to sleep in this separate space. As soon as they laid their babies down in the Co-Sleeper or bassinet, the babies woke up and started crying.

Carol, similar to Corinne, initially had great difficulty with breastfeeding due to inverted nipples that were undiagnosed during pregnancy.[28] Because of this condition, the nipple tissue needed to be drawn out and ultimately rebuilt to form a new nipple on the outside of the breast. While this process is painful in and of itself, it could have been completed gradually prior to the baby's birth using an electric breast pump. But since the condition was overlooked during pregnancy, Carol's baby was now using his suction to draw out the nipples while he was attempting to seek nourishment at the breast. In order to remedy the situation, multiple hospital staff members attempted to help but, according to Carol, did so in a rather aggressive form of "shoving" Jeremiah onto her, which caused Carol a great deal of pain. There was no good plan for how to proceed with breastfeeding beyond the discharge from the hospital, and yet multiple staff members suggested that she could simply supplement her breastmilk with formula. Carol resisted this advice, knowing that supplementation could undermine breastfeeding, and continued with breastfeeding when she returned home. This resulted in absolute agony—"toe-curling" pain—for Carol, and weight loss and enormous frustration for Jeremiah. At this critical juncture, Carol called a private lactation consultant, who assessed the baby and gave him formula while Carol expressed her breast milk using a pump. Justin, Carol's husband, then rented a hospital-grade pump so that she could continue to pump through the next day, enabling Carol's nipples to recover from extreme trauma. After that day, Carol was able to successfully breastfeed Jeremiah, and her nipples eventually fully healed.

It was in the midst of trying to breastfeed her baby in complete agony that Carol and Justin tried to figure out how to get Jeremiah to sleep. Carol, laughing, summed up their initial plans and their first night at home:

> You know, pre-baby 'Oh, the baby is not gonna sleep in *our* bed, the baby is gonna sleep in our room in the Co-Sleeper next to the bed.' So we get home and you swaddle him up, you know, you stick him into the Co-Sleeper, after ten min on the first night you hear WAAAH [we both laugh]. Baby comes out of the Co-Sleeper after about three of those cries into the bed between Justin and I. Really, he has not left. He pretty much sleeps stomach-to-stomach on this side or that side.[29]

Amidst the painful and frightening experience of feeding Jeremiah, the decision about where their baby would sleep was easy for Carol and Justin. Sleep and comforting Jeremiah was of the essence, and bringing him to bed offered an effective solution that soothed him and enabled everyone to get some rest.

Even when parents were able to get the baby to sleep on his/her own in a separate container for at least a short time, they themselves were sometimes unable to sleep. Although Leslie and Alex were exhausted after their hospital stay, both Leslie and Connor were adjusting to frequent breastfeeding throughout the day and night.[30] Leslie and Alex had looked forward to their return home. Yet, on their first night home, Leslie could not go to sleep while Connor slept in a portable play yard near their bed. Leslie anticipated the baby's next awakening, which might be just a few minutes from the last time he woke up, keeping her awake. Alex and Leslie both practiced putting Connor into the portable play yard after nursing, rocking him and getting him to fall asleep, even if briefly. But Leslie "couldn't relax" when her baby was away from her. Leslie explained: "When I had him in my arms it just didn't feel right to have him anywhere else." Leslie had planned to keep the baby in the portable play yard because she was very worried about the potential risks of sharing the same bed with her baby based on her readings during her pregnancy. As she was sitting up, unable to get to sleep, she and Alex exchanged glances and decided that bringing Connor to bed was what "works for our family." With the baby in the crook of Leslie's arm, all three were able to relax and fall asleep. This arrangement enabled Leslie to nurse Connor frequently throughout the night without him crying, without having to get up to soothe him, and without the worries that kept her awake. In each of the above cases the need for bodily proximity transcended the spatial separation in the couples' initial plans.

Three of the four parents who had surgical births via Cesarean section found that sleeping next to their babies was the only way that they could manage breastfeeding with the painful incision they had.[31] Paula had planned to have the baby in a bassinet next to their bed, but in the first few weeks she and her husband, Matthew, brought Isaac into their bed regularly in order to make it easier for Paula to breastfeed him.[32] Although by the end of the first month she moved Isaac into the bassinet for the night, Paula shared with me that the demands of nursing in that early period combined with the painful recovery from surgery were too much to manage in separate beds. In a similar vein, Camilla and Erik similarly planned to have their daughter, Robin, sleep in a Co-Sleeper. After Camilla's surgery Erik moved Robin in and out of the Co-Sleeper, since it was too painful for Camilla to do so. After Erik returned to work, however, this arrangement became too complicated and unsustainable, since it required too much getting up for both spouses. Camilla and Erik then decided to bring Robin into the bed, which made breastfeeding much simpler for Camilla and enabled Erik to get sufficient sleep for work the next day. In contrast to the above two couples, Angela and Oliver prepared for having their baby in bed with them, which made breastfeeding easier for Angela, who had also undergone a Cesarean section. They did not need to radically alter their plans in order accommodate this unanticipated complication. Although none of these three women had significant difficulties with breastfeeding, the recovery from major surgery combined with breastfeeding their babies frequently during the night made sharing a bed, at least for some time, a necessity for them regardless of their previous plans. When I visited each of them within a few weeks of birth, the pain of recovery—both physical pain and the emotional process of having to come to terms with surgery—could be seen in the careful way in which they moved their bodies as well as in the winces on their faces as they navigated breastfeeding positions that would not push on their surgical incisions.

As in the above couples' examples, the need to soothe a baby through frequent breastfeeding was one of the main reasons why parents slept next to their babies despite their previous plans. Although much of this co-sleeping took place in the parental bed, Corinne's example shows that beds and bedrooms were not the only spaces where co-sleeping occurred. Corinne and several other parents slept with their babies on their chests in a variety of places, including the couch and the guest bedroom. Mothers would sometimes take breaks from their babies while their spouses slept with their babies on their chests to allow mothers to get some rest. For some couples, this liminal period of sleeping in a variety of places within the house and in new, and often-changing, configurations lasted only a day or a few days. Most couples, like Carol and Justin and Leslie and Alex, found a routine that worked for them, at least temporarily. Others, like Corinne and Jacob, continued to struggle for several weeks. Ultimately, over the course of the first few weeks, patterns began to take clearer shape as about half of the parents in the study came to regularly share their bed with their baby, whereas the other parents regularly placed their baby on a separate surface close to their beds. The tremendous frequency with which parents brought their children into their beds, even if only for part of the night, reflected parental ability to use their sleeping spaces in a creative manner, producing unanticipated bodily proximity with their infants.

*Spatial Challenges within the Bedroom: Sleeping Together and Apart*

The group of parents who brought their babies to bed with them had to work out where exactly the baby would be located within the parental bed. As Carol indicated in her discussion of how their baby came to share the bed, their baby slept "stomach-to-stomach" on whichever side he last fell asleep after breastfeeding. Leslie had a different approach, where she was initially in the middle of the bed, with her husband and baby on each side.[33] In the middle of the night, she sometimes moved herself to the other side rather than moving the baby. She commented that it "seems funny to me that I do that." In Leslie's case, then, both her own and her baby's body might be reconfigured during the night, so that the baby would end up in the middle of the bed between Leslie and Alex. Thus, the arrangement of the parents' and child's bodies was often in flux during the night. Who went to bed first and which side the baby had fed on in the previous breastfeeding session would shape the specific arrangements. For parents whose babies slept in the bed for part of the night and slept in an attached bassinet or other surface next to the bed for the remainder of the night, the sleep arrangement might also vary. The fluidity of sleep arrangements throughout the night further highlights the significance of creative uses of sleep spaces and the equipment therein. Safety was of utmost concern to all bed-sharing parents and was negotiated in relation to biomedicalized notions of minimizing the risk of suffocation and SIDS (see chapter 2).

Parents who regularly shared their beds often made light of the additional equipment they had purchased that lay around the house but remained unused for its originally intended purpose. Many of these parents began to transform and/or move previous sleep equipment that they had planned to use for their babies. Rachel, for example, "felt bad" about someone having bought them a bassinet, since they quickly abandoned using it.[34] Nathan, however, jokingly reminded her that the bassinet will make a nice present for another couple who then will also use it for diaper storage instead of putting their baby to sleep in it. In a similar vein, Carol laughed when she first told me about the Co-Sleeper in which her son "slept, well, *laid* [Carol's emphasis] in ... for all of ten minutes on the first night."[35] This Co-Sleeper became a point of conversation for us in subsequent visits, as it filled different functions in different spaces of the house. At first, the empty Co-Sleeper was used mainly as storage: "It holds pillows. Not a whole lot else is going on with the Co-Sleeper. I don't know if much else will ever go on with the Co-Sleeper."[36] She also discovered that the Co-Sleeper created an edge for her side of the bed, which served as a barrier as Jeremiah was beginning to roll over. During this time, Carol and Justin used the crib in the nursery, which they had borrowed from Justin's cousin, for diaper changing. Later on, Carol moved the Co-Sleeper to the living room, where it was used for keeping various baby-related items on hand, such as extra diapers, toys, and Carol's sling in which she carried Jeremiah (see Figure 6.4). Ultimately, the Co-Sleeper was loaned to a friend who was expecting a baby.

Similarly, Kate and Joshua began using their Co-Sleeper for bedside storage in the early weeks postpartum.[37] When I first visited their home two weeks after Anna's birth, the Co-Sleeper held many different items, such as extra pillows to support the mother's hand and the baby's body during nighttime nursing sessions, a glass of water, and a book. In this sense, the Co-Sleeper's function was transformed into conveniently accessible space for the mother's use. Other couples made different adjustments to their sleeping spaces. Angela and Oliver, whose son slept in the middle of their bed in the Snuggle Nest, eventually detached the fourth wall of their crib and placed it directly adjacent to Angela's side of bed, forming an extension to their beds. Thus, Max spent part of the night in between them, and part of the night in the crib right next to Angela.

Just as the use and location of Co-Sleepers was modified, among bed sharing couples the parental bed itself came under scrutiny. This included the adjustment of pillows and blankets as well as the height of the bed in order to protect the baby from suffocation and

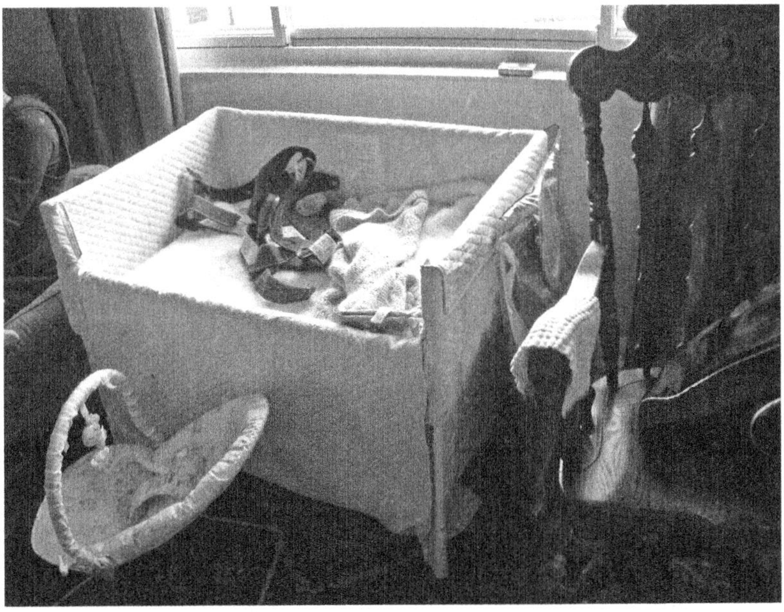

**Figure 6.4.** Carol's and Justin's Co-Sleeper. Originally designed to attach to the parents' bed, this Co-Sleeper, like Kate's and Joshua's, quickly turned into a place for storage and ended up in the living room, as pictured here. Photo by author.

falls (see chapter 2). Since most families slept on beds that were at least two feet off the ground, over time they became increasingly aware of their babies' potential to roll off the mattress. Camilla and Erik decided to avoid this situation simply by putting their mattress on the ground.[38] Because they were used to sleeping on a low bed and had slept on futons in the past, this caused no great difficulty or concern for them. However, they were unusual in their ease with such changes, reflecting the constraints of cultural ideologies that surround the parental bed as a reflection of middle-class propriety. Not having a "proper" bed on an elevated platform would lead to the bed touching the floor, which might be considered "dirty" and may signal poverty. Although in conversation several families considered lowering their mattress, their ultimate reluctance to lower the bed presented an example of the moral orders embodied in the object of the bed itself that they were unable to transcend, despite having overcome the barrier of sharing a bed with their children. For instance, Rachel, Nathan, and I had several discussions about their plans for how to deal with Maya's increasing mobility and potential falls from their bed, but they did not end up making any adjustments to the bed (nor did Maya ever fall out of the bed).

Other parents continued to share their bedroom with their children but did not share (or no longer shared) their beds with them. This arrangement enabled couples to retain bodily closeness to their child, while also retaining a degree of the culturally sanctioned separation enabled by separate sleep surfaces. They settled into more or less comfortable ways in which they could nurse their babies, return the babies to their own sleeping spaces, and go back to sleep. For instance, some couples used a Co-Sleeper attached to their bed or a bassinet or portable play yard, such as a Pack 'n Play, placed right next to the bed to place the baby in for sleep, picked up their babies to nurse them in their bed whenever they stirred, always placing them back in the separate sleep space thereafter. The need to make breastfeeding as easy and least burdensome as possible for the mother dominated these arrangements. Parents' early routines worked smoothly for about two-thirds of participants for the first few months at least. The main challenges to this arrangement arose from the difficulties of negotiating sleep equipment and from navigating sexual relations between spouses.

Petra and Julia had perfected a nightly routine in the first few months that entailed the couple using a bassinet next to their bed for bouts of sleep between nursing sessions. Julia slept next to the bassinet and picked up their baby and handed him to Petra, who breastfed Anders and then gave him back to Julia who soothed him back to sleep. This activity enabled Julia to touch, caress, and talk to the baby and also alleviated the burden of nighttime nursing, especially at times when Petra was delirious from sleep deprivation (see chapter 7).[39] When Anders quickly outgrew the bassinet, Petra and Julia faced the dilemma of whether they should move him to his crib in his own room.[40] Since they both enjoyed being close to Anders and did not feel ready to move him out of their room, the couple decided to replace the bassinet with a Pack 'n Play. This choice enabled Petra and Julia to contemplate their sleep arrangements and reformulate their plans for Anders, ultimately delaying their baby's move to his separate room until close to his first birthday.[41]

Petra and Julia's example illustrates the challenges of baby equipment. The bassinet, designed for very small babies, could not accommodate their desired pattern of sleeping next to their baby. While Petra and Julia were able to overcome these limits by their creative use of the portable play yard, they remained concerned that over time Anders would not have sufficient room in it and that he would ultimately be more comfortable in the crib. The crib could not be moved into the parental bedroom due to its large size. These thoughts, of course, not only reflected concerns about the limitations of the equipment, but also their concerns about how soon they would feel comfortable with moving their baby to his room, located across from the parents' bedroom. In this case, the spatial layout of their home as well as the equipment purchased for different rooms structured the couples' decisions about sleep arrangements. At the same time, the couple's changing choices of equipment and their delay in moving their son out of their bedroom reflect considerable ability to manipulate and challenge these structuring effects (see chapter 7 for more on Petra's and Julia's efforts to find a workable sleep arrangement for their family).

Paula and her husband, Matthew, shared similar concerns about the constraints of baby furnishings. As I described above, although they had not planned to share their bed with their baby, in the initial weeks Paula found it easier to nurse Isaac in their bed because she had a Cesarean section and was limited in her mobility.[42] After a few weeks, once her incision had healed and was no longer causing constant pain, they moved the baby into a bassinet next to their bed. Both of them felt more comfortable with Isaac being in the same room with them, where they could hear him and listen to his breathing and awakenings.[43] After the bassinet became too small, like Petra and Julia, they also moved their baby to a portable play yard next to the bed, knowing that this would again be a temporary solution until they figured out their next step.[44] Ultimately, although they had little extra space beyond their bed in their bedroom (albeit slightly more than Petra and Julia had in their bedroom), they moved the crib next to their bed.[45] This decision was inspired by the couple's desire to stay close to their child and their sense that this arrangement enhanced his safety. Matthew was relieved to hear Isaac's breathing at night, and Paula enjoyed the ease of breastfeeding Isaac within reach of their bed.

The couple buttressed their decision with their knowledge of Japanese cultural traditions of keeping children close to parents at night, according to which Matthew was raised, since his father was from Japan. They moved Isaac into a toddler bed in his room across from the master bedroom right before the end of the first year, partly motivated by preparations for the arrival of their second son a few months later.[46] Thus, while continuing to sleep in the same room with their baby and ultimately bringing the crib into the bedroom was not part of the couple's initial plans—in fact, this solution was discouraged by their pediatrician at the time—the couple made this significant spatial rearrangement and enjoyed this arrangement for many months. Paula's and Matthew's arrangements present another example of the challenges and limitations of equipment, but also their parental ability to use alternative cultural knowledge to circumvent them.

One of the challenges couples faced is how to be together and have sexual relations in the presence of a baby within the bedroom or the bed itself. Couples created a series of solutions. Some couples, for instance, put their babies to sleep in one room—either the parental bedroom or in the baby's room—for the early part of the night and then spent time together in a different room. For instance, Camilla and Erik enjoyed their family ritual of lying down next to Robin while Camilla nursed her to sleep. After Robin was asleep, they would plug in an infant monitor and move upstairs to another room in the house to spend time together. Rachel and Nathan had a similar strategy, although fatigue from the day's work could intervene and result in everyone going to sleep as they were putting their daughter to sleep.[47] Among participating couples, the fact that a large bed was located in the parental bedroom did not necessarily predict where couples spent time together or had sexual relations.

While many couples successfully worked out these arrangements to relocate for their time together, for other couples the baby's presence caused greater difficulties. For Joy the presence of her son,

Graham, was an obstacle to sex.[48] This sentiment also coincided with Joy's feelings that Graham's repeated awakenings for nursing were exhausting and limited her ability to have time to herself, to meet with friends, or engage in any activity other than caring for her baby. Joy and her husband, Jonathan, ultimately settled on a plan that enabled them to put Graham to sleep in his own room at the end of his first year, causing great relief for both parents.[49]

In spatially separating conjugal sexual relations from children's sleeping bodies, parents followed the pattern of relatively recent historical transformations described in chapter 2. Moving the child into a separate space for the night enabled couples to continue to have their sleep and sexual spaces in one room without concern. For others, separating family sleep spaces and couples' sexual spaces presented an alternative approach that decoupled the parental bed from its normative sexual association. In both cases, the spatial separation of children from sexual activity helped to restore the moral norms for sexuality within the house.

### *Waves of Migration from the Parental Bedroom to the Baby's Room*

Over the course of months after each baby's birth, I observed waves of movement out of the parental bedroom. Parents continued to discuss their sleep arrangements and often began to work on making changes that they felt would be helpful ways to prompt their babies to sleep separately from them, preferably in the baby's own room. The negotiation and implementation of these plans for moving the baby out of the parental bedroom while continuing to breastfeed the baby was a complex process that was often accompanied by temporary rearrangements and returns to the parental bedroom and even to the parental bed. The metaphor of ocean waves is particularly apt here, since the movement of waves back and forth captures the movements of children out of the bedroom that often went back and forth for some time before children eventually slept in their own bedroom for at least part of the night. Furthermore, the image of waves also helps to conceptualize the temporal quality of these movements.

Nearly all of the parents who moved their babies to another room had participated in extensive discussions of how to accomplish this goal both within the couple as well as with selected others (friends, parents, etc.). They had many friends and family who all moved their babies in the same pattern (bassinet in shared bedroom to crib in separate bedroom). Over time, the imperative to move the child to his or her room became more pressing for most couples. The spatial separation of children to a separate bedroom was always part of the process of "sleep training": methods parents could apply in order to align their children's bodies with cultural expectations of "sleeping through the night." The details of this process will be described in the next chapter.

Natalie was first to move their baby to a separate room within a few weeks after giving birth. This move was prompted by her husband's work schedule as well as her own preferences as described in detail in chapter 7. Despite the emphasis on preparations for the baby's room prior to the baby's arrival, only three other couples moved the baby out of the parental bedroom at the end of the first three months, with two of these couples retaining partial bed sharing or room sharing. After these first couples made a shift toward separate parental and child sleep spaces, it took several more months until the next couple did so at around six months postpartum. This change was prompted by Johanna's and Carl's move to a new house in a different state for Carl's new academic position.[50] In this case, the couple seems to have delayed the trajectory of moving their baby out of their room due to spatial constraints of their rental home in Green City. With the availability of the new house, which included the culturally desirable separate bedroom for their child, the couple was prompted to move their child into this new bedroom for the night (see chapter 7 on Johanna's and Carl's sleep training experiences).

While pediatrician advice about solitary sleep was an important concern in the early months due to the potential for endangering their young babies, couples became much less concerned about such advice over time. As I mentioned earlier, parents who continued to bring their babies into their beds employed a variety of strategies with pediatricians, from hiding their exact sleep arrangements, sharing as little information as possible, or switching to another practice (e.g., Paula and Matthew above). In general, parents found that pediatric practices that were supportive of breastfeeding were also more open to more diverse sleep arrangements. In fact, several participants chose the same practices, which were known for their supportive breastfeeding philosophy.

While most parents became more confident in their ability to negotiate pediatric experts' authority, Lynn and Gary had a different experience. Their son, Killian, was sleeping comfortably next to his parents in a portable play yard, having outgrown his Co-Sleeper. This arrangement suited both parents and made night-nursing easy for Lynn. Lynn was working full time and spent long hours away from home. Her office was located in a traditional business environment, where taking breaks was frowned upon, and there was no effort to facilitate Lynn's efforts to keep breastfeeding. Furthermore, her office walls were made of clear glass, as were all the walls in the building, making it even more challenging to secure privacy. She breastfed primarily in the mornings and evenings and nursed Killian two to three times a night. Over time, Lynn did not always wake up fully and could not actually recall how many times she nursed because she could simply reach over to feed him. When they visited their pediatrician for Killian's six-month checkup, however, the pediatrician asked them about their sleep arrangement and made an emphatic call for getting Killian out of his parents' bedroom and weaning him at night. The fact that they were "still" sharing a bedroom was the crux of his concern, although nursing at night was also problematic in his view. It was not entirely clear to me why Lynn and Gary felt compelled to follow the pediatricians' advice. It seemed that Lynn believed that this would be for the greater good of helping Killian learn how to sleep in a separate room, without nursing, for longer chunks of time. Nevertheless, Lynn and Gary did not follow through immediately, but eventually did move Killian to his room next to their bedroom around the seventh month and stopped night-nursing by the eighth month. By nine months, Killian slept alone in his own room and "weaned himself"; he had simply become uninterested in nursing.[51]

Although Lynn felt that this was simply her child's way of ending breastfeeding due to the lack of developmental need, multiple different factors seemed to have intersected to cause this shift. The lack of accommodation at her work could be seen as a marker of specific class status within the "middle class"; she did not have as much flexibility and support at work as some other women who returned to work in Green City. Furthermore, Lynn did not have the option to stop working, since the couple needed both incomes to support their family. She did not enjoy pumping (nor did most women in my study), and this sentiment was intensified by the inadequate pumping arrangements at her office. At the same time, she was also not as focused on pumping enough milk to supply her son with breastmilk alone. This may have been partly due to her suburban environment, where fewer people breastfed than in Green City, although couples approached these kinds of challenges in different ways. For instance, Petra, who had similarly challenging pumping arrangements, persisted with pumping regardless of these obstacles. While the above might also indicate that Lynn was ready to stop breastfeeding altogether, it was clear to me from our interactions that she enjoyed nursing Killian and was saddened by the pediatrician's advice. Well-established research suggests that the pediatrician's recommendation created a situation of very restricted access and a lack of stimulation for breastmilk production, both of which likely resulted in premature weaning (Ball, Hooker, and Kelly 1999).

This example highlights the fact that medical advice, even in the absence of evidence, can carry a high level of authority among parents. I believe that Lynn's and Gary's experience with the pediatrician was subtly interwoven into their comparatively lower middle-class position (among my participants). The careful selection of pediatricians, the ability to conduct research and come to a different conclusion from a biomedical expert's strong recommendation, and the environment in which such work is the norm are all markers and makers of class positions. Most families in the U.S. have little access to supportive pediatricians and far fewer resources to be able to counter authoritative biomedical advice. Lynn's and Gary's vulnerability to such advice indicates that ill-informed pediatricians assert significant influence over family sleep practices and thereby undercut breastfeeding relationships.

For most parents, the decision to move their babies out of the bedroom was difficult, fraught with anxiety, and entailed multiple phases. The struggles were often related to breastfeeding, since moving the baby away from the proximity of the mothers' body meant that some babies woke up more often during the night, cried more, and were more difficult to soothe back to sleep. While parents often got less sleep during the implementation of these new spatial arrangements, they eventually brought relief to parents. I believe that this sense of relief was due both to the success of developing a system that brought greater rest to parents and to the attainment of culturally desirable separate sleep arrangements for parents and children.

For Corinne and Jacob, however, the difficulties of transitioning their baby to his bedroom resulted in bringing him into the parental bed for the remainder of the study period. When, around the fourth and fifth month postpartum, Corinne attempted to move Finn to his own room because he had outgrown the bassinet-like hammock in which he was sleeping, she had trouble implementing this plan due to his frequent waking and crying.[52] Corinne contemplated moving the crib into the parental bedroom, but similar to Petra's and Julia's situation, the bedroom was too small to accommodate it. Corinne worked full time and felt that peaceful sleeping was more valuable than getting their son to go to sleep in a separate room. Thus, Corinne and Jacob ultimately lowered their bed to the floor by taking out the bedframe and brought Finn into the bed with them. This couple's example shows that even when parents are on a trajectory toward separate sleep arrangements for several months, the difficulties they encounter can prompt some to defy these conventions and radically rework their sleep arrangements.

At one year postpartum, two-thirds of participating families attained the culturally desirable norm of having their babies sleep apart from them for most of the night. In many of these families, however, babies still visited their parents' bed in the late morning or on the weekends. Four of these couples shared their bed with their children for part of the night and/or early morning periods on a regular basis. Finally, six couples continued to share their beds with their babies each night. Among these families, several had an early evening period where the baby slept alone and the couple was away from the family bedroom. Although all parents envisioned their children going to sleep in their own separate room in the long run, this latter group of parents significantly reworked the timeline for this norm (see chapter 7).

## Conclusion

As I worked with each family in my study, it became clear that the house served as a particularly important site for the production of children's personhood and the formation of kin relations. The construction of the baby's room initially anchored the child's personhood to this space, wherein kin relations from past generations joined with dreams for the child's future. Once children were born at the hospital and families returned home, however, the integration of children into these spaces met with significant unanticipated obstacles. The process of breastfeeding, which necessitated bodily proximity, challenged social practices and norms for domestic spaces that emphasized the separation of children from parents. By bringing their children into their beds, modifying sleep equipment, and delaying their children's move to a separate bedroom, couples transformed the house and the relations within as much as they replicated the moral order these spaces signified.

During the course of much of their child's first year of life, parents negotiated moral tensions between their desire to breastfeed and to comply with middle-class sleep conventions. Although the embodied practice of nighttime breastfeeding clearly disrupted parents' expectations for children's personhood and for parent-child kin relations, the resolution of these conflicts differed widely across participants. Overall, parents made significant spatial adjustments to their nighttime sleep practices to accommodate the bodily proximity induced by the breastfeeding relationship. Even as more parents moved away from this bodily proximity over time, they reworked the timeline for these transitions. These changes reflect a sense of emergent moralities that incorporate accounting for the perceived needs of the child while also simultaneously accommodating other obligations to spouses, work, and one's own body. These moralities were deeply felt, inhabited, and continually renegotiated in relation to the embodied experiences of the night and other social interactions. Through this process, parents substantively relocated and reworked their understanding of children's personhood as something that was produced over time through bodily engagement with one another. This processual model of personhood, however, remained in tension with more conventional ideologies of personhood that perceive the baby as, on the one hand, a much more fully formed, separate being from birth and even during pregnancy[53] and, on the other hand, in need of significant "training" to produce self-sufficiency and autonomy.[54] In Lynn's and Gary's case, this ideology received heavy emphasis from their encounter with a biomedical expert. The detrimental consequences of their pediatrician's advice served to highlight once again the privileges necessary to sustain breastfeeding over the long run, drawing attention to the multiple ways in which social class is evoked and remade through everyday parenting activities.

Those who habitually shared their beds with their children over the course of most of the first year made the most radical changes in relocating the site for producing children's personhood from a separate room to between the bodies of two parents for an extended period of time. This change entailed the greatest adjustment of parental bodies and domestic configurations of space compared with mainstream cultural conventions. On a sunny summer afternoon at Nathan's and Rachel's house seven months after their daughter's birth,[55] Nathan and I discussed the negative reactions he encountered among friends in response to their continued sharing of their bed with their breastfeeding daughter. Nathan recalled several conversations in which friends emphasized the importance of solitary sleep as a path for acquiring the value of independence for children, something he heard many times before. These friends argued that sharing the bed with their daughter would have long-term negative consequences—she might never leave their bed or move out of their house—something that Nathan found "ridiculous." Summing up these arguments, Nathan said, "I guess you have to push them out of nest early ... [laughs] and I don't know, eggs don't fly." Nathan suggested that pushing children out of the "nest" prematurely would leave them vulnerable, rather than prompting the development of greater precocity.

In comparing infants to eggs that have not yet hatched, Nathan renegotiated the familiar Bachelardian nest metaphor. While Nathan and his friends shared the sense that the family home offered a protective space for nurturance, Nathan located this "nest" within the bed the three of them shared, instead of the more conventional space of the baby's room occupied solely by the child. Nathan thereby challenged the spatial origins of children's personhood as well as the embodied relations entailed in their production. Nathan, along with other couples who continued to breastfeed and share their bed with their children, introduced a larger critique of U.S. ideologies of children's personhood that argued for a much more gradual formation of personhood over time. According to this model, dependence on one's parents and their constant nurturance are necessary, even desirable states that ultimately produce a successful adult—a good "flier." The production of this personhood necessitated reworking parental personhoods as well. Therefore, the dilemmas posed by nighttime breastfeeding stretched the limits of what was possible and reshaped the moral imagination. In the following chapter, I will explore the temporal dimensions of these negotiations and their effects.

## Notes

1. See Daniel 1984; Carsten and Hugh-Jones 1995; Carsten 2004; Bahloul 1996. For instance, breastfeeding in Malaysia played a key role in incorporating new children into webs of kinship through the process of sharing food cooked at the same hearth that linked the house with maternal bodies and the children they nourished (Carsten 1997).
2. Here, I am contrasting my analysis with that of Bourdieu's (1990), who famously assigned greater significance to the structuring effects of the spatiotemporal organization of everyday activities in and around the Kabyle house, especially in producing gendered inequities.

3. Bachelard argues that the symbolic power of a "nest" is rooted in creating a safe space to return to, not only in bodily form but also through dreaming of returning.
4. Bakhtin's ([1981] 1998) concept of the chronotope is helpful for developing the spatiotemporal implications of Bachelard's discussion of the nest. Bakhtin describes chronotopes as points wherein "time takes on flesh and becomes visible for human contemplation; likewise space becomes charged and responsive to the movements of time and history and the enduring character of a people" ([1981] 1998:7). Keith Basso (1996) has eloquently applied the concept of chronotopes to his analysis of the Western Apache landscape, in which "geographical features have served the people for centuries as indispensable mnemonic pegs on which to hang the moral teachings of their history" (1996:62). By teaching children to attend to this landscape through stories in which these features figure prominently, the landscape not only consolidates the past but enables the actualization of the Western Apache moral order in the present and in the future. Basso's insights demonstrate the analytical power of the concept of the chronotope to illuminate larger, mutually intertwined concepts of space, time, and morality (Bakhtin 1981:84; Basso 1996).
5. The median home sale price in Green City in 2006 was $251,000 (trulia.com). The range among neighborhoods, however, was very wide. The most desirable neighborhoods averaged approximately $500,000 (with specific houses much higher in this range, while the less desirable areas had median home sale prices in the low $110,000. This provides a rough guide for my participants, although each of their situations is far more complex, depending on when exactly they purchased their homes and with what resources (including family assistance) as well as the specific details of their streets, condition of their houses, etc. A larger study with greater attention to the details of property would be extremely helpful in gaining better insight into the differentiations of social class. Since the housing market's decline, which precipitated the larger financial crisis, all property values in the wealthier areas have declined, while some less expensive areas have been gaining in value as people were seeking less expensive options.
6. The median home sale price in Neighbor City in 2006 was $175,000, although with considerable variation among neighborhoods (trulia.com). All three other communities had lower, but more similar, median home sale prices compared with the figures for Green City (see below).
7. The median home sale in their general area in 2006 was $141,000 (trulia.com), with likely higher prices for their specific neighborhood, which had quiet, tree-lined streets and single-family homes.
8. The median home sale price in their area in 2006 was $135,000 (trulia.com). Within that area, however, they lived in a more desirable location with higher home values.

9. Paula and Matthew undertook a major project to expand their living space and later built their own house in a different neighborhood.
10. The median home sale price for this area was $160,000 (trulia.com). While Kristen and Daniel were most affected by the financial decline toward the end of my study by losing their jobs, they were able to recover more easily since they did not have a mortgage on their home.
11. Real estate sites, such as trulia.com provide information about school districts alongside property values.
12. Both of these new neighborhoods were in areas with higher property values and better schools, but the actual prices of homes were significantly declining by the time of their purchases due to the burst of the housing bubble.
13. Both of these families have since had their second children.
14. Since I shared a city apartment with four other members of my multi-generational family while growing up in Budapest, Hungary, I was often reminded of how much what is considered "adequate space" could vary across cultures. Compared with many Europeans, U.S. citizens often live in and aspire to live in much larger domestic spaces (Wilson and Boehland 2005; Gordon 2004; BBC News 2009). There is also considerable variation across countries in whether homes are owned or rented, and in occupying single-family homes versus attached townhouses or multi-story apartments.
15. The cultural value of houses played an important role in the recent economic crisis that began to unfold toward the end of my study. In the enormous rates of foreclosure due to cascading job losses, many families—disproportionately poorer and racial ethnic minorities—across the country not only lost their houses but also a particularly significant emblem of normative social class and the associated idealized family relations. At the same time, the crisis has also made the links between domestic economies and global financial markets clearer and has placed these issues and the inequalities they entail at the center of political debates.
16. See Hays 1996 on intensive caretaking and Zelizer 1994 on the growing focus on fewer children.
17. My own work clearly reflected these families' spatial practices. I spent considerably more time with mothers in their homes than with spouses who worked outside the home. While some of these spouses were present at most of our meetings, after long hours spent at work, evenings and weekends were usually times set aside for families to reconnect with one another and were not preferred meeting times with me.
18. In his work on Kaguru space, T. O. Beidelman (1986) has critiqued Bourdieu (1977) for his reductionist discussion of the Kabyle uses of space in terms of gendered dichotomies. In contrast to this reductionism, Beidelman cites diverse examples of Kaguru concepts and uses of space to demonstrate that while Kaguru culture is rich with gendered

oppositions, these ideals were constantly renegotiated, erased, and rebuilt in daily practice. Joelle Bahloul (1996), Erik Mueggler (2001), and others have made similar arguments based on their ethnographic evidence.
19. The rhythms of these separations and reconnections will be discussed further in the following chapter on temporality.
20. Johanna and Carl planned to have a separate room after their family's impending move due to Carl's new position.
21. For Carol and Justin, who purchased their home from another family with small children, the "nursery" was already set up, complete with brightly painted walls and stencils. Due to the convenient location of the nursery across from the parental bedroom, and the work the previous family had done, this couple spent comparatively less time on preparing their nursery. Furthermore, Carol and Justin, along with some others, also felt that they had more time to work on the room later, since they did not plan to have the baby sleep there for the first few months. This delay in completing the child's bedroom prior to their birth signaled a degree of temporal flexibility in accomplishing this culturally significant goal. Yet even such couples who delayed some preparations still invested some time in furnishing and/or decorating this space prior to the birth of their children.
22. Fieldnotes, August 22, 2007.
23. Fieldnotes, March 2, 2007.
24. See Dettwyler 1995; Smale 2001; Battersby 2007; Campo 2010; McKenna and McDade 2005.
25. Fieldnotes, March 13, 2007.
26. Colostrum, a thick, yellowish liquid that some lactation specialists call "liquid gold" for its immunological properties, is present at the moment a woman gives birth, but mature milk may take several days to arrive.
27. "Traumatized nipples" are technical terms that lactation specialists use to describe the damage to the breast tissue.
28. See Fieldnotes, February 27, 2007, for this account.
29. Fieldnotes, February 27, 2007.
30. See Fieldnotes, January 11, 2007, for this entire account.
31. Although Natalie also gave birth via Cesarean section, this did not motivate her to bring her baby into bed with her. See a more detailed discussion of Natalie's and Carsten's negotiation of nighttime sleep arrangements later in this chapter and in chapter 7.
32. See Fieldnotes, March 7, 2007, for this account.
33. Fieldnotes, January 11 and March 20, 2007.
34. Fieldnotes, March 8, 2007.
35. Fieldnotes, February 27, 2007.
36. Fieldnotes, April 18, 2008.
37. Fieldnotes, February 23, 2007.
38. Fieldnotes, May 14, 2007.
39. Fieldnotes, April 13, July 17, October 25, 2007.

40. Fieldnotes, July 17, 2007.
41. Fieldnotes, January 25, 2008.
42. Fieldnotes, March 17, 2007.
43. Fieldnotes, April 15, 2007.
44. Fieldnotes, August 21, 2007.
45. Fieldnotes, November 3, 2007.
46. Fieldnotes, March 15, 2008.
47. This kind of creative reworking of spatialized activities resembles couples' similar strategies in rural China as documented by Erik Mueggler (2001), who found that although two separate beds were set up for husbands and wives, most couples did not abide by the spatial norms embodied in the furniture (2001:78–81).
48. Fieldnotes, January 9, 2008.
49. Fieldnotes, April 18, 2008.
50. Fieldnotes, February 5, 2008.
51. Fieldnotes, May 3, 2008.
52. Fieldnotes, August 6, 2007.
53. See Morgan 1989; Ginsburg 1998; Kaufman and Morgan 2005; Layne 2000.
54. See, for instance, Shweder, Jensen, and Goldstein 1995; McKenna, Ball, and Gettler 2007.
55. Fieldnotes, June 24, 2007.

*Chapter 7*

# TIME TO SLEEP

## NIGHTTIME BREASTFEEDING AND CAPITALIST TEMPORAL REGIMES

Just as the embodied practice of breastfeeding disrupted the spatialized cultural expectations for children's personhood that I described in the previous chapter, it also upended aspects of personhood anchored to the rhythms of day and night. I found that parental experiences of fatigue, while seemingly a "natural" by-product of caring for young children, resulted from conflicts between competing pressures of capitalist time regimes that structured couples' lives and influenced ideologies of children's personhood, and the moral desire to fulfill cultural expectations to breastfeed. Parents' navigation of these pressures revealed different degrees of willingness and ability to adjust their own bodies to coordinate with those of their babies and to assert authority over their children's bodies in order to achieve desirable sleep patterns. These negotiations illuminate the profound ways in which capitalism shapes human experience while offering new insight into the formation of emergent embodied moralities that challenge and reshape capitalist regimes of temporality in personhood and kin relations.

### Time, Capitalism, and Children's Sleep

The profound changes in reckoning time since the rise of industrial capitalism have had a significant impact on families' sleep practices. While sleep could take place in multiple chunks under different labor conditions, industrial labor demanded a new kind of reckoning of time, one where continuous, maximally efficient work came to be emphasized (Ekirch 2005; Stearns, Rowland, and Giarnella 1996; Thompson 1967). This new kind of work regime, which emphasized discipline and efficiency, did not permit rest during the daytime and increasingly compressed available time for sleep for workers. Consequently, there were significant motivations for parents to regulate their children's sleep in order to conform to these new schedules.

Furthermore, these models of time dovetailed with mechanical models of human bodies espoused by biomedicine, wherein human bodies increasingly came to be seen within the framework of capitalist production. Emily Martin's (1987) and Davis-Floyd's (2004) work documented how tying the process of childbirth to time intervals was a key aspect of perceptions (and internalized self-perceptions) of women as failed machines requiring medical intervention. The clock played a major role in the undermining of breastfeeding in the twentieth century, since both mothers' lactating bodies and infants' feeding and sleep were tied to regulated, measured intervals of feeding schedules that interfered with the physiology of breastfeeding.[1] Fiona Dykes' (2005, 2006) ethnographic study of breastfeeding in a U.K. hospital maternity ward has shown that the clock, both through its use among health care workers and through its internalization among mothers themselves, continues to play a similarly problematic role in situating breastfeeding at the end of the hospital's production line and in setting up breastfeeding mothers as inefficient, failed machines that make supplementation with artificial formula milk necessary. In Dykes' (2009) more recent discussion of temporality in breastfeeding, she has further elaborated on the confusion and difficulties new mothers experience with the temporal rhythms of breastfeeding that contradict their expectations based on internalized models of linear clock-based time.[2]

Clock-based mechanical approaches toward children's sleep remain pervasive in pediatric advice.[3] Despite recent shifts toward more complex models of child development, these approaches continue to be justified by their ostensible role in producing self-regulation and self-efficacy, values that reflect characteristics of capitalist production. These legacies of temporal expectations for mothers and children cause significant challenges for contemporary U.S. families since they do not accommodate the embodied practices of breastfeeding,[4] particularly during the night, when children are expected to sleep away from their parents for long, uninterrupted periods of time.

In E.P. Thompson's (1967) classic study of temporality and industrial capitalism, Thompson noted that even before the full transition to factory labor and new reckonings of time took full effect, labor regimes had differential effects for mothers, fathers, and children. Among rural nineteenth-century English laborers, women bore the brunt of the time squeeze of daytime labor in the fields and nighttime care of their young children. Thompson argued that contemporary women's orientation to temporality remains conflicted between two temporal regimes: "despite school times and television times, the rhythms of women's work in the home are not wholly attuned to the measurement of the clock. The mother of young children has an imperfect sense of time and attends to other human tides. She has not yet altogether moved out of the conventions of 'pre-industrial'[5] society." (1967:79). These observations stand in direct opposition of historical evidence that mothers internalized clock-based models of time for their own reproductive processes while also becoming the primary agents of socializing their children into this new kind of temporality by scheduling their bodily processes such as feeding, sleeping, bathing, and toileting (Martin 1987; Apple 1987; Dykes 2009). Yet, Thompson's observation that children present challenges to work schedules, especially those dominated by capitalist labor practices for both parents, and that mothers play a role in attending to these challenges, merits further attention. I will argue that rather than mothers "stuck" in "pre-industrial" time regimes, contemporary families in my study negotiated these disruptions in gendered, but distinctly late capitalist ways.[6]

Finally, following Max Weber's (1958) footsteps, I situate my discussion of nighttime breastfeeding and temporality in the context of morality. Weber argued that a key characteristic of the Protestant ethic that propelled the rise of industrial capitalism was its approach to time, wherein time was equated with money and the inefficient use, or "wasting" of time, was considered a sin. I suggest that in the contemporary late capitalist U.S. context, cultural approaches to temporality possess similar moral characteristics that are deeply tied to capitalism through time regimes of labor and cultural expectations for the temporal regulation of mothers' and children's bodies, which are themselves infused with capitalist ideologies of production.

## Before the Baby: Middle-Class Couples' Time in Capitalist Work Regimes

Karl Marx and other scholars have argued that capitalist regimes of labor have produced distinct spatiotemporal separations between home and work, with important implications for the segregation of men's and women's labor.[7] With women's increasing participation in the labor force,[8] however, women's and men's spatiotemporal rhythms increasingly resemble one another, with both leaving the home for work and then returning to it afterward. For most middle-class workers, this schedule follows a (blurry) diurnal pattern with work during the daytime and leisure time and sleep at nighttime and weekends, but with a significant portion of work being performed beyond conventional time frames and from remote locations using the internet.

Although I got to know couples only during their pregnancies, conversations with them offered insight about their lives before their babies were born. Prior to their babies' birth, couples' views of time were dominated by their work schedules. Steady employment with health insurance coverage for the entire family supplied the family with adequate resources for maintaining a stable middle-class position, including the purchase of a home. This economic and geographic security was a pivotal element in couples' plans for a baby. Much of this stability derived from a high level of work commitment, demonstrated by lengthy work hours, often compounded by time for commuting to and from work.

The home and the workplace provided two interrelated poles of economic and spatiotemporal organization, but with considerable crossover between them. In most cases, at least one member of a couple had fairly strict work hours, to which the other member of the couple adjusted in order to ensure that they would spend time together. For example, after completing her master's degree, Camilla taught piano part time from their home. Erik, however, worked as an architect at a Green City firm.[9] Thus, the couples' schedule was framed around Erik's working schedule, since that was less flexible than teaching, which could be arranged to fit within this frame. The couple reunited in the evenings and shared the evening meal, household tasks, and leisure time together. Since Erik needed additional work hours beyond the workday in order to meet deadlines and to prepare for a series of important licensing exams, he often returned to his work tasks from home in the evening hours. Weekends could be spent in a more flexible manner since Erik did not have to go to the office, leaving more time for leisure as well as for larger household projects. During Camilla's pregnancy, this time was increasingly filled by preparations for their baby's arrival. In another similar example, Julia also worked as an architect with lengthy hours, some of which she completed from home late in the night.[10]

Petra was a teacher, with shorter daytime hours during the school year but, her work included considerable preparation and grading work beyond these hours. In order to coordinate their schedules, Petra completed much of this work by staying longer at school, enabling her to reunite with Julia in the evenings without the burden of additional work. During the summer months Petra took over the bulk of housework since she had a long break from teaching but Julia had few days off from work. These examples illustrate the blurry boundaries of where and when paid labor takes place as well as how couples coordinate their schedules to share leisure time and household labor.

The main departure from these time schedules included students and the one shift worker in the study. There were four students in the study: Nathan in a bachelor's program, Angela in a master's program, and Elise and Natalie in doctoral programs, both completing their theses. Although being students meant that, beyond attending classes and required events, they had greater flexibility in arranging their time to study, Angela and Natalie both adjusted their schedules to spend time with their full-time working spouses, who had more traditional working hours. Elise, a doctoral student, and her husband, Adam, probably had the least conventional timetables and greatest flexibility in daily schedules compared with other couples in the study since they both worked mainly out of their home. The lack of a rigid work schedule permitted them to divide their work time according to their needs.[11] In contrast, Nathan's and Rachel's schedules were probably the most complex in the study since he was a student who also worked part time, while Rachel was a nurse who primarily worked night shifts during the course of the study. In an attempt to minimize the financial burden of school, Nathan took on as much part-time labor as possible, leading to very long days of attending classes, studying, working, and commuting. Due to the combined demands of Rachel's shift work, which did not follow conventional diurnal patterns, and Nathan's extensive time commitments as a student and part-time worker, spending time together required careful planning even prior to their baby's birth.[12]

Even with long work hours and additional potential work commitments, however, couples found many opportunities to spend time together during evenings, weekends, and vacations prior to their babies' birth. Couples discussed this shared time in conversation with me as I got to know them better. Several couples discussed the importance of attending religious services and activities together. Photos of vacations or evidence of other shared interests were displayed within couples' homes, such as Camilla's and Erik's many musical instruments in their home, which would become starters of conversations about life before their baby's birth. Couples also discussed "going out" to restaurants and bars, to dance, or to see movies and performances together. Many of these activities took place in the evening and at night, usually toward the end of the week (e.g., Friday and Saturday nights). For instance, Joy and Jonathan enjoyed a very busy social life prior to their child's birth that included dance events and teaching dance as well. Paula and Matthew were very active in their local Baptist church community, with Sunday worship services, service in leadership committees, and regular prayer meetings. In accordance with contemporary ideologies of companionate marriage, spending time together and participating in joint activities built and reinforced emotional connections between spouses.[13] Members of couples also pursued activities on their own, such as reading, house projects, crafts, and gardening.

Couples' daily rhythms of work fit into larger temporal schemes of employment, which included planning for a baby. In particular, couples were aware of the high cost of raising children, from the cost of taking time off from work to the high cost of childcare and a college education. These costs necessitated attention to maintaining adequate employment as well as accumulating savings. Couples who were planning to have babies paid particular attention to having adequate leave for mothers and, in some cases, spouses after the birth as well as having health insurance for all members of the family. For the majority of women who worked full time prior to their children's birth, this meant planning maternity leave (usually six to eight weeks paid leave) and then any supplemental unpaid leave that the couple might agree upon, which could be taken by either or both members of the couple. Since this second kind of leave was unpaid, planning was essential to ensure that there were adequate financial resources for this period of time. For couples of whom one member planned to leave employment after birth, financial planning was essential in order to ensure that the family could live on a single income.

While babies could be added to spouses' health insurance plans under regulations that govern the acceptance of newborn babies within a certain time period, couples had to plan well so that mothers would not lose coverage should they decide to stop working after their babies' birth. For instance, Corinne and Jacob were each on employer-paid health insurance plans during Corinne's pregnancy.[14] Because Corinne had planned to return to work after a combination of paid and unpaid maternity leave of three months, she planned to add their baby to her health plan. If, however, Corinne decided to depart from her job after her parental leave was completed, she would have had to wait until the open enrollment period of her husband's health insurance plan in order to cover herself and her son.

In other couples' cases, health insurance could not be obtained from the spouse's employer, leaving few options for new mothers. Although Jocelyn also enjoyed her work, she wished for a lengthier maternity leave after her daughter's birth.[15] Jocelyn's employer-provided benefits, however, also covered her entire family and were a primary reason for the couple's decision for her to return to work full time immediately after her leave was completed and for Samuel to become the primary caregiver for their child. Finally, Petra's and Julia's planning was complicated by legal difficulties surrounding same-sex couples.[16] Petra held an employer-provided plan that covered herself and their son. If needed, Julia could add their son to her plan under a clause that included adopted children. She could not, however, cover Petra because the employer's plan did not provide benefits to same-sex couples. This situation forced Petra to continue to work even though she wished to take a more extended break from full-time employment after the birth of their son.

The above observations highlight how capitalist work regimes structured both the daily rhythms of couples' lives as well as the larger temporal framework within which they planned to have babies. In order to spend time together, couples had to coordinate their daily time schedules. Similarly, couples coordinated the greater arc of their working lives to accommodate plans for their children. Below I describe how the temporal frameworks of work regimes combined couples' ideologies and experiences of reproductive time to produce "a good time to have a baby."

## "A Good Time to Have a Baby"

For all the couples in my study, pregnancies were carefully planned and considered in relation to larger life plans. Among middle-class U.S. couples, this time frame has been under fierce negotiation, with the total time frame for being able to have a baby narrowing along the way (Moe and Shandy 2010; Simonds 2002). Many couples began dating after they had completed their schooling (often undertaking additional training/education after their bachelor's degree) and had gained experience in the labor market, getting married or making an exclusive commitment after several years. Most couples planned to have children only after these goals were met, when they were in their late twenties to early thirties.

Couples sought sufficient economic security to raise children, aware of the high cost of raising children in the U.S. This demanded that both members of the couple work for at least some time prior to the birth of their children. At the same time, couples were also concerned about the decline of fertility as well as potential problems with childbearing that become more frequent with age. These concerns were shaped by biomedicalized approaches toward reproduction, particularly a focus on women's bodies as the limiting factor on the window of time for fertility—a "biological clock" that begins with puberty and winds down toward the mid- to late thirties (Simonds 2002). This image of the bodily clock illustrates E.P. Thompson's (1967) point, extended by feminist scholars of reproduction, of how clocks that increasingly structured regimes of capitalist labor transformed subjective experiences of time, manifest in even women's own understanding of their bodies.[17]

Although women in my study tended to be younger than their spouses, women's bodies were thought to be primarily responsible for the regulation of fertility. Kristen and Daniel, for instance, did not originally plan to have children in the earlier years of their marriage.[18] With time, however, they changed their minds and began to plan their first pregnancy when Kristen was in her mid-thirties. Although they ultimately successfully gave birth to their daughter when Kristen was thirty-eight, they worried about whether they would be able to have a second child because of Kristen's age. These worries were compounded later by Kristen's diagnosis with an autoimmune disorder that necessitated taking medication that could harm a future pregnancy. Thus, Kristen and Daniel decided not to try a second pregnancy in the foreseeable future, unless changes were possible in Kristen's medications. Maternal age was a major factor even in the couple where two women could share the bodily tasks of pregnancy and lactation. Maternal age was the primary reason for prioritizing the first pregnancy for Petra, since she was the older member of the couple, thereby assuming that Julia would have more remaining fertile years for future pregnancies.

Couples who had experienced reproductive challenges faced additional difficulties as well as time pressures. Kate and Joshua, for instance, struggled with the memories of a previous miscarriage that made them no longer take a healthy pregnancy for granted.[19] Several couples struggled with infertility and the inability to conceive.[20] Angela experienced several years of infertility and underwent extensive medical examinations and interventions in order to achieve pregnancy.[21] In both of these cases, the ability to conceive and to have a healthy full-term pregnancy was located in women's bodies. In Camilla's and Erik's case and in Rachel's and Nathan's experience, physicians ultimately identified male infertility as the cause for the delay in getting pregnant. Even in these cases, however, male infertility was considered in the context of the limited total time women were likely to have. Thus, for Camilla, who was in her mid-thirties, there was a sense of a compressed time frame for being able to have children. Even though Rachel was a few years younger when she first got pregnant, because it took considerable time to conceive Maya, she was keenly aware that it might also take longer for them to become pregnant with their second child than for others who did not have fertility challenges, potentially limiting the number of children they would ultimately have. Thus, planning pregnancies and the length of breastfeeding must be viewed in relation to these larger fertility time frames, which are mainly considered in the context of women's biological temporal rhythms.

Angela and Oliver were the only ones to reconsider the larger frame of fertility time and change their approach toward reproduction.[22] After several years of major fertility difficulties and worries about the ability to have a successful pregnancy, the couple decided to take a different approach toward reproductive time. They were so grateful for their successful pregnancy that they decided not to worry about this time frame and to put themselves on the list at an adoption agency shortly after their first child was born in order to ensure that they would have the opportunity to raise a second child within a year or two. Their strategy considered the window of "good time" to raise children, but they made a conscious effort to step out of the pressures imposed by attempting to get pregnant by instead pursuing adoption. Ultimately, Angela unexpectedly got pregnant shortly thereafter and successfully gave birth to their second child, leading the couple to decide not to pursue adoption at that time.

As in the above cases, most participants wished to have more than one child. Breastfeeding to one year or beyond placed considerable pressure on this overall time frame. Camilla, Carol, and Joy each carefully considered the length of total breastfeeding time in relation to their larger family-planning time, either because of concerns over not getting their periods back due to breastfeeding, and/ or because they had hoped to have some reprieve from breastfeeding before beginning another pregnancy, which would place further demands on their bodies.

In sum, the temporal frame for "a good time to have a baby" was structured by couples' participation in the capitalist labor market in order to secure an economically stable middle-class life for themselves and for their children as well as by the combination of time constraints produced by these labor practices, gendered ideologies of biological reproduction, and physiological fertility challenges themselves. The following section on the daily negotiations of temporality after their babies' birth demonstrates that the capitalist regimes of time, which supported "a good time to have a baby," clashed with the temporal practices entailed in nighttime breastfeeding.

## Negotiating Nighttime after the Baby's Birth

In chapter 6, I described the acute fatigue parents experienced upon returning home from the hospital, already exhausted from giving birth, as they struggled with breastfeeding their babies throughout the day and night. Experiences of fatigue were also cumulative, especially when time for sleep was limited by work, when sleep arrangements were in flux, or when children experienced bouts of awakenings that parents could not reduce. Parents aligned their own and children's nighttime sleep patterns using primarily three spatiotemporal adjustments: 1) adjusting their own temporal rhythms to coordinate with their children's through bed sharing, 2) partially coordinating their bodily rhythms with their children's through room sharing or a mix of bed sharing and separate-surface sleeping, and 3) putting their babies in their own rooms to sleep through the night using "sleep training" techniques. These approaches offer insight into the diverse embodied temporal experiences for parents and children, highlighting the gendered effects of caring for breastfeeding babies. Furthermore, families' experiences illuminate the complexities, conflicts, and moral ambivalences that surround ideologies of children's personhood and kin relations.

*The Coordination of Nighttime Temporalities in Bed Sharing*
Parents who regularly shared their beds described three main shared experiences: breastfeeding took minimal effort, there was virtually no nighttime crying, and not only spouses but breastfeeding mothers themselves began to sleep through feedings and were no longer sure how often they were partially awake during the night.

First, all regularly bed-sharing parents noted how much easier they found breastfeeding their babies during the night. Kate and Joshua, for instance, quickly realized that nursing in bed and keeping Anna there throughout the night resulted in less labor, fewer interruptions, and better sleep for both of them. Bed sharing therefore not only made mothers' work easier, but also lightened the load on spouses who returned to their lengthy work schedules during the daytime. Carol, for instance, felt that since Justin returned to work soon after their son was born, developing an arrangement that enabled him to sleep was especially important since she could compensate by taking a nap during the day. Thus, bed sharing simultaneously facilitated breastfeeding while also accommodating the temporal demands of capitalist labor regimes.

Parents were clearly aware that bed sharing diminished or eliminated nighttime crying. See, for instance, Carol's and Justin's response of bringing Jeremiah into bed with them when he woke up crying several times in his Co-Sleeper in the previous chapter. The lack of crying was pivotal in producing the sense for parents that they experienced fewer disruptions during the night. Additionally, because their babies never reached a heightened state of being upset, the time it took to feed and soothe them back to sleep was further diminished. Without crying, even awakening multiple times a night to breastfeed felt more tolerable for these parents. Thus, for bed-sharing parents, these nighttime arrangements improved the quality and quantity of their own and their babies' sleep.

Furthermore, the presence or absence of crying was used to evaluate the baby's well-being both by parents and by others. For instance, when Rachel visited her grandmother, her cousin and her family was staying in the room next door, and they said that they didn't even notice that there was a baby next door. The lack of crying surprised her relatives because it did not align with cultural expectations of babies crying at night.[23] Maya virtually never cried and was described by all as a "happy" and healthy baby. Leslie's experience matched that of Rachel's. She was thrilled to watch Connor wake up cooing in the morning, smiling at her, and cooing at the mobile Alex took from Connor's room and attached to the head of their own bed. Having a "happy" baby provided evidence for parents of their child's well-being and was used to reinforce bed sharing that facilitated nighttime breastfeeding as a cornerstone of their parenting approach.

Bed sharing resulted in a tight coordination of mother-child sleep patterns wherein mothers often woke simultaneously or just ahead of their babies in anticipation of a feeding, and later would actually sleep through many breastfeeding sessions.[24] Leslie noticed that, while in the first few weeks of bed sharing she would wake up for each breastfeeding session, over time she began to not wake up fully for feedings and could no longer remember when she was up with her son.[25] Echoing Leslie, once Rachel and Nathan decided to share their bed with their daughter, Rachel quickly adjusted to sleeping through breastfeeding. Nathan described how he observed Maya latch on to Rachel's breast without assistance and without apparently waking Rachel.[26] Nathan's observation offered a rare glimpse into the details of nighttime breastfeeding since, most of the time, partners were asleep during these moments. For instance, in the early days of breastfeeding when she was more fully awake during feeding sessions, Leslie noticed that despite sharing a bed, Alex rarely woke up when she fed Connor, even though Leslie described their son as a very noisy eater.[27] Leslie saw that Alex would sometimes turn over in his sleep while she was nursing their son, but in the morning he would ask her if they were up during the night—he could not remember waking at all. These experiences were echoed by all the other fully bed-sharing mothers and their spouses.

Although bed-sharing families did not attempt to "sleep train" their babies, they did structure their babies' sleep to a certain degree. For instance, couples created time that they spent exclusively with each other during the early part of their children's sleep. Each mother, often joined by her partner, lay down and nursed her baby to sleep in the evenings, usually between 8:00 to 9:00 P.M., and then left the baby in the bed while the couple spent time together in another room of the house. Thus, their children's "night" was usually several hours longer than that of the parents, providing time for parents to reconnect with each other after the daytime they spent separately, taking care of their child or working outside the home. This was an example of mutual accommodations—parents helping their babies transition to sleep together, then leaving to spend time together, and returning to the baby at the time of the next awakening.

For most of these parents, sleeping together simply became the family routine. In fact, once these patterns were solidified, couples had little to say about sleep over the months of our meetings. They were happy with the arrangements and did not wish to modify them. Although nighttime nursing usually diminished over the course of the months, it never completely disappeared during the first year of their children's lives. Nonetheless, all members of the family were getting the most rest they felt they could get and were continuing to breastfeed as often as their children desired. For Corinne and Jacob and Adrianne and Doug, who both made the switch to fully sharing their beds with their children at later points in the study, the switch produced very similar experiences to the other bed-sharing parents of continued night-nursing but the sense of minimally interrupted sleep.

Parents felt that bed sharing resulted in more sleep for them, leaving them more rested to face the next day's work of taking care of their babies as well as working outside the home. Of this group of parents, only Carol and Justin ended up feeling the need to take a more active approach in regulating their child's sleep, in response to issues that developed later in the year. The above experiences echo biological anthropological and survey findings that while bed sharing is associated with increased frequency of breastfeeding, it also produces more sleep for mothers (McKenna, Ball, and Gettler 2007; Kendall-Tackett, Cong, and Hale 2010). In my study, it also appeared that bed sharing produced similar effects for spouses since they were not awakened by nighttime breastfeeding sessions. These experiences challenged dominant ideologies that portray continuous sleep as the most physiologically beneficial form of sleep, reflecting that the notion of continuity of sleep and its supposed healthfulness is tied up in cultural expectations for self-regulating bodies in accordance with capitalist time regimes.[28]

After the initial period of upheaval during which breastfeeding and sleep arrangements were worked out, the temporal coordination of parents' and children's bodies facilitated coping with the capitalist time regimes in which couples were immersed. For mothers who attempted to facilitate their own and their spouses' sleep, since their spouses had already returned to work, bed sharing offered a solution that accommodated all three parties while also enabling mothers and spouses to continue to share the same bed. For mothers who were employed outside the home during the study period, this arrangement also felt least cumbersome. After returning to her long shifts at University Hospital, for instance, Rachel felt that she was getting sufficient rest. She described sharing their bed as "so much easier" and much less disruptive than having her baby in the bassinet or crib. Leslie similarly felt that this arrangement enabled her to sleep the longest possible when she returned to work as a lawyer.

Bed sharing, however, required a renegotiation of the dominant models of personhood and kinship tied up in the spatiotemporal separation of parents and children, and the necessity of temporal regulation for the production of children. Through the mutual adjustment of bodies to accommodate the spatial proximity and temporal rhythms of the child, parents developed emergent ways of being, or new forms of *habitus* (Mauss [1935] 1973), that prompted them to question the above models. In Nathan's observation from the previous chapter, children were comparable to eggs that have not hatched—they were persons in the making that required this close embodied care instead of "sleep training."

Parents reflected on the affective dimension of this spatiotemporal closeness. Leslie, for instance, commented on how this arrangement helped her feel part of a "cozy little family."[29] Rachel highlighted the temporal dimension of this arrangement by noting that going to bed together constituted a "special time when she is falling asleep and we are all just hanging out."[30] In recognizing the affective significance of sharing nighttime with their children, these parents also reworked ideologies to include their babies in the concept of "spending time together," a category that previously worked to reinforce affective ties between the couple. Nighttime thereby became "family time" through the incorporation of a new form of *habitus*, a shared embodied practice.

### *The Partial Coordination of Temporalities in Mixed Sleep Arrangements*

Many parents found that either partial bed sharing and separate sleep, or room sharing but not bed sharing, worked for their families. Elise and Adam, for instance, were not able to get good rest when they attempted to sleep in the same bed with their son, Luke.[31] Elise, for instance, was hyperalert if she shared her bed in the beginning of the night. In biological anthropological terms, while Elise responded to Luke's awakenings with a coordination of her own patterns, her arousal level was higher than most mothers who shared their beds with their babies. In response, Elise and Adam decided to put Luke in his bassinet and later in his crib in another room for the first part of the night during which he usually did not awaken to feed, so Elise could get a few hours of uninterrupted sleep and then she or Adam would bring Luke into the bed where he remained for the rest of the night. Adam also facilitated any awakenings during this earlier portion of the night by transporting Luke back and forth to Elise when necessary. For Elise, this arrangement reduced the hyperalert sensation and ultimately enabled her to partially coordinate her sleep patterns with her baby, not fully awakening for the feedings during the latter portion of the night.

The above arrangement facilitated both Elise's and Adam's work schedules, producing adequate rest for Elise and relatively small disruptions for Adam, who could sleep through the latter portion of the night. Both parents could "sleep in"—sleep during late morning hours—because of their flexible work schedules. Elise and Adam did not describe this approach in terms of "sleep training," since they did not seek to remove Luke from their bedroom for the entire night or actively reduce nighttime breastfeeding sessions. Instead, this couple's system relied on Adam's willingness to distribute nighttime tasks in order to simultaneously facilitate rest for Elise and nighttime breastfeeding.

In families where parents did not share a bed with their children but were in close spatial proximity, there was a degree of embodied temporal coordination of sleep as well, especially in situations where the baby was right next to the bed in an attachable bassinet or a crib aligned with the surface of the bed. Several mothers remarked that they could anticipate when their children would wake up for nursing and that their children hardly ever cried during the night because they were quickly picked up and breastfed. This degree of coordination varied among parents, however, with some finding the awakenings during the night much more disruptive than others.

Although mothers in this group could not fully sleep through feedings, many experienced the sense that they were only half awake when they retrieved their babies for breastfeeding. Furthermore, many of these mothers experienced a diminishing number of breastfeeding sessions over time, with some reaching virtually no nighttime awakenings. Fathers in this group also reported a sense of coordination with their babies' rhythms. As I described in the previous chapter, for instance, the spatial adjustments that enabled continued sharing of the same room produced a sense of closeness and coordination for Matthew and Paula. Matthew was attuned to and reassured by the sound of Isaac's breathing during the night while Paula anticipated Isaac's increasingly less frequent nighttime awakenings.[32] This arrangement facilitated the parents' and child's mutual desire to be close to one another, accommodated nighttime feeding sessions, and provided sufficient rest for Matthew, who worked lengthy hours, and for Paula, who stayed home to care for their son during the daytime. Simultaneously, this bodily coordination also resulted in renegotiating models of children's personhood and parental relations that emphasized closeness and mutual interdependence instead of self-regulation and autonomy.

In the above examples, parents exercised a degree of control over their child's temporal rhythms using spatial adjustments. These spatial arrangements simultaneously facilitated breastfeeding while also providing some measure of bodily separation that appeared to increase the duration of continuous sleep for both parents during the night. For these parents, their sleep arrangements enabled them to successfully align their children's temporalities with their own, which was governed by capitalist labor regimes. In these arrangements parents retained certain elements of mainstream ideologies of children's sleep—e.g., having the baby sleep in his own room or own crib for a chunk of time—but they implemented these elements only in parts or in a circumscribed manner, and then complemented them with alternative practices. These renegotiations of sleep arrangements mirror a reworking of children's personhood that de-emphasized the importance of self-sufficiency and necessitated extensive embodied care and involvement of both partners. At the same time, the mixed strategies also revealed degrees of ambivalence and hesitation about a fuller coordination of children's and adults' temporality. This was certainly the case with Paula and Matthew, who could not envision sharing a bed with their child in the long run. In Elise's and Adam's case, the challenges of closer coordination are more difficult to decipher but may also reflect an embodied response to violating morally laden social norms. These findings point toward the formation of a *habitus* that facilitated a more limited, but nonetheless substantial, reworking of prevailing models of personhood and kinship.

In contrast to these couples who successfully used the mixed strategies over the course of the year, other parents felt increasingly exhausted by being woken up to breastfeed. For some of these parents, the sense of exhaustion derived from the cumulative weight of being regularly disrupted even if this was only a few times each night, while others experienced a significant increase in nighttime awakenings at some point along the way. For most of these parents, sharing their room was a short-term experience along the way toward separate sleep arrangements, leaving only the specific approach and its timing in question. These parents' efforts reveal a mounting desire to curtail their own bodily adjustment and instead to more fully align their babies' bodies with separate, continuous sleep regimes and ideologies of a more self-sufficient personhood.

### "Sleep Training"

Parents in this group employed a variety of techniques to actively regulate children's sleep rhythms. The most prominent feature of these cases was parents' belief that they had the power and ability to regulate children's sleep in order to accomplish the specific goal of producing a continuous stretch of parental sleeping time. This goal was largely accomplished by separating children from their parents and limiting nighttime breastfeeding sessions for at least part of the night. In the following section, I highlight both the diversity as well as the common themes in their approaches. Temporality was key in each of these cases with regard to the timing and specific implementation of these approaches. The vignettes below span the entire period of my study—from three weeks postpartum in Natalie's and Carsten's case, all the way to the end of the first year with Petra's and Julia's experiences. Each of these cases illustrates how specific couples negotiated the challenges of adjusting breastfeeding babies' bodies to capitalist labor regimes while also accommodating cultural ideologies of self-sufficiency in children's personhood.

### Natalie's and Carsten's Pioneering Move: A Delayed Response Approach

Natalie and Carsten were the pioneers in the study for actively working to change the sleep patterns of their child, attempting to maximize the time for their own sleep between awakenings.[33] When their son, Alexander, was two weeks old, Carsten went back to work. Natalie and Carsten decided that the "fussiness" of their child at night was too disruptive for their sleep, and Natalie, in particular, worried about Carsten's ability to get enough sleep in light of a lengthy commute early in the morning. She felt that a "screaming baby in the room" at night was no longer acceptable when he was working full time, which prompted her to move Alexander to his own room for the night. Thus, a major aim of this change was to help align Alexander's body to Carsten's work schedule, which demanded uninterrupted nighttime sleep, while also maintaining the couple's ability to spend each night in the same bedroom.

The approach of taking Alexander out of the bedroom was reinforced by Carsten's colleagues, whom he asked about how they put their babies to sleep. Although Carsten had expected to have the baby stay in their room for a longer period of time, he was reassured when he learned that some of his colleagues had their babies in a separate room from the very beginning. Carsten's ambivalence was therefore put to rest by his colleagues' voicing of mainstream cultural ideologies about separate sleep arrangements between children and parents, even though their practice might have been quite different from how they represented it to him in conversation.

Natalie told me that when they shared a room and she heard Alexander crying in the portable crib (similar to a Pack 'n Play), she would think "Oh, baby, he is *crying*" [emphasis original] and rush to pick him up.³⁴ But when he was in the other room and she heard crying, she would think, "Oh, baby, it's not so bad, I'll be right there," but would take her time. She would choose not to respond right away, but hoped that he would calm down. Natalie developed a strategy for interpreting her son's behavior: she learned that if Alexander stopped making sounds, she would not go in the room, but if her son would not calm down, then she interpreted his sounds as a "hungry cry," and this cry would prompt her to go and feed him. She would go to the nursery and breastfeed her son there and put him back to sleep. Natalie's approach to produce a greater stretch of uninterrupted sleep time involved spatiotemporal changes in parenting. First, the baby needed to be removed from the parental bedroom. It was this spatial separation that enabled Natalie to delay responding to each sound the child made and also to begin creating different categories of sounds: those that would prompt a response and those that were deemed non-urgent. These changes were implemented to reduce their son's crying so that his parents could sleep for longer uninterrupted stretches. Although this solution was ostensibly designed to help align their baby with capitalist regimes of temporality centering around Carsten's work days, sleep training also fulfilled dominant ideologies of children's personhood that valued the production of autonomy and self-regulation.

The results of this approach were initially mixed. On the one hand, Natalie could delay or potentially forego responding to Alexander's sounds from the other room as she described above. On the other hand, initially it would take Natalie a longer time to put him back to sleep in the nursery. Furthermore, in a conversation about three months after this approach was implemented,³⁵ I learned that, in the first month and a half to two months, Alexander cried frequently, especially in the evening hours after he initially went to sleep for the night, around 8:00 P.M. Natalie said that Alexander would often wake up every half an hour or so in the evenings, and there were long bouts of crying that sometimes escalated and extended over time. At these times Natalie handed the baby to her husband, who would walk around with Alexander, carrying him in his arms in an upright position that he preferred. She also described that with each awakening at night, she was unsure about what would happen, whether her son would go back to sleep easily or whether he would cry and have difficulty being soothed. Therefore, it was not clear to me that removing Alexander to the other room and delaying responding to him produced more sleep in the early months, since the interruptions of nighttime feedings, soothing back to sleep, and comforting a crying baby took considerable time for both Natalie and Carsten.

Natalie herself did not link these lengthy disruptions to the family's approach to sleep. Instead, she attributed the extensive periods of crying to a developmental phase, as she read in some articles from a variety of parenting sources, which would disappear by three months of age. By locating the crying as an internal characteristic of her son, she removed the context of the crying from the analysis, reflecting an ideology of children's personhood that unfolded according to developmental progress with the passage of time.[36] In actual parenting practice, however, Natalie's approach continued to focus on the mechanistic regulation of her son, although this regulation was omitted as an explanatory factor in her accounts. The pattern of crying did change between two and three months, and Natalie felt that her son was much less "fussy" before nighttime and even before naps.[37] She felt that he was much "less afraid of going to sleep" and that he was learning that at night, after feedings, he would simply go back to sleep. Once again, the notion that Alexander was previously "afraid" of going to sleep was not linked to sleep arrangements, reinforcing Natalie's understanding of children's personhood.

Natalie began to be able to put Alexander back to sleep at night much faster than in the past. By three months of age, Natalie reported that her son had learned not to cry for food.[38] Natalie told me that he could go for five hours or more without food and he did not usually cry. She felt that he learned not to cry for food because he developed a certainty that he would receive it without crying. She told me, for instance, that even in the morning, when she knew that Alexander woke up hungry, she did not feed him right away. Instead, she greeted him, turned on his mobile, washed her face, and took some time to wake up before she fed him. Natalie reasoned that this approach helped encourage her son to develop confidence that he would receive a feeding in a few minutes and to anticipate this delay without crying. The lack of crying was interpreted as a sign that Alexander mastered the embodied skills of separate, continuous sleep and a degree of self-sufficiency that no longer demanded parental contact for large chunks of the night.

By our meeting a couple of weeks into the fourth month postpartum,[39] Alexander woke up only about twice each night, and sometimes not at all from 8:00 P.M. to 7:00 A.M. Alexander came to have a more predictable pattern, and "like clockwork," he would begin to nurse by about 7:30 P.M. and would be asleep by 8 P.M., having fallen asleep at the breast and then woken up by being burped and placed into his crib in his room. Although Natalie enjoyed the extra sleep, she preferred that Alexander woke up at least once during the night because her breasts got too full overnight, uncomfortably engorged and leaking by the morning. During these longer nights, he sometimes "cried a little" but Natalie said that the crying would stop by the time she would get to the door or got out of bed. By this time, she felt that her son's nighttime crying greatly diminished and that he usually only "complained" at night—making small sounds, but not crying. In fact, she knew that something was wrong when Alexander cried at night the week before, and she discovered that he had gotten a cold and developed a fever. The temporal regularity and predictability of her son's sleep patterns were welcomed by Natalie as Alexander increasingly adjusted to a bodily rhythm that conformed to parental time regimes and expectations of a self-sufficient personhood.

It is notable here that the goal of Natalie's approach was not necessarily to produce fewer episodes of awakening on the baby's behalf, but rather to reduce episodes of crying. For instance, although she reported that Alexander slept five hours or more in continuous stretches at night, she also stated that he made "sounds," which were interpreted to be non-crying sounds, periodically during the night. It is possible that Alexander awakened multiple times during the night, but rarely cried during these awakenings. Since Natalie and her husband slept through these sounds or were only occasionally awoken by them, they were interpreted as being made while Alexander was asleep—something that could not be verified by observation. Nonetheless, in Natalie's experience, her approach of removing Alexander to a separate room and changing her pattern of responding to him ultimately—if not at first—resulted in a longer continuum of uninterrupted time for sleep for both Natalie and her husband. Both she and her husband were satisfied with this arrangement. Carsten's only complaint was that he wished that Alexander would go to bed later in the evening, since he had little time to spend with him after he arrived home from work.[40]

How did this approach affect Natalie's breastfeeding? In order to increase her own and Carsten's sleeping time, Natalie's strategy clearly reduced the number of feeding sessions at night. Recall that Carsten shared with me his relief when he learned that his colleagues also used similar approaches to their babies' sleep. When I asked whether these parents were breastfeeding, Carsten said that he thought so, although he sounded rather uncertain. Although it is possible that these colleagues' children were breastfed, I was skeptical that they were either exclusively breastfed in the first six months or that they could sustain breastfeeding for the recommended one-year period based on my review of the literature. Few parents would be able to maintain breastfeeding using Natalie's approach since frequent nursing sessions during both day and night are essential to the successful establishment of breastfeeding (McKenna, Ball, and Gettler 2007; Ball 2003) and, later on, mothers who do not breastfeed at night usually need to compensate with additional daytime breastfeeding sessions in order to maintain breastfeeding. Lynn's breastfeeding, for instance, ended around the eighth month due to the implementation of such an approach.

Unlike most women, however, Natalie had an exceptionally abundant milk supply. Furthermore, in contrast to Lynn, who worked full time outside the home, Natalie worked from home as a doctoral student and could nurse Alexander during the day. I believe that it was this unusual combination of circumstances that enabled her to continue to breastfeed her son successfully without any difficulties despite the institution of early nighttime separation. In fact, Natalie's milk supply continued to be very abundant, and Alexander's weight was in the 98$^{th}$ percentile during most of the study period. Thus, despite the fact that Natalie and Carsten were by far the first parents to move their child out of the bedroom for the entire duration of the night (which lasted about twelve hours for their son), this approach toward nighttime did not have any discernible negative consequences for Natalie's breastfeeding.[41]

The clash of capitalist work regimes that dictated Carsten's work and the bodily rhythms of their baby initially motivated Natalie's and Carsten's plan, thereby revealing the gendered challenges of negotiating conflicting temporal rhythms. An analyst can argue that this example illustrates a couple's response to a mother being split between her husband's and child's nighttime temporality. My conversations with Natalie, however, indicate that this plan also suited Natalie's own schedule, enabling her to spend time with her husband in the evenings as well as for her to sleep longer in the mornings. In fact, Natalie was ultimately in charge of both developing and implementing this plan, although Carsten sought and received support and encouragement from his colleagues as well. The spatial separation wherein Natalie relied on aural perception only—instead of the proximate visual, touching, and aural perception within the bedroom—enabled Natalie to feel more removed from these cues and to be able to delay responding to her son. This then led to increasing stretches of time that Natalie could use for sleeping. Consequently, Natalie became the ultimate arbiter of when her son's night began and ended, accommodating her own needs as well as limiting disturbance for her husband.

The fact that no other solutions were considered to address the potential nighttime disturbances—e.g., sharing the bed with the baby or having Natalie sleep next to the baby in a separate room—reflect the cultural primacy of the couple's sharing of the same bed and the importance of having children placed in separate rooms for the night. Although Natalie did not have the same cultural background for preparing the baby's room prior to his birth as most of the other participants, she quickly embraced the cultural value of creating a separate nighttime space for her child—a transition that was reinforced by Carsten's family's approach to children as well as his colleagues. This couple's approach illustrates that in aligning children with capitalist time regimes, the construction of spatiotemporal separation that reinforces the emphasis on self-sufficiency and autonomy remains a primary cultural objective. Because Natalie's and Carsten's approach did not produce any conflicts with continued breastfeeding, these ideologies of children's personhood were reproduced without any major revisions.

### Johanna's and Carl's "Crying It Out" Approach

Johanna and her husband began with a Co-Sleeper next to their bed in order to facilitate breastfeeding, but neither she nor her husband, Carl, felt comfortable sharing their bed with their baby, Haden.[42] Each time Johanna nursed her son, she would pick him up from the Co-Sleeper and then soothe him back to sleep and place him back into the Co-Sleeper. This was a strategy I described earlier that enabled Johanna to anticipate Haden's awakenings to a degree, but did not permit her to sleep through them. Johanna stayed at home to care for their son and thus could partly compensate for this sleep arrangement with daytime sleep, but she largely conformed her activity patterns to her husband's schedule, who worked full time outside the home. Although the frequency of their son's awakenings greatly diminished over time, the continuation of these regular awakenings began to wear Johanna down.

After an extended visit with her family, the couple settled in their new home in another city, where Johanna's husband began a new position. When they moved to their new home, they had a separate room for Haden, something they did not have in their rented home in Green City. The couple decided to use this as an opportunity to move Haden to his own room, motivated by the frequent awakenings Johanna experienced due to breastfeeding. They realized that although so-called "gentle" approaches to sleep training appealed to them, such as the book "The No-Cry Sleep Solution" (Pantley 2002), they did not feel that they had the "resolve" to follow through with such a "time consuming" strategy. They joked that this approach would have been better titled "The No-Sleep Cry Solution"—referring to parents crying over their lost sleep. Thus, they decided to put Haden in his crib and "let him cry for half an hour" without coming into the room to pick him up or feed him in response to the crying. This period lasted for a week, with the crying diminishing each day. In these early attempts this couple chose an authoritative method of conditioning their baby in order to train his body to comply with their own desires. The choice of this approach both stemmed from the fatigue of inadequate coordination of sleep as well as from the desire to adopt mainstream models of separate, continuous sleep for children.

Johanna and Carl developed a routine they both liked for getting Haden ready for bed, with one or the other of them using a bottle of expressed breastmilk to feed Haden and then rocking him, reading to him, and putting him to bed in his own room. This routine worked quite well for most of the next three months, with only one or two awakenings at night. Johanna "tried not to nurse" at night, instead asking Carl to go into Haden's room if he woke up before 7:00 A.M. This system therefore relied on Johanna's and Carl's willingness to work together and share the responsibilities of nighttime parenting. Bedtime crying disappeared quickly and, according to Johanna, "he got really good at going to sleep" on his own, laying down to bed wide awake, and smiling. In Johanna's language, their baby was acquiring a useful skill in being able to sleep on his own. Furthermore, similar to bed-sharing parents, Haden's behavior of smiling as he was placed in his crib was interpreted as evidence of the success of the parents' approach. Johanna's relief that the plan succeeded and her own sense of improved happiness and wellbeing indicated that this system also accommodated her own need for longer uninterrupted periods of sleep. [43]

Although the above routine worked well for the most part, there were also periods when she adjusted the system. Between five and six months, when Haden began to wake up more often, there were times when she, or sometimes her husband, slept with the baby for part of the night in his room since it had a single bed in addition to a crib. After a long time of being worried about sharing a bed with the baby because of safety concerns, Johanna became more comfortable with sleeping next to their baby because he had grown and matured over the months. But during one night when she breastfed many times during the night, something she referred to as "a marathon breastfeeding session," she pulled a muscle in her neck and had significant neck and shoulder pain for several days.[44] This discouraged her from sharing a bed and reinforced the importance of the separate sleep routine.

After a holiday visit to see family, however, the routine got derailed. Johanna had a much more difficult time putting her son to sleep awake and "got into the bad habit of putting him down asleep." In addition, Haden then also got sick, which made her worried about "letting" her baby cry for fear that his coughing would get worse. Thus, in this case Johanna accommodated her baby's temporal rhythm and adjusted her own body to it. During this visit, however, she also had the baby in bed with her for part of the night and re-injured her neck muscle due to a combination of the sleep position and tired back from carrying her baby in a front pack during the day. This is what ultimately prompted Johanna and her husband to revisit their sleep arrangements and change their approach once again.

Johanna and Carl decided to "let him cry in the middle of the night" without feeding or comforting Haden. On the first night, he cried for two hours and woke up crying again later. At this second awakening, Carl went in and helped put him back to sleep. After this night, Johanna no longer fed Haden at night. Johanna said that she would not have had difficulty getting up once during the night, but felt that there was no way to accomplish this without having to get up more frequently to soothe the baby back to sleep. Johanna's husband also felt that it would be too much work for him to soothe him back to sleep each time when she was not breastfeeding him. This example echoes the conflict between husbands' capitalist labor regimes and babies' nighttime temporality and the consequent fatigue women experience as they aim to accommodate both. Because Carl could not take on the nighttime burden of waking up regularly and soothing their son to sleep, the couple settled on no feedings at night.

On the second night, their son woke up and cried for twenty minutes and then went back to sleep, and on the third night he cried a bit and Carl held him to soothe him. Ultimately, after this third night Haden did not wake up crying at night. Johanna felt that breastfeeding at night was a "crutch" that impeded his ability to sleep longer.

Using the language of the crutch, a temporary device that people use to walk on their own, was particularly revealing about the sense that breastfeeding was something that interfered with their son's ability to develop independence. According to Johanna, once that "crutch" was removed, Haden was able to sleep and they were all much happier—once again providing justification for the approach in not only producing independent, self-sufficient sleep but happiness as well.

Johanna also instituted a similar approach at nap time, and systematically avoided nursing Haden to sleep before each nap. This reinforced the couple's overall approach, which emphasized the separation of breastfeeding from sleeping, encouraging their son to become increasingly self-sufficient in going to sleep. Johanna then monitored her breastmilk production, adjusting her pumping schedule to maintain a good milk supply. She felt that getting a full night of sleep was essential to her ability to maintain breastfeeding in the long run, which she was successfully continuing at thirteen months postpartum—well beyond the average time spent breastfeeding in the U.S.[45]

Johanna's and Carl's case introduces us to a much longer process of sleep training compared with Natalie's and Carsten's technique, wherein multiple different approaches are tried at different times to produce desired results. Unlike the couples whose use of mixed strategies of partial bed or room sharing led to a sustainable partial coordination of adults' and children's temporality, for this couple the degree of coordination was inadequate and, to a degree, undesirable. Like Natalie and Carsten, Johanna and Carl never planned to share their bed with their child and did not feel comfortable doing so. The delay in moving their child to a separate room was heavily influenced by spatial constraints in their rental home prior to their move to their own house. But unlike Natalie, Johanna's breastfeeding was much more tied up in spatiotemporal coordination. Even after their baby was in a separate room, Johanna accommodated frequent awakenings with frequent breastfeeding in response. Johanna's milk supply was also dependent on continued nighttime nursing as reflected by her need to monitor her supply and increase milk expression once night weaning took place. Finally, Johanna and her husband were more ambivalent about both the timing and desirability of attaining separate, continuous sleep than Natalie and Carsten.

Johanna's ambivalence was most clearly expressed in her episodes of sharing a bed with her son, first in his room, and later during a visit to her family. During these times, she experienced greater coordination of their sleep patterns and recalled enjoying being able to sleep next to him and breastfeed with ease, especially when Haden was frequently waking up to nurse. In both episodes of sharing a bed with Haden, and especially in leaving the bed she shared with her husband to sleep next to her son, Johanna challenged mainstream ideologies of sleep arrangements for parents and children. At the same time, each of these episodes ended with an embodied response that made it virtually impossible for Johanna to share a bed with Haden and prompted the couple to re-introduce the "cry-it-out" sleep training plan to readjust his sleep patterns toward a more culturally normative model. I suggest that Johanna's inability to share a bed with her baby was the result of the embodied moral ambivalence she felt toward this practice. The alternation between training their baby's body to perform continuous, separate sleep with episodes of coordinating parents' and their child's nighttime temporality also suggest the emergence of contingent embodied moralities—moments of change and renegotiation in light of conflicting ideologies of personhood and kinship. This ambivalence was shared by both members of the couple, echoed in Carl's own approach, wherein he also occasionally shared a bed with Haden but then also participated in instituting the sleep training plan (see chapter 5). Thus, although Johanna and Carl eventually largely reproduced dominant ideologies of personhood in their final success in sleep training, their embodied moral ambivalence resulted in the delaying of this process and the maintenance of conflicted or even multiple, situationally emergent modes of *habitus*.

This case illustrates that there is indeed fatigue resulting from the mismatch between the couple's temporality that is aligned with capitalist labor regimes and their temporality that embodies aspects of nighttime breastfeeding. The resolution of this misalignment involves careful negotiations of both members of the couple and underlines the cultural primacy of self-sufficiency in ideologies of children's personhood as well as in parents' authoritative role in producing this personhood.

*Seeking Rest Between the "Human Pacifier" and "Crying it Out"*

In chapter 6 I described how Petra and Julia renegotiated their sleep plans, extending Anders' stay in their bedroom by incorporating the Pack 'n Play, thereby delaying moving him to his own room for the night. At this time, they were generally satisfied with their sleep arrangements, although they did think about whether their approach ultimately would become problematic since they had heard from pediatricians and relatives that children need parents' help to sleep well. This "help" entailed getting the baby to sleep on his own instead of nursing him to sleep, moving him out of the room, and eliminating nighttime feedings. Their own resistance to this advice surprised Petra and Julia, since they had envisioned quickly moving their baby to his own room, which they had lovingly prepared for him. Now that their baby was born, however, they could not imagine being separated from him during the night. Petra and Julia were both willing to compromise their sleep in order to sustain the closeness they desired. Their reluctance thus challenged the couple's own understanding of their child's personhood as a relatively self-sufficient, already separate being as well as their own models of caring for their son that now entailed much more emphasis on proximate bodily interaction.

Similar to Johanna's and Carl's experiences, Anders also went through a period when he began waking up significantly more than he had done so before. This period coincided with Petra returning to her usual school teaching schedule after summer vacation.[46] Petra had been dreading this time, since she cherished the weeks she spent with her son without working outside the home. In fact, both Petra and Julia would much rather have stayed home with their son than worked full time. Petra's teaching position was a stressful job with many responsibilities that escalated over the course of the fall semester. To add to the stress of returning to work, Anders was also growing new teeth at this time. Because of the coincidence of several different sources of difficulty, it was impossible for Petra to tell which, if any, of these played the most important role in their son's new sleep pattern.

Petra reflected on her state of exhaustion: "I can't believe how little sleep I'm living on right now. To know that we were getting to the point that he was getting more sleep. I would get up to four hours [or] five hours [of] sleep in a row."[47] But now Anders was waking up regularly, almost mimicking the time when he was a newborn: "When I went back to work he was waking up one or two [times] a night, now he wakes up three or four times." Petra was willing to get up to breastfeed during the night, but the time squeeze from having to get up early for her work was making her delirious. "If I go to bed really early it doesn't bother me to get up three times, but some nights I am literally close to insanity." She was beginning to fear driving to work exhausted in the morning. Petra's description most clearly illustrates the conflict between capitalist time regimes and their baby's nighttime temporality. Because Petra was no longer able to compensate by following her son's bodily rhythms and taking naps or sleeping later into the morning as she did during her maternity leave, her body simply could not accommodate the stresses of an inflexible daytime work schedule compounded by commuting and the frequent nighttime awakenings that she could not sleep through. This example shows most acutely how mothers who themselves have to return to the work force shortly after birth are squeezed by the incompatible temporalities of capitalist labor and infants' breastfeeding needs.

Petra was clearly reaching her very limit in being able to cope. Julia was also growing concerned about her partner's wellbeing, and they began to contemplate a change in their sleep plan. One night they decided to act upon Petra's sister's and her pediatrician's advice and put Anders in his own room and let him cry instead of getting up to nurse him. This approach only produced more agony for them as they found it impossible to listen to his crying. They described this experience as "horrible." On another exhausting night, Petra found herself having fallen asleep with Anders in her arms. While they enjoyed having him near, they found that this arrangement resulted in nearly constant nursing at night, which prompted Petra to comment on how her son used her as a "human pacifier." Additionally, neither of them was able to sleep well with him in the bed.

During this period of employing different sleep strategies, competing ideologies of personhood clearly came to a head. The couple found the crying that was entailed in achieving solitary continuous sleep unbearable; to them the crying indicated that their son needed his parents and the comfort of breastfeeding. This pushed the couple back toward a model of emerging personhood that must be nurtured by intimate bodily care. Sharing their bed with their child, however, posed new problems. I believe that similar to Johanna's experience, Petra's and Julia's inability to sleep "well" next to their child was due to their embodied sense of moral ambivalence toward this practice, which they had not planned on and which was not supported by either their families or their pediatrician. Petra eloquently verbalized this ambivalence: "We're kind of at a loss because we tried to have him cry it out for a night and it's not our personalities ... we are lost in the middle. It's not our personalities to have him co-sleep with us in bed and it's not our personalities to have him cry it out." Petra's statement shows that parents' personhood is thoroughly enmeshed with that of their child's—producing the culturally sanctioned self-sufficient person also requires the production of a particular kind of parental personhood. Petra and Julia felt that they could neither accomplish this kind of personhood, nor the one that explicitly challenged the dominant model.

Toward the end of the year, during the holiday break, Petra and Julia began to put their son to sleep in his own room.[48] During the night Petra nursed him there instead of bringing Anders to their bedroom. Julia also went in for some awakenings and soothed Anders instead of Petra offering to nurse him. They both said that their son was generally happy with this arrangement, crying only occasionally and only for a few minutes. Petra felt that part of the success of this transition was due to the fact that she had been putting Anders down for naps in his crib all along, creating a familiar space for him in anticipation of this future transition. Anders began to sleep for longer stretches of time, giving Petra much-needed relief from the exhaustion.[49] In this final part of the sleep plan, the couple moved toward the dominant model of separate, continuous sleep, but only gradually so nearly a year after their son's birth. The production of continuous sleep was spatialized by removing Anders to another room and reinforced by Petra's similar nap-time routines. But the removal to another room occurred without separating the child from continued parental presence and care in response to awakenings, which was similar to some of the strategies employed by other couples using mixed arrangements. While separation and self-sufficiency were eventually accomplished during the night, the couple's embodied moral ambivalence offered the opportunity for significant reshaping and temporal delays in the culturally desirable mode of children's personhood as well as their own embodied parental relations with their child.

## Conclusion

In this chapter I described how couples' expectations of temporality were disrupted by the embodied praxis of nighttime breastfeeding. These disruptions were most often experienced as fatigue, resulting from the mismatch of parental spatiotemporal expectations and the embodied realities of frequent breastfeeding during the course of the night. Building on Thompson's observations, I highlighted the gendered dimensions of parental negotiations of these challenges, showing that mothers continue to bear a greater weight of the need to reconcile the temporal conflicts between capitalist work regimes and the caring of children. This conflict was heightened by the fact that only women can breastfeed,[50] and in this cultural setting breastfeeding is the sole responsibility of the biological mother. At the same time, I also showed that rather than women belonging to a pre-industrial time, similar to the characterization of non-western people by observers (Trouillot 2003), mothers and their partners navigated these temporal challenges in culturally specific ways in late capitalist U.S. society. Breastfeeding in this setting was not simply a matter of following "human tides," to use Thompson's phrase (1967: 79). Instead, breastfeeding was made possible by making a conscious commitment to it, which entailed the mobilization of a wealth of resources, including the relational resources of partners who were not physically breastfeeding but actively supported this embodied process.

Capitalism was implicated in the temporal aspects of breastfeeding and sleep in a multitude of ways, including the economic and biomedical construction of a "good time to have a baby," the daily rhythms of capitalist labor practices, and the embodiment of the biomedical temporal regimentation of women's lactation, infant feeding, and sleep. These temporal aspects of life have moral salience in how they are embedded in cultural expectations for children's personhood and parental personhoods, which are constructed in and through social interaction with one another.

The experiences of nighttime breastfeeding and sleep highlighted conflicts among these moral realms and revealed moments of moral ambivalence that produced substantial shifts in most participants' parental expectations for children as well as for themselves. Even when dominant ideologies were upheld, few parents were willing to implement the changes they perceived were necessary to conform to them within their previously anticipated time frame. I described how parents experienced moral ambivalence on an embodied level, manifested in difficulties with specific sleep arrangements, and suggested that multiple kinds of *habitus* emerged, were negotiated, and cultivated among parents in their attempts to reconcile these dilemmas. In conclusion, even amidst powerful constraints, these tensions gave rise to competing ideologies of personhood and kinship that subtly renegotiated the effects of capitalism in everyday life.

## Notes

1. See Apple 1987; Millard 1990; Stearns, Rowland, and Giarnella 1996; Simonds 2002. See also Whitaker 2000 for a comparative Italian example.

2. Dykes' (2009:212) ethnographic data includes a description of a mother's anxiety about getting her child to conform to a predictable pattern of feeding that would also facilitate placing her in a separate room.
3. McKenna, Ball, and Gettler 2007; McKenna and Ball 2010; Henderson et al. 2010.
4. Or other aspects of reproduction per Simonds 2002; McCourt 2009; McCourt and Dykes 2009; Dykes 2009.
5. Thompson explained that he put "pre-industrial" in quotes in order to show that such a division between pre-industrial and industrial societies in a nineteenth-century English context is a problematic one, since social and economic transformations associated with industrial capitalism were well on their way by that time period (1967:79–80). Nonetheless, the use of the term "pre-industrial" (even in quotation marks) to label women's temporal regimes warrants close analytical attention.
6. Many other scholars have commented and expanded upon Thompson's treatment of women's work and temporality. See for instance Everingham 2002; Maher 2009; McCourt 2009; McCourt and Dykes 2009.
7. Lefebvre 2000.
8. Moe and Shandy 2010.
9. Fieldnotes, January 7, 2007.
10. Fieldnotes, April 13, 2007.
11. Fieldnotes, May 25 and June 22, 2007.
12. Fieldnotes, February 13 and March 8, 2007.
13. See Hirsch and Wardlow 2006.
14. Fieldnotes, April 13 and August 6, 2007.
15. Fieldnotes, February 4 and May 20, 2008.
16. Fieldnotes, July 16, 2007.
17. McCourt and Dykes 2009; McCourt 2009; Dykes 2009, 2005, 2006; Davis-Floyd and Sargent 1997; Simonds 2002; Millard 1990; Martin 1987.
18. Fieldnotes, September 27, 2007, May 4 and November 30, 2008.
19. See Layne 2000.
20. See Inhorn and Van Balen 2002.
21. Fieldnotes, November 23, 2007.
22. Fieldnotes, July 10 and September 18, 2008.
23. Fieldnotes, September 26, 2007.
24. It was through discussions about the sleeping/feeding log that I first realized how little bed-sharing mothers awoke during night-nursing. This also led me to use any logs as points of discussion for experiences of the night (rather than its measurement in clock-bound modes) and to ultimately curtail the use of logs in the study in order to avoid tying participants' accounts to this framework.
25. Fieldnotes, July 19, 2007.
26. Fieldnotes, June 24, 2007.
27. Fieldnotes, March 20, 2007.

28. See Ekirch 2005; Thompson 1967; and chapter 2.
29. Fieldnotes, March 20, 2007.
30. Fieldnotes, March 8, 2007.
31. Fieldnotes, October 16 and December 20, 2007; April 18, 2008; see also chapter 4 for a detailed description of Jocelyn's experience.
32. Fieldnotes, June 19, 2007.
33. Fieldnotes, October 5 and 27, 2007.
34. Fieldnotes, October 5, 2007.
35. Fieldnotes, December 11, 2007.
36. This understanding itself did not replicate capitalist, mechanistic theories of child development, but instead approximated an organicist perspective described by Harkness, Super and colleagues (1996), but with significant modification of the erasure of environmental interaction in that model.
37. Fieldnotes, December 11, 2007.
38. Ibid.
39. Ibid.
40. Fieldnotes, October 27 and December 11, 2007.
41. Fieldnotes, June 4, 2008.
42. Fieldnotes, June 1 and 26, 2007.
43. Fieldnotes, February 5, 2008.
44. Ibid.
45. Fieldnotes, June 2, 2008.
46. Fieldnotes, October 25, 2007.
47. Ibid.
48. Fieldnotes, January 25, 2008.
49. Fieldnotes, July 10, 2008.
50. With some rare exceptions, see Giles 2003.

# Conclusion

In this book I have drawn on a diverse set of approaches to develop deeper insights into how middle-class U.S. parents negotiate the cultural complexities that surround breastfeeding and related sleep arrangements. I began by tracing the origins of why breastfeeding and related sleep arrangements are problematic in the U.S. and investigated the contradictory role of biomedicine in this process and feminist responses to this involvement. I then turned to my own ethnographic evidence to examine how the moral dilemmas of breastfeeding, especially nighttime breastfeeding, are shaped and negotiated by middle-class families in Green City. Using the ethnographic study of lived experiences of my participants as the core of my analysis, I shed light on how breastfeeding and sleep participate in making persons and kin relations, reproducing inequalities and local-global political economic relations. Throughout, I have insisted that paying close attention to the embodied moral dilemmas of breastfeeding and sleep illuminates not only how these larger processes constrain my participants' lives, but also how they actively shape and reformulate the social relations of which they are a part.

My research provides important new perspectives on conceptualizing the local and global landscapes of breastfeeding. My study points to the importance of considering diversity within biomedicine toward breastfeeding, especially to transform dogmatic approaches to infant sleep. The work of biological anthropologists continues to play a minor role in mainstream biomedical advice for breastfeeding and infant sleep and has been taken up in some problematic as well as helpful ways in breastfeeding promotion. Yet, biological anthropologists are in a unique position to appreciate the deep historical origins of breastfeeding and human sleep as well as contemporary biological variation in a cross-cultural context. Thanks to researchers' openness to insights from other areas of anthropology, such as that evidenced in the work of Ball, McKenna, and colleagues, I see this work as a locus of possibility for interdisciplinary collaboration that enables the production of more sophisticated scientific and biomedical work and ultimately leads to the provision of better support for new parents. The Infant Sleep Information Source (ISIS) website in the U.K., http://www.isisonline.org.uk/—a collaboration of Prof. Helen Ball and her research team at Durham University, La Leche League International, National Childbirth Trust (NCT), and UNICEF UK Baby Friendly Initiative, supported by a grant from the Economic and Social Research Council—is a pioneering example of this kind of work, which provides both professionals and parents with anthropologically-grounded research on infant sleep with a thorough consideration of its evolutionary context and relationship with breastfeeding. This research and its applications could be enhanced by greater participation of sociocultural anthropologists, who could help situate the study of embodied physiological interactions in the context of studies of social relationships. These collaborations could have a significant impact in transforming biomedical approaches to breastfeeding and infant sleep.

Another implication of my work concerns the role of public health efforts that promote breastfeeding. I have argued that advocacy that focuses solely on the product of breastfeeding and its biological properties and on mothers' moral responsibility to deliver these properties to their children fail on multiple levels. These approaches simultaneously make it easier to commodify breastmilk and replace it with other commercial products (e.g., the "human-like" milk made from Chinese transgenic cows) and perpetuate existing inequalities among families through the stratification of women who can or cannot meet these moral obligations. Unlike other scholars who believe that advocacy should be removed because of its problematic moral implications, I believe that such an approach would deny women's and their families' access to vital knowledge about their children's and their own bodies while also making them vulnerable to further exploitation via commercial interests. Both of these effects would significantly contribute to further reproductive stratification and embodied inequalities. Instead, I propose to reshape approaches to breastfeeding that focus on fostering and enabling the breastfeeding relationship within local cultural contexts while also providing rigorous scientific information about the role of breastfeeding in health. This approach necessitates a much more intense focus on social policies that reduce growing economic inequities in the U.S. by incorporating legislation that ensures access to adequate health care, work policies that account for the gendered dimensions of motherhood, and legislation that limits the unfettered proliferation of increasingly biocapitalistic regimes that facilitate corporate interests seeking profits from breastmilk substitutes.

Present-day U.S. politics serve as a powerful reminder of why academic discussions of breastfeeding should not simply be confined to esoteric ivory-tower debates but can have important social implications. Recent debates about breastfeeding in the U.S. have emerged in the larger context of the new and hotly debated Patient Protection and Affordable Care Act and the Health Care and Education Reconciliation Act, signed into law in March 2010 and upheld by the Supreme Court in June of 2012 after numerous legal challenges. These laws, which are at the core of the Obama administration's efforts to institute major health care reform in the U.S., aim to improve access to health care primarily through health insurance reform. The new law provides access to breaks and separate spaces for expressing breastmilk at the workplace (United States Breastfeeding Committee 2011)—provisions that have received increasing publicity since the law was signed into effect. Furthermore, due to letters written to the Internal Revenue Service (IRS) by a group of democratic senators, the IRS reversed a previous ruling, released in March 2011, which excluded breast pumps and related supplies from its tax deductible flexible health spending accounts. In the context of these two prior changes, Michelle Obama's mention of breastfeeding advocacy as a priority during a 2011 celebration of the completion of the first year of the "Let's Move" campaign targeting childhood obesity became a lightning rod for conservative criticism of government policies (Good Morning America 2011; Parnes 2011). Michelle Obama's effort to promote breastfeeding drew comment from Michele Bachmann (R-Minnnesota), who argued the tax break is an example of "social engineering" (Good Morning America 2011).

While Bachmann did not directly dispute the value of breastfeeding, since she emphasized that she breastfed her own five children, her response reflects significant resistance from Republicans and Tea Party supporters to state-sponsored advocacy and policies that aim to reduce social inequalities and thereby improve health. By claiming that breastfeeding is a matter of "choice" that should take place without state interference, Bachmann erased her privilege of being able to "choose" to breastfeed her five children and undermined the possibility of enacting social policies that would enable others to make similar "choices." Similar criticism has plagued New York City's recent "Latch On NYC" initiative, which provides support to mothers who choose to breastfeed, discontinues hospitals' routine use of infant formula unless medically indicated or requested by the mother, and prohibits the distribution of promotional infant formula (which usually arrive in hospital "goodie bags" and in "free samples") (Farley 2012). While some of the concerns about the program were raised by mothers who felt that the initiative interfered with their decision to feed their babies with infant formula, other criticism has targeted Mayor Bloomberg as the latest incarnation of the "Nanny State" that limits individual freedom and "choice" (Limbaugh 2012). Notably absent from this latter critique is a concern about the corporate influence asserted through the distribution of infant formula at hospitals or the acknowledgment of the role of support in producing better health outcomes for poor women and their babies.

In light of these political appropriations of the discourses of "choice" in debates about government-sponsored breastfeeding promotion efforts, it is essential that academics contribute a grounded and thoughtful perspective on breastfeeding. This perspective, as Penny Van Esterik has argued (1989, 2002, 2012), emerges from close study of the nexus of social relationships in which breastfeeding is engaged and incorporates attention to data from multiple realms, including branches of anthropology and biomedical research. Such an approach is particularly relevant for examining the role of breastfeeding in attempts to reduce racial and socioeconomic inequalities in health in the U.S. as well as in similar efforts to address global health disparities.

Anthropologically grounded research also has implications for global breastfeeding initiatives. Similar transformations in promotional efforts that I have suggested above are necessary to avoid reductionist approaches to breastfeeding (Gottschang 2007). These transformations must take place with close attention to the local cultural histories of breastfeeding and contemporary negotiations of infant feeding in the context of social relationships, including the dynamics of kinship, personhood, morality, the politics of reproduction and social divisions, and their entailments in political economic realms. These concerns remain salient for HIV prevention efforts as well. Although the 2010 World Health Organization guidelines are helping to restore an emphasis on protecting breastfeeding while reducing transmission of HIV from mothers to children, greater attention to the social context of breastfeeding will remain crucial as many women continue to lack access to appropriate HIV treatment during breastfeeding and beyond.

This book presents one possible approach, grounded in the experiences of a small set of participants, to the sustained anthropological study of nighttime breastfeeding and related sleep arrangements. Much more research is needed to provide comparative perspectives among different groups of participants from diverse racial, ethnic, and socioeconomic groups. The role of gender and sexuality in nighttime breastfeeding and sleep also warrants a great deal more attention. A similar ethnography among lesbian couples would be a very productive direction for investigating gender roles and division of labor in relation to nighttime breastfeeding. Additionally, while sexuality figures into breastfeeding and sleep arrangements in numerous ways—through the sexual objectification of breasts in the media and popular culture, the role of breasts in sexual practices as well as in the nourishment of children, concerns over inappropriate sexuality in breastfeeding and shared sleep arrangements, and the spatiotemporal location of sexual activities—I was not able to develop a systematic approach to the study of these issues. This was mainly motivated by desire to respect my participants and their concerns over maintaining their privacy; I was careful (perhaps overly so) not to cross these boundaries. Studies that more explicitly address sexuality in breastfeeding and sleep in their aims are necessary to explore this important dimension of the cultural ambivalence toward nighttime breastfeeding and bed sharing.

An ethnographic anthropological study of breastfeeding and sleep practices in the U.S. can yield rich insights that offer important opportunities for anthropological engagement with public health breastfeeding advocacy and provide new directions for future research. Scholars may find this study useful for opening new paths for investigating the landscapes of embodied social and moral relationships when parents embark on a journey to breastfeed their children. For parents who encounter this book, anthropological perspectives can shed light on some of the most challenging aspects of nighttime breastfeeding and sleep and offer an alternative to the polarized, and often hostile, discussions of these issues in the media. Ultimately, this book adds another voice to the growing chorus advocating for reforms that would help create a more equal, compassionate social and cultural environment, wherein all families are able to enjoy better support for these intimate, embodied ways of caring for their children.

# Appendix I
## Sleeping/Feeding Log

| Time | Sleeping (Y/N) | Sleep Location | Feedings | Other Activities, Notes |
|---|---|---|---|---|
| 6:00 p.m. | | | | |
| | | | | |
| 7:00 p.m. | | | | |
| | | | | |
| 8:00 p.m. | | | | |
| | | | | |
| 9:00 p.m. | | | | |
| | | | | |
| 10:00 p.m. | | | | |
| | | | | |
| 11:00 p.m. | | | | |
| | | | | |
| 12:00 p.m. | | | | |
| | | | | |
| 1:00 a.m. | | | | |
| | | | | |
| 2:00 a.m. | | | | |
| | | | | |

| 3:00 A.M. | | | | |
| --- | --- | --- | --- | --- |
| | | | | |
| 4:00 A.M. | | | | |
| | | | | |
| 5:00 A.M. | | | | |
| | | | | |
| 6:00 A.M. | | | | |
| | | | | |
| 7:00 A.M. | | | | |
| | | | | |
| 8:00 A.M. | | | | |
| | | | | |
| 9:00 A.M. | | | | |
| | | | | |

## Instructions for Infant Sleeping and Feeding Log

**Sleeping:** Please note whether your child is sleeping Y=yes N=no during the hours listed.

**Sleep location:** Please note where the child is sleeping, e.g. in crib, in parents' bed, etc. If another person(s) is sleeping next to the child, please note that person/those persons as well.

**Feedings:** Please note the approximate times when the child is being fed and what is being fed to the child, e.g. breastfeeding, formula, water, baby foods, etc.

**Other activities, notes:** Please note any other important activities and circumstances, such as if your child is sick, he or she is crying, he or she is awake and playing during the night, and any other circumstances you would like me to know about that might have affected your arrangements for the night.

# APPENDIX II

## TABLE OF DEMOGRAPHIC CHARACTERISTICS OF THE COUPLES INVOLVED IN THE STUDY[1]

| Race | |
|---|---|
| Euro-American (White) | 35 |
| Asian American | 1 |
| **Ethnicity** | |
| White, non-Hispanic | 35 |
| Hispanic | 1 |
| **Native Country of Origin** | |
| United States | 31 |
| Other (Canada, Europe) | 5 |
| **Residence** | |
| Green City | 30 |
| Surrounding towns | 6 |
| **Home Ownership** | |
| Own single family home[2] | 36 |
| **Education Level** | |
| Some college coursework | 1 |
| College | 17 |
| Advanced coursework or degree | 18 |

1. This table reflects demographic characteristics of both spouses from each couple, including those of the three spouses who did not formally participate in the study.
2. I am including Johanna and Carl in this category, since they bought a house during the course of the study.

| **Age** | | |
|---|---:|---|
| | 25–29 | 8 |
| | 30–34 | 22 |
| | 35–39 | 5 |
| | 40–44 | 1 |
| **Sexual Orientation** | | |
| | Heterosexual | 34 |
| | Lesbian | 2 |

# Appendix III
## Biographical Sketches of the Core Participants

Rachel and Nathan, a white couple in their late twenties, resided in their small home on a tree-lined street in Neighbor City with their cat. Most of Rachel's family lived close to the couple, and they regularly interacted with one another, although some of these relations were challenging. The couple was quite close to Nathan's family, who lived on the West Coast, and moved closer to them after the conclusion of the study. Rachel was a nurse at University Hospital, while Nathan completed his bachelor's degree in Green City and worked part time as a computer programmer. Rachel's and Nathan's desire for a child was complicated by male-factor infertility, which was ultimately resolved after some time. Rachel and Nathan attended childbirth education courses at Family Center and gave birth to their daughter Maya under the supervision of certified nurse-midwives at University Hospital with the assistance of morphine and epidural analgesia. Rachel breastfed Maya exclusively for the first six months and then continued for several months past the one-year mark. After a brief stay in a bassinet nearby, their daughter spent the remainder of the study period in their bed. Rachel returned to work part time after her three-month maternity leave, transitioning to full time later on. Nathan also shared the care of their daughter while working and studying. Since the conclusion of the study, Rachel and Nathan have welcomed their second and third children.

Leslie and Alex, a white couple in their early thirties, were Canadian transplants to Green City, where they owned a spacious home in a subdivision, which they shared with their cats. They moved here because of Alex's job as a highly qualified engineer in the auto industry in a nearby city, and Leslie, a lawyer, found a job at the university in Green City. Leslie and Alex attended childbirth education classes at Holistic Center and had their son, Connor, at University Hospital, attended by an obstetrician with the assistance of epidural analgesia and the support of a doula. Leslie breastfed Connor exclusively for six months and was continuing to breastfeed him at the study's conclusion. Connor slept in a bassinet only for a little while before Leslie and Alex decided to share their bed with him, where he remained for the majority of the night during the study period. After an extended leave, Leslie returned to her work full time at five months postpartum but eventually left it when she could not negotiate a part-time arrangement. She was studying for a master's degree in law during her hiatus from wage labor. Leslie's mother spent several weeks with the couple during Leslie's initial transition to work. Alex also took substantial additional time off to care for Connor when Leslie initially returned to work. Since the conclusion of my study Leslie and Alex welcomed their second child.

Petra (35) and Julia (33), both Euro-Americans, owned an older home that they had updated with their own touches at the end of a tree-lined street in Green City. Their family also included their very friendly dog. Both Petra and Julia were part of large families, and they were particularly close to Petra's mother and sisters. They married in a formal ceremony with their families and friends in attendance, although their union was not recognized in this Midwestern state. Petra commuted to her work as a schoolteacher in a nearby community, while Julia was an architect at a Green City firm. Petra conceived their son through artificial insemination with sperm from a donor with whom the couple has a personal relationship. Petra and Julia did not attend the longer childbirth education series but did take a breastfeeding course at Family Center. Petra's and Julia's son, Anders, was born with their family physician in attendance at University Hospital after Petra was unexpectedly diagnosed with preeclampsia and induced with Pitocin. Petra breastfed Anders exclusively for six months and was continuing with breastfeeding well beyond the first year at the end of the study period. Petra returned to work full time after her nine-week maternity leave, and Julia worked condensed hours to share the care of their son. Anders slept in a bassinet and later a Pack 'n Play in Petra's and Julia's room for the majority of the study period, transitioning to a crib in his room at the end of our time together. Anders also spent some time sleeping in the same bed with his parents during the course of the study and continued to do so during early mornings and on weekends. Petra and Julia were planning another pregnancy at the end of the study with the same donor, but Petra experienced complications that prevented her from trying again for some time. They were contemplating whether Julia would try for a pregnancy next or whether they would wait until Petra could try getting pregnant again.

Carol (31) and Justin (34), a white couple, owned a home in a subdivision in Green City that was filled with new parents and growing families. The community had a playground at its center and parks nearby. Justin's family lived nearby, and his cousin with her family lived in the same community. Carol was a social worker who also did part-time consulting prior to the birth of their son, Jeremiah, but took a break from employment to raise a family. Justin was a college-educated worker with additional qualifications in the auto industry and tested equipment. They were active in a local progressive Christian church. Carol transferred her care from an obstetrics practice to the certified nurse-midwives at University Hospital after a change in her insurance plan. Carol and Justin attended courses at Holistic Center and gave birth to Jeremiah without major interventions at University Hospital (they also received support from a young doula-in-training). Carol briefly introduced infant formula during a major breastfeeding crisis but otherwise went on to exclusively breastfeed Jeremiah for six months and continued breastfeeding for several months into his second year and began a second pregnancy. After a brief attempt at having Jeremiah sleep in a Co-Sleeper, Jeremiah mostly slept with his parents, later transitioning to part-time sleep on a mattress in his own room followed by returning to the parental bed for a large part of the night. Carol and Justin welcomed the birth of their second son a few months after the conclusion of my study.

Corinne and Jacob, a white couple in their early thirties, owned a home in Neighbor City that they shared with their cat and several other small pets. Corinne and Jacob both worked at the University in Green City, as a librarian and as a programmer, respectively. Corinne's mother and sister (with her own husband and children) both lived nearby, and they maintained a very close relationship with one another. Corinne and Jacob attended courses at Holistic Center and gave birth to their son, Finn, at University Hospital, attended by an obstetrician and supported by a doula. Corinne's labor was induced with prostaglandin gel because she was considered to have gone beyond the normal period of pregnancy. Corinne exclusively breastfed Finn for six months and continued to breastfeed him well into his second year of life. Corinne returned to work full time after her three-month maternity leave, with her mother caring for Finn throughout the study. After spending many days in his mother's and father's arms, several months of using a special hammock bed, and trying out sleep in a crib in his own room, Finn ended up sharing a bed with his parents. Corinne and Jacob have welcomed the birth of twins since the conclusion of this study.

Paula and Matthew, both in their late twenties, owned a home in a community within about half an hour driving distance to Green City. The home they shared with their dog and cat stood across from a large park and an elementary school. Paula was Euro-American, while Matthew was Asian American, with a Japanese father and a Euro-American mother. Both branches of the family resided in the state and maintained a close connection to the couple. Paula had taken some college courses but did not complete her degree and earned money as a nanny after marrying Matthew, who worked as a computer programmer. Paula and Matthew were very active in a local Baptist church and were unusual among participants in their conservative religious and political orientation. Paula had planned to take time off to raise a family. Paula and Matthew took childbirth education classed at Holistic Center. They were attended in labor by certified nurse-midwives and supported by a doula, but later received additional physician care for epidural analgesia and a Cesarean section. Paula exclusively nursed their son, Isaac, for six months and was continuing to breastfeed him at thirteen months while beginning her second pregnancy. After a few weeks of sharing his parents' bed, Isaac spent the first year sleeping within arm's reach of his parents in a bassinet, Pack 'n Play, and later a crib. Paula and Matthew moved Issac's crib into his own room toward the end of the study. Paula gave birth to the couple's second son (via an unmedicated vaginal birth after Cesarean section) a few months after the conclusion of the study.

Kate and Joshua, a white couple in their late twenties, owned a home in Neighbor City, where they were active in their local community organization. Kate was especially close to her sister and her family as well as her parents, all of whom lived nearby. Kate worked as a teacher prior to Anna's birth, but took an extended leave to care for their daughter and to work toward the completion of her master's degree. After completing his bachelor's degree, Joshua was employed as an ecologist at a local environmental center. Kate and Joshua experienced the loss of their first pregnancy a year earlier. In light of that difficult experience, they were both thrilled but also anxious about their second pregnancy. Kate and Joshua attended courses at Holistic Center and birthed Anna at University Hospital with certified nurse-midwives and their doula. Pitocin was used to speed up Kate's labor. During the course of the study, Kate's and Joshua's lives were profoundly affected by the illness and death of Kate's mother. Kate was intensely grieving while also raising her daughter. Kate exclusively breastfed Anna for six months and continued to breastfeed her in her second year. After some brief negotiations of the Co-Sleeper, Anna slept in Kate's and Joshua's bed. Joshua was one of the men in the study who took substantial time off to share their child's care. Kate and Joshua are now parents of three young children, two of whom were born after the conclusion of our study.

Bridget, in her late twenties, and Roland, in his late thirties, owned a home in Green City. Both Euro-American, Roland's roots were in Spain, where he still had a large family. Bridget's parents lived close by, and her mother was especially involved in trying to help Bridget during her difficulties after the birth of their daughter. Bridget worked as an administrator for the University in Green City, and Roland was a purchaser with long hours and a long commute. Roland's difficult work schedule did not permit him to formally participate in the study, but he was supportive of the project and welcomed my presence when we saw each other. The couple was thrilled that Roland was able to find a local job in Green City, which he started at the end of the study. Bridget followed Roland's faith tradition, and they attended Catholic church services regularly. Bridget and Roland enrolled in Holistic Center for their childbirth education courses and gave birth to their daughter, Angelina, at University Hospital with no major medical interventions, attended by nurse-midwives and their doula. Bridget used expressed breastmilk as well as infant formula during a very challenging start to breastfeeding but transitioned to exclusive breastfeeding by seven weeks postpartum. Bridget then exclusively breastfed Angelina until six months postpartum and continued with breastfeeding well into her second year. Angelina slept in multiple different configurations but mostly shared a bed with her parents throughout the duration of the study. Bridget returned to her job after three months of maternity leave, first part time (for four months), then full time. Since then, Bridget and Roland celebrated the birth of their second daughter.

Camilla and Erik, a white couple in their mid-thirties, shared a home and a large yard with their cats on the edge of Green City, next to a progressive church in which Erik's family actively participated. Camilla completed a master's degree at the university in Green City and taught piano part time. She took a break from students for the majority of the study period but began to teach more later on. Erik worked as an architect at a Green City firm. After challenges with infertility, Camilla and Erik successfully conceived and attended Holistic Center's courses. They gave birth to their daughter, Robin, at University Hospital, attended by midwives and a physician who was a close friend of Camilla's. Camilla had a very difficult labor and eventually received Pitocin and an epidural to facilitate progress, but the labor ended with a Cesarean section. Camilla exclusively breastfed Robin for six months and then went on to nurse her well into Robin's second year as she began a second pregnancy. After some time in the Co-Sleeper, Robin spent the remainder of the study period in her parents' bed. Camilla gave birth to the couple's second child via a successful unmedicated vaginal birth after a Cesarean section (VBAC).

Joy and Jonathan, a Euro-American couple in their early thirties, resided in their home in Green City, located on a tree-lined street across from a park accessed by (but away from) a major city road. Both of them had extensive family networks living nearby, including parents and siblings. Both college educated, Joy worked as an administrator at the university in Green City, while Jonathan had a relatively short commute to his work in the environmental field. Joy and Jonathan attended Holistic Center's courses and gave birth to their son, Graham, at Private Hospital, attended by certified nurse-midwives and their doula. Joy received Pitocin to speed up her labor and an epidural to reduce the pain. Joy exclusively breastfed Graham for six months and continued to breastfeed him for a few more months into his second year. Graham spent most of the first year in a Pack 'n Play in the same room with his parents, transitioning to sleeping in a crib in his own room toward the end of the study. Graham also spent some time in his parents' bed, particularly in the early mornings and on weekends. Joy took an extended unpaid leave from her work for six months and then quit her job when she was not able to negotiate a part-time arrangement. Joy and Jonathan celebrated the birth of their daughter (without medical interventions, attended by different midwives at University Hospital) a year after the study's conclusion.

Lynn and Gary, a white couple in their early thirties, lived in their small home in a community near a major interstate highway between Green City and the state's large industrial city. They lived nearlarge family networks, with Gary's parents living within blocks of their house, and Lynn's parents and sister close by. This couple differed significantly from most of my other participants in several respects. First, although they lived in a quiet area set off from the highway with sidewalks and tree-lined streets, this was a significantly more working-class neighborhood than those where other participants resided. Second, Gary worked as a welder in the nearby large metropolis and thereby held a blue-collar job, although one that paid relatively well. Gary had a previous marriage from which he had two other children, and his ex-wife and children lived in Green City. Due to his work hours and commitments to both sets of children, Gary did not participate in the study. In contrast to Gary, Lynn was a college-educated, white-collar administrator working at a nearby large corporation. Lynn and Gary attended Holistic Center's courses and gave birth to their son, Killian, at an alternative birthing center near their home with certified nurse-midwives and no interventions. Lynn breastfed Killian exclusively for six months but then had trouble maintaining her milk supply, and Killian became uninterested in breastfeeding by nine months. Killian spent his night in a Co-Sleeper next to his parents, then later in a Pack 'n Play as well as in bed with his mother (after Gary left for work), and then was moved to a crib in his own room around eight months. Lynn returned to her work full time after three months of maternity leave, and Gary took a substantial chunk of time off to ease this transition and care for Killian. Lynn kept in touch with me after our study meetings ended to share the birth of her second son and her decision to become a stay-at-home mother thereafter.

Johanna and Carl, a white couple in their early thirties, resided in a rented home in Green City. Carl, a postdoctoral fellow, was in the middle of an academic job search during the study period and was unable to participate due to his extensive commitments. Neither member of the couple had family networks in Green City, although Johanna maintained a close relationship with her family on the West Coast, visiting and talking to them regularly. Johanna was an elementary school teacher who took a break from employment to have a baby in this period of transition before the couple's move to a state in the South during our study period. I scheduled several meetings during Johanna's pregnancy as well as in the early months after their son's birth, and later followed Johanna through several long telephone conversations after their move halfway through the study period. Thus, my work with Johanna was partly ethnographic, but did not have the same degree of ethnographic continuity as I had experienced with other couples. Nevertheless, Johanna helped me compensate for this lack as best as she could, and I was able to follow her breastfeeding and sleep practices for thirteen months postpartum.

Johanna and Carl attended Holistic Center's courses, and gave birth at University Hospital, attended by certified nurse-midwives and a doula, with the aid of epidural analgesia. Johanna breastfed their son, Haden, exclusively for six months and was breastfeeding at our last conversation at thirteen months. Haden initially slept next to Johanna in a Co-Sleeper, followed by several transitional periods of sleeping in a crib in a separate room and sharing a bed with Johanna and Carl, eventually transitioning fully to sleeping in a crib in his own room. Johanna and Carl were planning on adding another child to their family at the time of our last conversation.

Adrianne and Doug, a white couple nearing their mid-thirties, lived in an older renovated home in Green City. Doug, an industrial scientist, worked nearby. Adrianne, a junior professor at the university in Green City, took unofficial time off in between her academic semesters to have their son, Cameron. This couple was the most highly educated among my participants, with both parents holding doctorate degrees from prestigious universities. Adrianne and Doug attended Holistic Center's classes and had Cameron at University Hospital, attended by an obstetrician with the support of a doula. Adrianne's labor was induced with Cervidil, but she received no further interventions. Adrianne exclusively breastfed Cameron for six months, continuing breastfeeding into his second year. Cameron slept in a Co-Sleeper next to Adrianne and, over time, began spending more time in the couple's bed, eventually fully transitioning to sharing the bed for the night. Since the conclusion of the study, Adrianne gave birth to the couple's second son.

Elise and Adam, a white couple just beginning their thirties, lived in their townhouse in Green City with their dog. Both had their family networks nearby and relied on the support of their parents, especially Elise's mother, during the study period. Elise, a doctoral student at the University, gave birth to the couple's son, Luke, between her semester of teaching and writing her book. Adam worked from their home in the music industry with a highly flexible schedule. Elise and Adam attended Holistic Center's courses and had Luke at University Hospital, with certified nurse-midwives and a friend in attendance and without any major interventions. Elise breastfed Luke exclusively for six months and was continuing breastfeeding in Luke's second year. Elise and Adam shared their bed with Luke for a few weeks before arriving at a part-time bassinet/bed-sharing arrangement, later transitioning to Luke sleeping in a crib in his own room for a few hours, followed by bed sharing with his parents. Since the ending of our study, Elise and Adam have welcomed the birth of their second child.

Angela and Oliver, both in their early thirties, grew up in Eastern Europe before immigrating to the United States. They resided in Green City in a spacious home on the side of a hill, surrounded by similar homes and tree-lined streets. When I first met them, they shared their home with Oliver's sister and her family. Although this family later moved to their own apartment, Angela and Oliver regularly hosted their parents and other visitors at their home. Angela and Oliver were delighted by their pregnancy, which came after major reproductive difficulties with in vitro fertilization. Angela was enrolled in a master's program in social work at the university in Green City and was working part time as a researcher. She took a semester off to care for the couple's son, Max, and then continued her studies and research part time. Oliver was a purchaser for a large corporation with a local branch in Green City. Angela and Oliver enrolled in Holistic Center's courses and decided to have a home birth attended by a certified practicing midwife (CPM) during that time. During labor, however, Angela developed a fever, which led the midwife to recommend a transfer to University Hospital, where she gave birth to Max via Cesarean section. Angela exclusively breastfed Max for six months and continued to breastfeed him in his second year of life. Max spent his early weeks in a Snuggle Nest in his parents' bed, followed by spending part of his time in a three-sided crib placed next to the edge of their bed and the rest of his time in between the couple. Angela and Oliver were surprised and delighted by an unexpected pregnancy and the birth of their daughter while in the process of beginning an adoption.

Jocelyn, who just turned thirty, and Samuel, who was in his late-thirties, were a Euro-American college-educated couple who lived in Green City in their small home on a tree-lined street with their cats. Jocelyn and Samuel also had family in the area, but most of their family members did not have a significant role in their everyday lives. In anticipation of future children, toward the end of the study they moved from this home to a more spacious one in a neighborhood located on a hillside close to an elementary school with less traffic nearby and lots of families with children. Jocelyn worked as an administrator at Green City's university and returned to work full time after eight weeks of maternity leave. Samuel worked at a local delicatessen and reduced his hours after the birth of their daughter, Deirdre, to care for her. He compensated by working from home, including during the night when Jocelyn was home and on the weekends. He was also able to take Deirdre to work with him for some work meetings. Of all spouses, Samuel spent the most time caring for his child and later went on to be a full-time stay-at-home Dad after the birth of their second child. Jocelyn and Samuel attended Family Center's courses and gave birth to Deirdre at Private Hospital, attended by certified nurse-midwives and a doula. Jocelyn received Pitocin to accelerate her labor but did not use additional interventions. Jocelyn breastfed Deirdre for six months exclusively and continued to breastfeed her at the end of the study. Jocelyn and Samuel experimented with various configurations of sleep arrangements, all of which entailed some degree of bed sharing, in combination with a bassinet next to their bed and a crib in another room, before arriving at a part crib/part bed-sharing arrangement that worked for them. Jocelyn and Samuel welcomed their second child, a son, after the conclusion of my study.

Kristen and Daniel, a Euro-American couple, resided in a community approximately fifteen to twenty minutes away from Green City, where they shared their home with their dog. They lived in a hundred-year-old house that had been in Kristen's family since it was built, and they had family networks nearby, including Kristen's mother, who cared for their daughter after Kristen returned to work. Kristen, in her late thirties, worked as a project manager at a large corporation, while Daniel, in his mid-forties, worked in information technology in a similar corporate setting. The couple actively participated in their Catholic church and had a large network of support from this community. Kristen and Daniel had not initially planned to have children but changed their mind and were thrilled by their pregnancy and the birth of their daughter, Simone. They attended Family Center's courses and gave birth at Private Hospital with an obstetrician. Kristen had difficulties with establishing and maintaining her milk supply, despite sustained effort and additional stimulation from an electric breast pump. Therefore, the couple supplemented breastfeeding with infant formula from early on. Kristen was later diagnosed with an autoimmune disorder, which likely contributed to these difficulties. Nevertheless, Kristen continued to breastfeed Simone until her eighth month, when she had to take medication that was potentially harmful for her daughter. Kristen struggled a great deal with this decision and only after researching the medications and postponing them for as long as possible did she decide to stop breastfeeding. Simone slept in a bassinet next to the couple's bed for the first two months, and then Kristen and Daniel moved her to a crib in her own room right next to their bedroom where she slept for the remainder of the year. She did, however, spend short periods of time in her parents' bed during the early weeks.

This couple experienced the effects of the financial crisis that was beginning to unfold toward the end of my study and resulted in large numbers of corporate layoffs. After returning to work from a brief eight-week maternity leave, which proved a very difficult transition for Kristen, she was laid off from her job midway through my study. A few months later, Daniel was also laid off from his company. At the time of our last meeting, Daniel thankfully secured a new position, while Kristen was unable to do so. While Kristen thoroughly enjoyed her unexpected time with Simone, this change caused some worries about the long-term financial implications of the lack of a second job in the family.

Natalie and Carsten, the final couple in my study, were Euro-American homeowners in their late twenties/early thirties, residing in a quiet, tree-lined Green City neighborhood with a park nearby. Natalie grew up in Eastern Europe and was completing her dissertation at the university during the study period. Carsten grew up part of a large, close-knit family that mostly still lived nearby (about forty minutes from Green City) and worked as a businessman at a corporation within commuting distance of their home. The couple enrolled in Family Center's courses and had their baby at University Hospital, attended by an obstetrician. After Natalie's labor did not progress, doctors first ruptured her membranes in an effort to facilitate labor. Natalie opted for an epidural because of exhaustion and pain and then received Pitocin as well, but the labor ultimately stalled and ended with a Cesarean section. Natalie exclusively breastfed Alexander for six months and continued to breastfeed him at the end of the first year. Alexander spent a short period of time sleeping in a bassinet near his parents' bed but was quickly moved to a crib in a separate room where he remained for the duration of the study. The couple planned to have more children after Natalie completed her studies.

# Bibliography

Abbott, Susan. 1992. "Holding On and Pushing Away: Comparative Perspectives on an Eastern Kentucky Child-Rearing Practice." *Ethos* 20 (1): 33–65.
Abu-Lughod, Lila. 1990. "The Romance of Resistance: Tracing Transformations of Power through Bedouin Women." *American Ethnologist* 17 (1):41–55.
Ajao, Taiwo I., Rosalind P. Oden, Brandi L. Joyner, and Rachel Y. Moon. 2011. "Decisions of Black Parents about Infant Bedding and Sleep Surfaces: A Qualitative Study." *Pediatrics* 128 (3):494–502.
AAP (American Academy of Pediatrics) Task Force on Sudden Infant Death Syndrome. 2005. "The Changing Concept of Sudden Infant Death Syndrome: Diagnostic Coding Shifts, Controversies Regarding the Sleeping Environment, and New Variables to Consider in Reducing Risk." *Pediatrics* 116 (5):1245–55.
———. 2011. "SIDS and Other Sleep-Related Infant Deaths: Expansion of Recommendations for a Safe Infant Sleeping Environment." *Pediatrics* 128 (5):E1341–67.
AAP (American Academy of Pediatrics) Work Group on Breastfeeding. 1997. "Breastfeeding and the Use of Human Milk." *Pediatrics* 100 (6):1035–39.
———. 2005. "Breastfeeding and the Use of Human Milk." *Pediatrics* 115 (2): 496–506.
ACOG (American College of Obstetricians and Gynecologists). 2008. "Home Births in the United States: ACOG Statement of Policy." http://www.acog.org [Accessed 20 April 2011].
ACOG (American College of Obstetricians and Gynecologists) Committee on Obstetric Practice. 2011. "Committee Opinion Number 476: Planned Home Birth." *Obstetrics & Gynecology* 117 (2):425–28.
Apple, Rima D. 1987. *Mothers and Medicine: A Social History of Infant Feeding, 1890–1950.* Wisconsin Publications in the History of Science and Medicine. No. 7. Madison: University of Wisconsin Press.
———. 2006. *Perfect Motherhood: Science and Childrearing in America.* New Brunswick, N.J.: Rutgers University Press.

Arber, Sara, Jenny Hislop, Marcos Bote, and R. Meadows. 2007. "Gender Roles and Women's Sleep in Mid and Later Life: A Quantitative Approach." *Sociological Research Online* 12 (5):3.
Arber, Sara J., and Susan Venn. 2011. "Caregiving at Night: Understanding the Impact on Carers' Sleep." *Journal of Aging Studies* 25 (2):155–65.
Armbruster, Heidi, and Anna Laerke. 2009. *Taking Sides: Ethics, Politics, and Fieldwork in Anthropology.* New York: Berghahn Books.
Asad, Talal. 1997. "Remarks on the Anthropology of the Body." In *Religion and the Body: Comparative Perspectives on Devotional Practices,* edited by S. Coakley. Cambridge, U.K.: Cambridge University Press.
Attachment Parenting International. 2008. "What Is API All about? API's Eight Principles of Parenting." http://attachmentparenting.org/principles/principles.php [Accessed 5 June 2011].
———. 2011. "Bottle Feeding." http://www.attachmentparenting.org/parentingtopics/bottlefeeding.php [Accessed 5 June 2011].
Avishai, Orit. 2004. "At the Pump: Lactating Bodies At Work." *Journal of the Motherhood Initiative For Research and Community Involvement* 6 (2): 138–49.
———. 2007. "Managing the Lactating Body: the Breast-Feeding Project and Privileged Motherhood." *Qualitative Sociology* 30 (2):135–52.
———. 2011."Managing the Lactating Body: the Breastfeeding Project in the Age of Anxiety." *Infant Feeding Practices, A Cross-Cultural Perspective,* edited by Pranee Liamputtong, 23–38. New York: Springer.
Bachelard, Gaston. [1958] 1994. *The Poetics of Space.* Boston, M.A.: Beacon Press.
Bahloul, Joelle. 1996. *The Architecture of Memory: A Jewish-Muslim Household in Colonial Algeria, 1937–1962.* Cambridge, U.K.: Cambridge University Press.
Bakhtin, Mikhail Mikhailovich. [1981] 1998. *The Dialogic Imagination: Four Essays.* Austin: University of Texas Press.
Baldwin, Peter C. 2002. "'Nocturnal Habits and Dark Wisdom': the American Response to Children in the Streets at Night, 1880–1930." *Journal of Social History* 35 (3):593–611.
Ball, Helen L. 2003. "Breastfeeding, Bed-Sharing, and Infant Sleep." *Birth* 30 (3):181–88.
———. 2007. "Bed-Sharing Practices of Initially Breastfed Infants in the First 6 Months of Life." *Infant and Child Development* 16 (4):387–401.
———. 2009. "Bed-Sharing and Co-Sleeping: Research Overview." *NCT New Digest* 48:22–27.
Ball, Helen L., Elaine Hooker, and Peter J. Kelly. 1999. "Where Will the Baby Sleep: Attitudes and Practices of New and Experienced Parents Regarding Cosleeping with their Newborn Infants." *American Anthropologist* 101 (1):143-151.
———. 2000. "Parent-Infant Co-Sleeping: Fathers' Roles and Perspectives." *Infant and Child Development* 9 (2): 67–74.

Ball, Helen L., and Kristin P. Klingaman. 2007. "Breastfeeding and Mother-Infant Sleep Proximity: Implications for Infant Care." In *Evolutionary Medicine and Health*, edited by W.R. Trevathan, E.O. Smith, and J.J. McKenna. Oxford, U.K.: Oxford University Press.

Ball, Helen L., and Lane E. Volpe. 2012. "SIDS Risk Reduction and Infant Sleep Location: Moving the Discussion Forward." *Social Science & Medicine* 79: 84–91.

Ball, Helen L., Martin P. Ward-Platt, Emma Heslop, Stephen J. Leech, and Kath A. Brown. 2006. "Randomised Trial of Infant Sleep Location on the Postnatal Ward." *Archives of Disease in Childhood* 91 (12):1005–10.

Barlow, Kathleen, and Bambi L. Chapin. 2010. "The Practice of Mothering: An Introduction." *Ethos* 38 (4):324–38.

Barry, Herbert, and Lenora M. Paxson. 1971. "Infancy and Early Childhood: Cross-Cultural Codes 2." *Ethnology* 10 (4):466–508.

Bartick, Melissa. 2006. "Bed Sharing with Unimpaired Parents Is Not an Important Risk for Sudden Infant Death Syndrome: To the Editor." *Pediatrics* 117 (3):992.

Bartle, Carol. 2010. "Going with the Flow: Contemporary Discourses of Donor Breastmilk Use and Breastmilk in a Neonatal Intensive Care Setting." In *Giving Breastmilk: Body Ethics and Contemporary Breastfeeding Practices*, edited by A. Bartlett and R. Shaw. Toronto: Demeter Press.

Bartlett, Alison. 2005. "Maternal Sexuality and Breastfeeding." *Sex Education: Sexuality, Society and Learning* 5 (1):67–77.

Bartlett, Alison, and Rhonda Shaw. 2010. "Mapping the Ethics and Politics of Contemporary Breastmilk Exchange: An Introduction." In *Giving Breastmilk: Body Ethics and Contemporary Breastfeeding Practice*, edited by R. Shaw and A. Bartlett. Toronto: Demeter Press.

Basso, Keith H. 1996. *Wisdom Sits in Places: Landscape and Language among the Western Apache*. Albuquerque: University of New Mexico Press.

Battersby, Susan. 2007. "Not in Public Please: Breastfeeding as Dirty Work in the UK." In *Exploring the Dirty Side of Women's Health*, edited by M. Kirkham. London: Taylor & Francis.

BBC News. 2009. "Room to Swing A Cat? Hardly." *BBC News Magazine*, 15 August 2009. http://news.bbc.co.uk/2/hi/8201900.stm [Accessed 20 October 2012].

Beasley, Annette Noble. 1996. *Breastfeeding for the First Time: A Critical-Interpretative Perspective on Experience and the Body Politic*. Palmerston North, N.Z.: Dept. of Social Anthropology, Massey University.

Beidelman, Thomas O. 1986. *Moral Imagination in Kaguru Modes of Thought*. Indianapolis: Indiana University Press.

Ben-Ari, Eyal. 1996. "From Mothering to Othering: Organization, Culture, and Nap Time in a Japanese Day-Care Center." *Ethos* 24 (1):136–64.

———. 2008. "'It Is Bedtime' in the World's Urban Middle Classes: Children, Families and Sleep." In *Worlds of Sleep*, edited by L. Brunt and B. Steger. Berlin: Frank & Timme.

Betran, Ana P., Mario Merialdi, Jeremy A. Lauer, Wang Bing-Shun, Jane Thomas, Paul Van Look, and Marsden Wagner. 2007. "Rates of Caesarean Section: Analysis of Global, Regional and National Estimates." *Paediatric and Perinatal Epidemiology* 21 (2):98–113.

Bharadwaj, Aditya. 2010. "Reproductive Viability and the State: Embryonic Stem Cell Research in India." In *Globalization, Reproduction and the State: New Theoretical and Ethnographic Perspectives*, edited by C. Browner and C. Sargent. Durham, N.C.: Duke University Press.

Bianchera, E., and S. Arber. 2007. "Caring and Sleep Disruption among Women in Italy." *Sociological Research Online* 12 (5):4.

Blair, Peter S. 2010. "Perspectives on Bed-Sharing." *Current Pediatric Reviews* 6 (1):67–70.

Blair, Peter S., Jon Heron, and Peter J. Fleming. 2010. "Relationship between Bed Sharing and Breastfeeding: Longitudinal, Population-Based Analysis." *Pediatrics* 126 (5):E1119.

Blum, Linda M. 1999. *At the Breast: Ideologies of Breastfeeding and Motherhood in the Contemporary United States*. Boston, M.A.: Beacon Press.

Bobel, Chris G. 2001. "Bounded Liberation: A Focused Study of La Leche League International." *Gender and Society* 15 (1):130–51.

———. 2002. *The Paradox of Natural Mothering*. Philadelphia: Temple University Press.

Borst, Charlotte. 1995. *Catching Babies: The Professionalization of Childbirth, 1870–1920*. Boston: Harvard University Press.

Bourdieu, Pierre. 1977. *Outline of a Theory of Practice*. No. 16, *Cambridge Studies in Social Anthropology*. Cambridge, U.K.: Cambridge University Press.

———. 1990. *The Logic of Practice*. Palo Alto, C.A.: Stanford University Press.

Bradley, Robert A. 2008. *Husband-Coached Childbirth: The Bradley Method of Natural Childbirth*. 5th ed. New York: Bantam Books.

Bridges, Khiara M. 2011. *Reproducing Race: An Ethnography of Pregnancy as a Site of Racialization*. Oakland: University of California Press.

Britton, Cathryn. 1998. "'Feeling Letdown': An Exploration of an Embodied Sensation Associated with Breastfeeding." In *The Body in Everyday Life*, edited by S. Nettleton and J. Watson. New York: Routledge.

Brody, Howard. 2010. "Professional Medical Organizations and Commercial Conflicts of Interest: Ethical Issues." *The Annals of Family Medicine* 8 (4):354.

Brondo, Keri Vacanti, Linda Bennett, Harmony Farner, and Cindy Martin. 2009. "Work Climate, Gender, and the Status of Practicing Anthropologists." Report Commissioned by the Committee on the Status of Work.

Brown, Tamara Mose, and Erynn Masi de Casanova. 2010. "Mothers in the Field: How Motherhood Shapes Fieldwork and Researcher-Subject Relations." *WSQ: Women's Studies Quarterly* 37 (2):42–57.

Browner, Carole H., and Carolyn F. Sargent. 2011. "Toward Global Anthropological Studies of Reproduction: Concepts, Methods, Theoretical Approaches." In *Reproduction, Globalization, and the State: New Theoretical and*

*Ethnographic Approaches*, edited by C. Browner and C. Sargent. Durham, N.C.: Duke University Press.
Brunt, Lodewijk, and Brigitte Steger, eds. 2008. *Worlds of Sleep*. Berlin: Frank & Timme.
Bryant, Joanne, Maree Porter, Sally K. Tracy, and Elizabeth A. Sullivan. 2007. "Caesarean Birth: Consumption, Safety, Order, and Good Mothering." *Social Science & Medicine* 65 (6):1192–1201.
Bryant, Kristen. 2010. "The Role of Consumption in Constructing the Moral Identity of a 'Parent.'" *The Berkeley McNair Research Journal* 17:15–27.
Bunzl, Matti. 2004. "Boas, Foucault, and the 'Native Anthropologist': Notes toward a Neo-Boasian Anthropology." *American Anthropologist* 106 (3): 435–42.
Burgard, S.A. 2011. "The Needs of Others: Gender and Sleep Interruptions for Caregivers." *Social Forces* 89 (4):1189–1215.
Burns, E., Virginia Schmied, A. Sheehan, and J. Fenwick. 2009. "A Meta-Ethnographic Synthesis of Women's Experience of Breastfeeding." *Maternal & Child Nutrition* 6 (3):201–19.
Calnen, Gerald. 2007. "Paid Maternity Leave and Its Impact on Breastfeeding in the United States: An Historic, Economic, Political, and Social Perspective." *Breastfeeding Medicine: The Official Journal of the Academy of Breastfeeding Medicine* 2 (1):34–44.
———. 2010. "The Impact of Maternity Leave on Breastfeeding Rates." *Breastfeeding Medicine: The Official Journal of the Academy of Breastfeeding Medicine* 5 (5):233–34.
Campo, Monica. 2010. "The Lactating Body and Conflicting Ideals of Sexuality, Motherhood and Self." In *Giving Breastmilk: Body Ethics and Contemporary Breastfeeding Practice*, edited by R. Shaw and A. Bartlett. Toronto: Demeter Press.
Carrithers, Michael, Steven Collins, and Steven Lukes. 1985. *The Category of the Person: Anthropology, Philosophy, History*. Cambridge, U.K.: Cambridge University Press.
Carsten, Janet. 1995. "The Substance of Kinship and the Heat of the Hearth: Feeding, Personhood, and Relatedness among Malays in Pulau Langkawi." *American Ethnologist* 22 (2):223–41.
———. 1997. *The Heat of the Hearth: The Process of Kinship in a Malay Fishing Community*. Oxford, U.K.: Oxford University Press.
———. 2004. *After Kinship*. Cambridge, U.K.: Cambridge University Press.
Carsten, Janet, and Stephen Hugh-Jones. 1995. *About the House: Levi-Strauss and Beyond*. Cambridge, U.K.: Cambridge University Press.
Carter, Pam. 1995. *Feminism, Breasts and Breast-Feeding*. New York: St. Martin's Press.
Cassidy, Tanya, and Abdullahi El-Tom. 2010. "Comparing Sharing and Banking Milk: Issues of Gift Exchange and Community in the Sudan and Ireland." In *Giving Breastmilk: Body Ethics and Contemporary Breastfeeding Practice*, edited by R. Shaw and A. Bartlett. Toronto: Demeter Press.

Caudill, William, and David W. Plath. 1966. "Who Sleeps by Whom? Parent-Child Involvement in Urban Japanese Families." *Psychiatry: Journal for the Study of Interpersonal Processes* (4):344–66.

CDC (Centers For Disease Control and Prevention). 2010a. "Breastfeeding among U.S. Children Born 1999–2007." CDC National Immunization Survey. http://www.cdc.gov/breastfeeding/data/nis_data/index.htm [Accessed 20 April 2010].

———. 2010b. "Breastfeeding Report Card: United States, 2010." Centers For Disease Control and Prevention. http://www.cdc.gov/breastfeeding/data/reportcard/reportcard2010.htm [Accessed 22 October 2012].

———. 2010c. "Racial and Ethnic Differences in Breastfeeding Initiation and Duration, by State. National Immunization Survey, United States, 2004–2008." *Morbidity Mortality Weekly Report* 59 (11):327–34.

———. 2012. "Breastfeeding Report Card: United States 2012." Department of Health and Human Services, Centers For Disease Control and Prevention. http://www.cdc.gov/breastfeeding/pdf/2012breastfeedingreportcard.pdf [Accessed 16 September 2012].

———. 2013a. "Breastfeeding Report Card: United States 2013. Department of Health and Human Services, Centers For Disease Control and Prevention. http://www.cdc.gov/breastfeeding/pdf/2013breastfeedingreportcard.pdf [Accessed 18 April 2014].

———. 2013b. "Progress in Increasing Breastfeeding and Reducing Racial/Ethnic Differences — United States, 2000–2008 Births." *Morbidity Mortality Weekly Report* 62 (05):77–80.

Charles, Camille Z. 2003. "The Dynamics of Racial Residential Segregation." *Annual Review of Sociology* 29:167–207.

Chianese, J., D. Ploof, C. Trovato, and J.C. Chang. 2009. "Inner-City Caregivers' Perspectives on Bed Sharing with their Infants." *Academic Pediatrics* 9 (1):26–32.

Clarke, Adele E., Janet K. Shim, Laura Mamo, Jennifer Ruth Fosket, and Jennifer R. Fishman. 2003. "Biomedicalization: Technoscientific Transformations of Health, Illness, and U.S. Biomedicine." *American Sociological Review* 68:161–94.

Clarke, Alison J. 2004. "Maternity and Materiality: Becoming a Mother in Consumer Culture." In *Consuming Motherhood*, edited by J.S. Taylor and L.L. Layne. New Brunswick, N.J.: Rutgers University Press.

Cohen, Lawrence. 2005. "Operability, Bioavailability, and Exception." In *Global Assemblages: Technology, Politics and Ethics as Anthropological Problems*, edited by A. Ong and S.J. Collier. New York: Blackwell.

Collier, Jane F., and Sylvia J. Yanagisako. 1987. *Gender and Kinship: Essays toward a Unified Analysis*. Palo Alto, C.A.: Stanford University Press.

Collier, Stephen J., and Aihwa Ong. 2005. "Global Assemblages, Anthropological Problems." In *Global Assemblages: Technology, Politics and Ethics as Anthropological Problems*, edited by A. Ong and S.J. Collier. Malden, M.A.: Wiley-Blackwell.

Collins, Jane L., Brett Williams, and Micaela di Leonardo. 2008. *New Landscapes of Inequality: Neoliberalism and the Erosion of Democracy in America.* Santa Fe, N.M.: School for Advanced Research Press.
Cone, Thomas E. 1981. *History of American Pediatrics.* New York: Little, Brown.
Cook, Emma. 2010. "Mothers Who Breastfeed Beyond Babyhood: Can Breastfeeding Really Be Good For Older Children? Emma Cook Meets Mothers Who Keep Going Up to School Age and Beyond." *The Guardian,* 9 January 2010. http://www.theguardian.com/lifeandstyle/2010/jan/09/breastfeeding-older-children [Accessed 4 March 2011].
Craven, Christa. 2010. *Pushing For Midwives: Homebirth Mothers and the Reproductive Rights Movement.* Philadelphia: Temple University Press.
Creed, Gerald W. 2000. "'Family Values' and Domestic Economies." *Annual Review of Anthropology* 29:329–55.
Crook, Thomas. 2008. "Norms, Forms and Beds: Spatializing Sleep in Victorian Britain." *Body & Society* 14 (4):15–35.
Crossley, Nick. 2007. "Researching Embodiment by Way of 'Body Techniques.'" *The Sociological Review* 55 (S1):80–94.
Crowther, Stefania M., Lois A. Reynolds, and Tilli M. Tansey. 2009. *The Resurgence of Breastfeeding, 1975–2000.* London: Wellcome Trust Centre for the History of Medicine at University College London.
Csordas, Thomas J. 1990. "Embodiment as a Paradigm for Anthropology." *Ethos* 18 (1):5–47.
———. 1994. *Embodiment and Experience: The Existential Ground of Culture and Self.* Cambridge, U.K.: Cambridge University Press.
———. 2002. *Body/Meaning/Healing.* New York: Palgrave Macmillan.
Cunnigham, F. Gary, Kenneth L. Leveno, Steven L. Bloom, John Hauth, Dwight Rouse, and Catherine Spong. 2009. "Pregnancy Hypertension." In *Williams Obstetrics,* edited by F.G. Cunnigham, K.L. Leveno, S.L. Bloom, J. Hauth, D. Rouse, and C. Spong. New York: McGraw-Hill.
D'Emilio, J., and E.B. Freedman. 1998. *Intimate Matters: A History of Sexuality in America.* Chicago: University of Chicago Press.
Daniel, Valentine E. 1984. *Fluid Signs: Being a Person the Tamil Way.* Berkeley: University of California Press.
Davis-Floyd, Robbie. 2004. *Birth as an American Rite of Passage.* 2nd ed. Berkeley: University of California Press.
Davis-Floyd, Robbie, and Melissa Cheyney. 2009. "Birth and the Big Bad Wolf: An Evolutionary Perspective." In *Childbirth Across Cultures: Ideas and Practices of Pregnancy, Childbirth and the Postpartum,* edited by H. Selin and P.K. Stone. New York: Springer.
Davis-Floyd, Robbie, and Carolyn Fishel Sargent, eds. 1997. *Childbirth and Authoritative Knowledge: Cross-Cultural Perspectives.* Berkeley: University of California Press.
Declercq, Eugene. 2011. "Where We Stand in Improving Maternity Care. Keynote Presentation." In *Reframing Birth and Breastfeeding: Moving Forward Symposium.* Chapel Hill: University of North Carolina.

Declercq, Eugene, Miriam H. Labbok, Carol Sakala, and M.A. O'Hara. 2009. "Hospital Practices and Women's Likelihood of Fulfilling their Intention to Exclusively Breastfeed." *American Journal of Public Health* 99 (5):929.

Dettwyler, Katherine A. 1988. "More than Nutrition: Breastfeeding in Urban Mali." *Medical Anthropology Quarterly* 2 (2):172–83.

———. 1995. "Beauty and the Breast: The Cultural Context of Breastfeeding in the United States." In *Breastfeeding: Biocultural Perspectives*, edited by K.A. Dettwyler and P. Stuart-Macadam. New York: Aldine.

Di Leonardo, Micaela. 1987. "The Female World of Cards and Holidays: Women, Families, and the Work of Kinship." *Signs* 12 (3):440–53.

Donohue-Carey, Patricia. 2002. "Solitary or Shared Sleep: What's Safe?" *Mothering Magazine* 114 (September/October):39–45.

Dudgeon, M.R., and M.C. Inhorn. 2009. "Gender, Masculinity, and Reproduction: Anthropological Perspectives." In *Reconceiving the Second Sex: Men, Masculinity, and Reproduction*, edited by M.C. Inhorn, T. Tjornhoj-Thomsen, H. Goldberg, and M. La Cour Mosegaard. New York: Berghahn Books.

Durkheim, Emile. [1895] 1982. *The Rules of Sociological Method*. New York: Simon & Schuster.

Dykes, Fiona. 2005. "'Supply' and 'Demand': Breastfeeding as Labour." *Social Science & Medicine* 60 (10):2283–93.

———. 2006. *Breastfeeding in Hospital: Mothers, Midwives and the Production Line*. Oxon, O.X.: Routledge.

———. 2009. "'Feeding All the Time': Women's Temporal Dilemmas around Breastfeeding in Hospital." In *Childbirth, Midwifery and Concepts of Time*, edited by C. McCourt. New York: Berghahn Books.

Eats on Feets. 2011. "About Eats on Feets." http://www.eatsonfeets.org/ [Accessed 20 June 2011].

Edelman, Marc, and Angelique Haugerud. 2005. *The Anthropology of Development and Globalization: From Classical Political Economy to Contemporary Neoliberalism*. Malden, M.A.: Wiley-Blackwell.

Eidelman, Arthur I., and Lawrence M. Gartner. 2006. "Bed Sharing with Unimpaired Parents Is Not an Important Risk for Sudden Infant Death Syndrome: To the Editor." *Pediatrics* 117 (3):991.

Ekirch, A. Roger. 2005. *At Day's Close: A History of Nighttime*. London: Weidenfeld & Nicolson.

Elias, Marjorie F., Nancy A. Nicolson, Carolyn Bora, and Johanna Johnston. 1986. "Sleep/Wake Patterns of Breast-Fed Infants in the First 2 Years of Life." *Pediatrics* 77 (3):322.

England, Pam, and Rob Horowitz. 1998. *Birthing from Within: An Extra-Ordinary Guide to Childbirth Preparation*. Albuquerque, N.M.: Partera Press.

Everingham, Christine 2002. "Engendering Time Gender Equity and Discourses of Workplace Flexibility." *Time & Society* 11 (2–3):335–51.

Faircloth, Charlotte. 2009. "Mothering as Identity-Work: Long-Term Breastfeeding and Intensive Motherhood." *Anthropology News* 50 (2):15–17.

---. 2010a. "'If They Want to Risk the Health and Well-Being of their Child, That's Up to them': Long-Term Breastfeeding, Risk and Maternal Identity." *Health, Risk & Society* 12 (4):357–67.

---. 2010b. "'What Science Says Is Best': Parenting Practices, Scientific Authority and Maternal Identity." *Sociological Research Online* 15 (4):4.

Fallone, Gahan, Judith A. Owens, and Jennifer Deane. 2002. "Sleepiness in Children and Adolescents: Clinical Implications." *Sleep Medicine Reviews* 6 (4):287–306.

Farley, Thomas. 2012. "Latch On NYC: A Hospital-Based Initiative to Support a Mother's Decision to Breastfeed." New York City Department of Health and Mental Hygiene. http://www.nyc.gov/html/doh/downloads/pdf/ms/initiative-description.pdf [Accessed 22 September 2012].

Faubion, James D. 2011. *An Anthropology of Ethics.* New York: Cambridge University Press.

Feeley-Harnik, Gillian. 2001. "The Ethnography of Creation: Lewis Henry Morgan and the American Beaver." In *Relative Values: Reconfiguring Kinship Studies,* edited by S. Franklin and S. McKinnon. Durham, N.C.: Duke University Press.

Ferber, Richard. 2006. *Solve Your Child's Sleep Problems.* rev. ed. New York: Fireside.

Ferguson, J. 2010. "The Uses of Neoliberalism." *Antipode* 41 (S1):166–84.

Foss, Katherine A. 2012. "'That's Not A Beer Bong, It's A Breast Pump!' Representations of Breastfeeding in Prime-Time Fictional Television." *Health Communication* 28(4):329–40.

Foster, Anneke. 2010. "Cafe Manager Berates Breastfeeding Mom." *ABC News,* 13 May 2010. http://abcnews.go.com/WhatWouldYouDo/breastfeeding-mom-harrassedrestaurant/story?id=10627999 [Accessed 20 April, 2011].

Foucault, Michel. 1990. *The History of Sexuality Vol. 1.* New York: Vintage.

Franklin, Sarah. 1997. *Embodied Progress: A Cultural Account of Assisted Conception.* New York: Routledge.

Franklin, Sarah, and Margaret Lock, eds. 2003. *Remaking Life & Death: Toward an Anthropology of the Biosciences.* Santa Fe, N.M.: School of American Research Press.

Franklin, Sarah, and Susan McKinnon, eds. 2001. *Relative Values: Reconfiguring Kinship Studies.* Durham, N.C.: Duke University Press.

Fraser, Gertrude J. 1998. *African American Midwifery in the South: Dialogues of Birth, Race, and Memory.* Cambridge, M.A.: Harvard University Press.

Galtry, Judith. 2000. "Extending the 'Bright Line': Feminism, Breastfeeding, and the Workplace in the United States." *Gender and Society* (2):295–317.

---. 2001. "Suckling and Silence in the USA: The Costs and Benefits of Breastfeeding." *Feminist Economics* 3 (3):1–24.

---. 2003. "The Impact on Breastfeeding of Labour Market Policy and Practice in Ireland, Sweden, and the USA." *Social Science & Medicine* 57 (1):167–77.

Galtry, Judith, and Paul Callister. 2005. "Assessing the Optimal Length of Parental Leave For Child and Parental Well-Being: How Can Research Inform Policy?" *Journal of Family Issues* 26 (2):219–46.

Gartner, Lawrence M. 1994. "Neonatal Jaundice." *Pediatrics in Review* 15 (11):422.

Gatrell, Caroline Jane. 2007. "Secrets and Lies: Breastfeeding and Professional Paid Work." *Social Science & Medicine* 65 (2):393–404.

———. 2011. "Managing the Maternal Body: A Comprehensive Review and Transdisciplinary Analysis." *International Journal of Management Reviews*.

Gerson, Kathleen. 1993. *No Man's Land: Men's Changing Commitments to Family and Work*. New York: Basic Books.

Gessner, Bradford D., and Thomas J. Porter. 2006. "Bed Sharing with Unimpaired Parents Is Not an Important Risk for Sudden Infant Death Syndrome: Letter to the Editor." *Pediatrics* 117 (3):990.

Gettler, Lee T., and James J. McKenna. 2010. "Never Sleep with Baby? Or Keep Me Close But Keep Me Safe: Eliminating Inappropriate Safe Infant Sleep Rhetoric in the United States." *Current Pediatric Reviews* 6 (1):71–77.

———. 2011. "Evolutionary Perspectives on Mother-Infant Sleep Proximity and Breastfeeding in a Laboratory Setting." *American Journal of Physical Anthropology* 144 (3):454–62.

Giles, Fiona. 2003. *Fresh Milk: The Secret Life of Breasts*. New York: Simon and Schuster.

Ginsburg, Faye D. 1998. *Contested Lives: The Abortion Debate in an American Community*. Berkeley: University of California Press.

Ginsburg, Faye D., and Rayna Rapp. 1995. *Conceiving the New World Order: The Global Politics of Reproduction*. Berkeley: University of California Press.

Goffman, Erving. [1963] 1986. *Stigma: Notes on the Management of Spoiled Identity*. New York: Touchstone.

Golden, Janet L. 1996. *A Social History of Wet Nursing in America: From Breast to Bottle*. New York: Cambridge University Press.

Good Morning America. 2011. "Michele Bachman vs. First Lady." ABC News video, 5:52, 17 February 2011. http://abcnews.go.com/Gma/Video/Michele-Bachmann-At-Odds-with-First-Lady-12939201 [Accessed 18 February 2011].

Gordon, Robert J. 2004. "Two Centuries of Economic Growth: Europe Chasing the American Frontier." Chicago: CEPR Discussion Papers.

Gottlieb, Alma. 2004. *The Afterlife Is Where We Come From: The Culture of Infancy in West Africa*. Chicago: University of Chicago Press.

Gottschang, Suzanne Zhang. 2007. "Maternal Bodies, Breast-Feeding, and Consumer Desire in Urban China." *Medical Anthropology* 21 (1):64–80.

Gowen, Gwen. 2009. "Breast-Feeding Past Infancy: 'I'm Comforting Him.'" ABC News, 2 January 2009. http://abcnews.go.com/Health/story?id=6551439 [Accessed 20 October 2012].

Gram, David. 2009. "Airlines sued after throwing breast-feeding passenger off plane." *Seattle Times*, 9 October 2009. http://seattletimes.nwsource.com

/html/travel/20100345 l 2_webbreastfeedpassenger09.html [Accessed 20 April 2011].
Granju, Kate A. 2001. "Did 'America's Pediatrician' Sell Out? Attachment Parenting Guru Dr. William Sears Is Found to Have Ties to the Infant-Formula Industry." *Salon*, 25 January 2001. http://www.salon.com/Life/Feature/2001/01/25/Formula/index.html [Accessed 15 October 2012].
Gray, Richard. 2011. "Genetically Modified Cows Produce 'Human' Milk." *The Telegraph* (U.K.), 2 April 2011. http://www.telegraph.co.uk/earth/agriculture/geneticmodification/8423536/Genetically-Modified-Cows-Produce-Human-Milk.html [Accessed 10 June 2011].
Grumet, Jamie Lynn. 2012. "Our Experience with TIME." *I Am Not the Babysitter* (blog), 7 August 2012. http://www.iamnotthebabysitter.com/time-cover/ [Accessed October 15 2012].
Grummer-Strawn, Laurence M., and Katherine R. Shealy. 2009. "Progress in Protecting, Promoting, and Supporting Breastfeeding: 1984–2009." *Breastfeeding Medicine: The Official Journal of the Academy of Breastfeeding Medicine* 4 Suppl 1:S31–39.
Hackett, Martine. 2007. *Unsettled Sleep: The Construction and Consequences of a Public Health Media Campaign*. New York: The City University of New York.
Halley, Jean O'Malley. 2007. *Boundaries of Touch: Parenting and Adult-Child Intimacy*. Chicago: University of Illinois Press.
Han, Sallie. 2006. "The Baby in the Body: Pregnancy Practices as Kin and Person Making Experience in the Contemporary United States." Ann Arbor: University of Michigan.
———. 2009a. "Making Room for Daddy: Men's 'Belly Talk' in the Contemporary United States." In *Reconceiving the Second Sex: Men, Masculinity, and Reproduction*, edited by M.C. Inhorn, T. Tjornhoj-Thomsen, H. Goldberg, and M. La Cour Mosegaard. New York: Berghahn Books.
———. 2009b. "Men At Home: The Work of Fathers in the House and the Nursery." *Phoebe: Journal of Gender & Cultural Critiques* 21 (2):21.
———. 2013. *Pregnancy in Practice: Expectation and Experience in the Contemporary US*. New York: Berghahn Books.
Harding, Kate. 2009. "Lactate on Your Own Time, Lady." *Salon*, 28 August 2009. http://www.salon.com/2009/08/28/fired_for_pumping/ [Accessed 2 March 2011].
Hardyment, C. 2007. *Dream Babies: Childcare Advice from John Locke to Gina Ford*. London: Frances Lincoln.
Harkness, Sara, Charles M. Super, Constance H. Keefer, Chemba S. Raghavan, and Elizabeth Kip Campbell. 1996. "Ask the Doctor: The Negotiation of Cultural Models in American Parent-Pediatrician Discourse." In *Parents' Cultural Belief Systems: Their Origins, Expressions, and Consequences*, edited by S. Harkness and C.M. Super. New York: Guilford Press.
Harmon, Amy. 2005. "And Baby Makes Three in One Bed." *New York Times*, 29 December 2005. http://www.nytimes.com/2005/12/29/fashion/thursdaystyles/29sleep.html [Accessed 5 March 2011].

Hartigan, John. 1999. *Racial Situations: Class Predicaments of Whiteness in Detroit.* Princeton, N.J.: Princeton University Press.

———. 2005. *Odd Tribes: Toward A Cultural Analysis of White People.* Durham, N.C.: Duke University Press.

Harvey, Travis A., and Lila Buckley. 2009. "Childbirth in China." In *Childbirth across Cultures: Ideas and Practices of Pregnancy, Childbirth and the Postpartum,* edited by H. Selin and P.K. Stone. New York: Springer.

Hashimoto, Naoko, and Christine McCourt. 2009. "From 'To Learn' to 'To Know': Women's Embodied Knowledge of Breastfeeding in Japan." In *Infant and Young Child Feeding: Challenges to Implementing A Global Strategy,* edited by F. Dykes and V.H. Moran. Sussex, U.K.: Wiley-Blackwell.

Hassan, Narin. 2010. "Milk Markets: Technology, the Lactating Body, and New Forms of Consumption." *WSQ Women's Studies Quarterly* 38 (3): 209–28.

Hauck, Fern R., S.M. Herman, M. Donovan, S. Iyasu, C.M. Moore, E. Donoghue, R.H. Kirschner, and M. Willinger. 2003. "Sleep Environment and the Risk of Sudden Infant Death Syndrome in an Urban Population: The Chicago Infant Mortality Study." *Pediatrics* 111 (5):1207–1214.

Hauck, Fern R., John M.D. Thompson, Kawai O. Tanabe, Rachel Y. Moon, and Metchild M. Vennemann. 2011. "Breastfeeding and the Reduced Risk of Sudden Infant Death Syndrome: A Meta-Analysis." *Pediatrics* 128 (1):1–8.

Hausman, Bernice L. 2003. *Mother's Milk: Breastfeeding Controversies in American Culture.* New York: Routledge.

———. 2007. "Things (Not) to Do with Breasts in Public: Maternal Embodiment and the Biocultural Politics of Infant Feeding." *New Literary History* 38 (3):479–504.

———. 2008. "On the topic of Breastfeeding: A Review of Three Books." *Journal of Medical Humanities* 30 (1):77–81.

———. 2009. "Motherhood and Inequality: A Commentary on Hanna Rosin's 'The Case Against Breastfeeding.'" *Journal of Human Lactation: Official Journal of International Lactation Consultant Association* 25 (3):266–68.

———. 2010. "Risk and Culture Revisited: Breastfeeding and the 2002 West Nile Virus Scare in the United States." In *Giving Breastmilk: Body Ethics and Contemporary Breastfeeding Practice,* edited by R. Shaw. Toronto: Demeter Press.

———. 2011. *Viral Mothers: Breastfeeding in the Age of HIV/AIDS.* Ann Arbor: University of Michigan Press.

Hausman, Bernice L., Paige H. Smith, and Miriam H. Labbok. 2012. "Introduction: Breastfeeding Constraints and Realities." In *Beyond Health, Beyond Choice: Breastfeeding Constraints and Realities,* edited by P.H. Smith, B. Hausman, and M.H. Labbok. New Brunswick, N.J.: Rutgers University Press.

Hays, Sharon. 1996. *The Cultural Contradictions of Motherhood.* New Haven, C.T.: Yale University Press.

Heath, Deborah, Rayna Rapp, and Karen-Sue Taussig. 2004. "Genetic Citizenship." In *A Companion to the Anthropology of Politics*, edited by D. Nugent and J. Vincent. Malden, M.A.: Blackwell.

Heinig, Jane M. 2007. "The Burden of Proof: A Commentary on 'Is Breast Really Best: Risk and Total Motherhood in the National Breastfeeding Awareness Campaign.'" *Journal of Human Lactation* 23 (4):374–76.

Heintz, Monica. 2009. *The Anthropology of Moralities*. New York: Berghahn Books.

Henderson, Jacqueline M.T., Karyn G. France, Joseph L. Owens, and Neville M. Blampied. 2010. "Sleeping through the Night: The Consolidation of Self-Regulated Sleep across the First Year of Life." *Pediatrics* 126 (5):E1081.

Hess, Amanda. 2011. "Public breastfeeding advocates stage 'nurse-in' at Hirshhorn Museum." *ABC News*, 8 February 2011. http://www.tbd.com/blogs/amanda-hess/2011/02/nurse-in-planned-at-hirshhorn-to-promote-public-breastfeeding--8216.html [Accessed 20 April 20 2011].

Hirsch, Jennifer S., and Holly Wardlow. 2006. *Modern Loves: The Anthropology of Romantic Courtship and Companionate Marriage*. Ann Arbor: University of Michigan Press.

Hochschild, Arlie R., with Anne Machung. 1989. *The Second Shift: Working Parents and the Revolution at Home*. New York: Viking.

Hopkinson, Judy M. 2007. "Response to 'Is Breast Really Best? Risk and Total Motherhood in the National Breast-Feeding Awareness Campaign.'" *Journal of Health Politics, Policy and Law* 32 (4):637–48.

Hrdy, Sarah B. 1999. *Mother Nature: A History of Mothers, Infants, and Natural Selection*. New York: Pantheon.

Inhorn, Marcia C. 2003. *Local Babies, Global Science: Gender, Religion, and in Vitro Fertilization in Egypt*. New York: Routledge.

———. 2010. "Globalization and Gametes: Islam, Assisted Reproductive Technologies, and the Middle Eastern State." In *Reproduction, Globalization and the State*, edited by C. Browner and C. Sargent. Durham, N.C.: Duke University Press.

Inhorn, Marcia C., Tine Tjornhoj-Thomsen, Helene Goldberg, and Maruska La Cour Mosegaard. 2009. "Introduction: The Second Sex in Reproduction? Men, Sexuality, and Reproduction." In *Reconceiving the Second Sex: Men, Masculinity, and Reproduction*, edited by M.C. Inhorn, T. Tjornhoj-Thomsen, H. Goldberg, and M. La Cour Mosegaard. New York: Berghahn Books.

Inhorn, Marcia C., and Frank Van Balen. 2002. *Infertility Around the Globe: New Thinking on Childlessness, Gender, and Reproductive Technologies*. Berkeley: University of California Press.

Institute of Medicine. 2004. *Safety of Genetically Engineered Foods: Approaches to Assessing Unintended Health Effects*. Washington, DC: The National Academies Press.

Jacobs-Huey, Lanita. 2002. "The Natives Are Gazing and Talking Back: Reviewing the Problematics of Positionality, Voice, and Accountability among 'Native' Anthropologists." *American Anthropologist* 104 (3):791–804.

Jenni, Oskar G., and Bonnie B. O'Connor. 2005. "Children's Sleep: An Interplay between Culture and Biology." *Pediatrics* 115 (1):204–16.

Johansen, Shawn. 2001. *Family Men: Middle-Class Fatherhood in Early Industrializing America.* New York: Psychology Press.

Johnson, Sally, Dawn Leeming, Iain Williamson, and Steven Lyttle. 2013. "Maintaining the 'Good Maternal Body': Expressing Milk as a Way of Negotiating the Demands and Dilemmas of Early Infant Feeding." *Journal of Advanced Nursing* 69 (3): 590-599.

Johnson, Sally, Iain Williamson, Steven Lyttle, and Dawn Leeming. 2009. "Expressing Yourself: A Feminist Analysis of Talk around Expressing Breast Milk." *Social Science & Medicine* 69 (6):900–907.

Jojo329. 2009. "OSHA Regulation on Breastmilk Stored in Fridge at Work?" *Fertile Thoughts* forum, 7 August 2009. http://www.fertilethoughts.com/forums/general-parenting/659679-osha-regulation-breastmilk-stored-fridge-work-seriously-update-32-a.html [Accessed 5 June 2011].

Jordan, Brigitte. [1978] 1993. *Birth in Four Cultures: A Crosscultural Investigation of Childbirth in Yucatan, Holland, Sweden, and the United States*, 4th ed., revised and expanded by R. Davis-Floyd. New York: Waveland Press.

———. 1997. "Authoritative Knowledge and Its Construction." In *Childbirth and Authoritative Knowledge: Cross-Cultural Perspectives*, edited by R. Davis-Floyd and C.F. Sargent. Berkeley: University of California Press.

Joyner, Brandi L., Rosalind P. Oden, Taiwo I. Ajao, and Rachel Y. Moon. 2010. "Where Should My Baby Sleep: A Qualitative Study of African American Infant Sleep Location Decisions." *Journal of the National Medical Association* 102 (10):881.

Kassirer, Jerome P. 2007. "Professional Societies and Industry Support: What Is the Quid Pro Quo?" *Perspectives in Biology and Medicine* 50 (1):7–17.

Kaufman, Sharon R., and Lynn M. Morgan. 2005. "The Anthropology of the Beginnings and Ends of Life." *Annual Review of Anthropology* 34:317–41.

Kelleher, Christa M. 2006. "The Physical Challenges of Early Breastfeeding." *Social Science & Medicine* 63 (10):2727–38.

Keller, Meret A., and Wendy A. Goldberg. 2004. "Co-Sleeping: Help or Hindrance for Young Children's Independence?" *Infant and Child Development* 388:369–88.

Kendall-Tackett, Kathleen, Zhen Cong, and Thomas W. Hale. 2010. "Mother-Infant Sleep Locations and Nighttime Feeding Behavior." *Clinical Lactation* 1:27–31.

Khatib-Chahidi, Jane. 1992. "Milk Kinship in Shi'ite Islamic Iran." In *the Anthropology of Breast-Feeding*, edited by V. Maher. Oxford, U.K.: Berg.

Kleinman, Arthur, and Rachel Hall-Clifford. 2009. "Stigma: A Social, Cultural and Moral Process." *Journal of Epidemiology and Community Health* 63 (6):418.

Klingaman, Kristin Patricia. 2009. "Breastfeeding after a Caesarean Section: Mother-Infant Health Trade-offs." Doctoral thesis, Durham University, U.K.

Knaak, Stephanie. 2010. "Contextualising Risk, Constructing Choice: Breast-feeding and Good Mothering in Risk Society." *Health, Risk & Society* 12 (4): 345–55.

Knowles, Barbara. 2012. Woman says she was asked to leave Covington Applebee's while breast-feeding her son. *Rockdale Citizen*, 18 September 2012. http://www.rockdalecitizen.com/news/2012/sep/18/woman-says-she-was-asked-to-leave-covington/ [Accessed 5 October 2012].

Krieger, Nancy. 2010. "The Science and Epidemiology of Racism and Health: Racial/Ethnic Categories, Biological Expressions of Racism, and the Embodiment of Inequality, an Ecosocial Perspective." In *What's the Use of Race? Modern Governance and the Biology of Difference*, edited by I. Whitmarsh and D.S. Jones. Cambridge, M.A.: MIT Press.

Krugman, Paul. 2010. "Eating the Irish." Op-ed, *New York Times*, 25 November 2010. http://www.nytimes.com/2010/11/26/Opinion/26krugman.html [Accessed 5 March 2011].

Kukla, Rebecca. 2005. *Mass Hysteria: Medicine, Culture, and Mothers' Bodies*. New York: Rowman & Littlefield Publishers.

———. 2006. "Ethics and Ideology in Breastfeeding Advocacy Campaigns." *Hypatia* 21 (1):157–80.

La Leche League International. 2007. "Should I Sleep with My Baby?" Last edited 14 October 2007. http://www.llli.org/faq/cosleep.html [Accessed 20 October 2011].

———. 2011. "Online Store: Parenthood" http://store.llli.org/public/category/3 [Accessed 20 April 2011].

Lambek, Michael. 2010. *Ordinary Ethics: Anthropology, Language, and Action*. Bronx: Fordham University Press.

Lambert, Helen. 2000. "Sentiment and Substance in North Indian Forms of Relatedness." In *Cultures of Relatedness: New Approaches to the Study of Kinship*, edited by J. Carsten. Cambridge, U.K.: Cambridge University Press.

Lands, Leeann. 2009. *The Culture of Property: Race, Class, and Housing Landscapes in Atlanta, 1880–1950, Politics and Culture in the Twentieth-Century South*. Athens: University of Georgia Press.

Lane, Sandra D. 2008. *Why Are Our Babies Dying? Pregnancy, Birth, and Death in America*. Boulder, C.O.: Paradigm Publishers.

Layne, Linda L. 1996. "'How's the Baby Doing?' Struggling with Narratives of Progress in A Neonatal Intensive Care Unit." *Medical Anthropology Quarterly* 10 (4):624–56.

———. 1999. *Transformative Motherhood: On Giving and Getting in a Consumer Culture*. New York: New York University Press.

———. 2000. "'He Was A Real Baby with Baby Things': A Material Culture Analysis of Personhood, Parenthood and Pregnancy Loss." *Journal of Material Culture* 5 (3):321–45.

———. 2003. *Motherhood Lost: A Feminist Account of Pregnancy Loss in America*. New York: Routledge.

Leavitt, Judith Walzer. 1986. *Brought to Bed: Childbearing in America, 1750–1950*. New York: Oxford University Press.

Lee, Ellie. 2007. "Health, Morality, and Infant Feeding: British Mothers' Experiences of Formula Milk Use in the Early Weeks." *Sociology of Health & Illness* 29 (7):1075–90.

———. 2008. "Living with Risk in the Age of 'Intensive Motherhood': Maternal Identity and Infant Feeding." *Health, Risk & Society* 10 (5):467–77.

———. 2011. "Feeding Babies and the Problems of Policy." Centre for Parenting Culture Studies, University of Kent. http://blogs.kent.ac.uk/parentingculturestudies/files/2011/02/CPCS-Briefing-on-feeding-babies-FINAL-revised.pdf [Accessed 26 March 2014].

Lee, Ellie, Jan Macvarish, and Jennie Bristow. 2010. "Risk, Health and Parenting Culture." *Health, Risk & Society* 12 (4):293–300.

Lee, Sang-Il, Young-Ho Khang, and Moo-Song Lee. 2004. "Women's Attitudes toward Mode of Delivery in South Korea: A Society with High Cesarean Section Rates." *Birth* 31 (2):108–16.

Lee, Sang-Il, Young-Ho Khang, Sungcheol Yun, and Min-Woo Jo. 2004. "Rising Rates, Changing Relationships: Caesarean Section and Its Correlates in South Korea, 1988–2000." *BJOG: An International Journal of Obstetrics & Gynaecology* 112 (6):810–19.

Lefebvre, Henri. 2000. *The Production of Space*. Malden, M.A.: Wiley-Blackwell.

Lepore, Jill. 2009. "Baby Food: If Breast Is Best, Why Are Women Bottling Their Milk?" *New Yorker*, 29 January 2009. http://www.newyorker.com/reporting/2009/01/19/090119fa_fact_lepore [Accessed 13 March 2011].

Li, Ruowei, Natalie Darling, Emmanuel Maurice, Lawrence Barker, and Laurence M. Grummer-Strawn. 2005. "Breastfeeding Rates in the United States by Characteristics of the Child, Mother, or Family: The 2002 National Immunization Survey." *Pediatrics* 115 (1):E31–37.

Liamputtong, Pranee. 2011. *Infant Feeding Practices: A Cross-Cultural Perspective*. New York: Springer.

Limbaugh, Rush. 2012. "The Nanny of New York Strikes Again." *The Rush Limbaugh Show*, 30 July 2012. http://www.rushlimbaugh.com/Daily/2012/07/30/the_Nanny_of_New_York_Strikes_Again [Accessed 22 September 2012].

Litt, Jacquelyn S. 2000. *Medicalized Motherhood: Perspectives from the Lives of African-American and Jewish Women*. New Brunswick, N.J.: Rutgers University Press.

Lock, Margaret M. 1993. "Cultivating the Body: Anthropology and Epistemologies of Bodily Practice and Knowledge." *Annual Review of Anthropology* 22:133–55.

Lock, Margaret M., and Patricia A. Kaufert, eds. 1998. *Pragmatic Women and Body Politics, Cambridge Studies in Medical Anthropology*. New York: Cambridge University Press.

Lock, Margaret M., and Vinh-Kim Nguyen. 2010. *An Anthropology of Biomedicine*. Malden, M.A.: Wiley-Blackwell.

Lowen, Linda. 2012. "TIME's Breastfeeding Cover Promotes Controversy Over Parenting." *About.com Women's Issues*, 14 May 2012. http://wom

ensissues.about.com/b/2012/05/14/times-breastfeeding-cover-prom otes-controversy-over-parenting.htm [Accessed 5 October 2012].

Lozoff, Betsy, Abraham W. Wolf, and Nancy S. Davis. 1984. "Cosleeping in Urban Families with Young Children in the United States." *Pediatrics* 74 (2):171.

Lu, Michael C., Julia Prentice, Stella M. Yu, Moira Inkelas, Linda O. Linge, and Neal Halfon. 2003. "Childbirth Education Classes: Sociodemographic Disparities in Attendance and the Association of Attendance with Breastfeeding Initiation." *Maternal and Child Health Journal* 7 (2):87–93.

Lupton, Deborah. 1995. *The Imperative of Health: Public Health and the Regulated Body.* London: Sage Publications.

———. 2000. "'A Love/Hate Relationship': the Ideals and Experiences of First-Time Mothers." *Journal of Sociology* 36 (1):50.

Mabilia, Mara. 2005. *Breast Feeding and Sexuality: Behaviour, Beliefs and Taboos among the Gogo Mothers in Tanzania, Fertility, Reproduction, and Sexuality;* New York: Berghahn Books.

MacDorman, Marian F., Fay Menacker, and Eugene Declercq. 2008. "Cesarean Birth in the United States: Epidemiology, Trends, and Outcomes." *Clinics in Perinatology* 35 (2):293–307.

———. 2010. "Trends and Characteristics of Home and Other Out-of-Hospital Births in the United States, 1990–2006." *National Vital Statistics Reports: From the Centers for Disease Control and Prevention, National Center for Health Statistics, National Vital Statistics System* 58 (11):1.

Maher, JaneMaree. 2009. "Accumulating Care: Mothers beyond the Conflicting Temporalities of Caring and Work." *Time & Society* 18 (2–3):231– 45.

Maher, Vanessa. 1992. *The Anthropology of Breast-Feeding: Natural Law or Social Construct, Cross-Cultural Perspectives on Women.* Oxford, U.K.: Berg.

Maisels, M. Jeffrey, and Anthony F. McDonagh. 2008. "Phototherapy for Neonatal Jaundice." *New England Journal of Medicine* 358:920–28.

Martin, Emily. 1987. *The Woman in the Body: A Cultural Analysis of Reproduction.* Boston, M.A.: Beacon Press.

———. 1994. *Flexible Bodies: The Role of Immunity in American Culture from the Days of Polio to the Age of AIDS.* Boston, M.A.: Beacon Press.

Mauss, Marcel. [1935] 1973. "Techniques of the Body." *Economy and Society* 2 (1):70–88.

McBride-Henry, Karen, and Rhonda Shaw. 2010. "Giving Breastmilk as Being-with." In *Giving Breastmilk: Body Ethics and Contemporary Breastfeeding Practice*, edited by R. Shaw and A. Bartlett. Toronto: Demeter Press.

McCourt, Christine. 2009. "Cosmologies, Concepts and Theories: Time and Childbirth in Cross-Cultural Perspective." In *Childbirth, Midwifery and Concepts of Time*, edited by C. McCourt. New York: Berghahn Books.

McCourt, Christine, and Fiona Dykes. 2009. "From Tradition to Modernity: Time and Childbirth in a Historical Perspective." In *Childbirth, Midwifery and Concepts of Time*, edited by C. McCourt. New York: Berghahn Books.

McCoy, Rosha Champion, Carl E. Hunt, Samuel M. Lesko, Richard Vezina, Michael J. Corwin, Marian Willinger, Howard J. Hoffman, and Allen A Mitchell. 2004. "Frequency of Bed Sharing and Its Relationship to Breastfeeding." *Journal of Developmental and Behavioral Pediatrics* 25 (3):141–49.

McKenna, James J. 1986. "An Anthropological Perspective on the Sudden Infant Death Syndrome (SIDS): The Role of Parental Breathing Cues and Speech Breathing Adaptations." *Medical Anthropology* 10 (1):9–53.

———. 2002. "Breastfeeding & Bedsharing Still Useful (and Important) after All These Years." *Mothering Magazine* 114 (September/October):28–37.

McKenna, James J., and Helen L. Ball. 2010. "Early Infant Sleep Consolidation Is Unnecessary Barrier to Breastfeeding: E-Letter in Response to Henderson et al." *Pediatrics* 126 (5):E1081.

McKenna, James J., Helen L. Ball, and Lee T. Gettler. 2007. "Mother-Infant Cosleeping, Breastfeeding and Sudden Infant Death Syndrome: What Biological Anthropology Has Discovered about Normal Infant Sleep and Pediatric Sleep Medicine." *American Journal of Physical Anthropology Supp* 45:133–61.

McKenna, James J., and Thomas McDade. 2005. "Why Babies Should Never Sleep Alone: A Review of the Co-Sleeping Controversy in Relation to SIDS, Bedsharing and Breast Feeding." *Paediatric Respiratory Reviews* 6 (2):134–52.

McKenna, James J., Sarah S. Mosko, and Chris A. Richard. 1997. "Bedsharing Promotes Breastfeeding." *Pediatrics* 100 (2):214.

———. 1999. "Breast Feeding and Mother-Infant Cosleeping in Relation to SIDS Prevention." In *Evolutionary Medicine,* edited by W.R. Trevathan, E.O. Wilson, and J.J. McKenna. New York: Oxford University Press.

McKenna, James J., Evelyn Thoman, Thomas F. Anders, Abraham Sadeh, Vicki L. Schechtman, and Steven F. Glotzbach. 1993. "Infant-Parent Co-Sleeping in an Evolutionary Perspective: Implications for Understanding Infant Sleep Development and the Sudden Infant Death Syndrome." *Sleep* 16 (3):263–82.

McMillen, Sally G. 1997. *Motherhood in the Old South: Pregnancy, Childbirth, and Infant Rearing.* Baton Rouge: Louisiana State University Press.

Meadows, Robert, Sara Arber, Susan Venn, and Jenny Hislop. 2008. "Unruly Bodies and Couples' Sleep." *Body & Society* 14 (4):75–91.

Meadows, Robert, Sara Arber, Susan Venn, Jenny Hislop, and Neil Stanley. 2009. "Exploring the Interdependence of Couples' Rest-Wake Cycles: An Actigraphic Study." *Chronobiology International* 26 (1):80–92.

Metzl, Jonathan, and Anna Rutherford Kirkland. 2010. *Against Health: How Health Became the New Morality.* New York: New York University Press.

Millard, Anne V. 1990. "The Place of the Clock in Pediatric Advice: Rationales, Cultural Themes, and Impediments to Breastfeeding." *Social Science & Medicine* 31 (2):211–21.

Miller, Daniel. 1987. *Material Culture and Mass Consumption.* New York: Blackwell.

———. 1998. *A Theory of Shopping.* Ithaca, N.Y.: Cornell University Press.

———. 2001. *Consumption: Critical Concepts in the Social Sciences.* New York: Routledge.

Moe, Karine S., and Dianna J. Shandy. 2010. *Glass Ceilings and 100-Hour Couples: What the Opt-Out Phenomenon Can Teach Us about Work and Family.* Athens: University of Georgia Press.

Morelli, Gilda A., Barbara Rogoff, David Oppenheim, and Denise Goldsmith. 1992. "Cultural Variation in Infants' Sleeping Arrangements: Questions of Independence." *Developmental Psychology* 28 (4):604–13.

Morgan, Lynn 1989. "When Does Life Begin? A Cross-Cultural Perspective on the Personhood of Fetuses and Young Children." In *Abortion Rights and Fetal Personhood,* edited by E. Doerr and J. W. Prescott. Long Beach, C.A.: Centerline Press.

Morton, Christine H., and Clarissa Hsu. 2007. "Contemporary Dilemmas in American Childbirth Education: Findings from a Comparative Ethnographic Study." *The Journal of Perinatal Education: An ASPO/Lamaze Publication* 16 (4):25–37.

Mosko, Sarah, James J. McKenna, Michael Dickel, and Lynn Hunt. 1993. "Parent-Infant Cosleeping: The Appropriate Context for the Study of Infant Sleep and Implications for Sudden Infant Death Syndrome (SIDS) Research." *Journal of Behavioral Medicine* 16 (6):589–610.

Mosko, Sarah, Christopher Richard, James J. McKenna, and Sarah Drummond. 1996. "Infant Sleep Architecture during Bedsharing and Possible Implications for SIDS." *Sleep* 19 (9):677.

Mueggler, Erik. 2001. *The Age of Wild Ghosts: Memory, Violence, and Place in Southwest China.* Berkeley: University of California Press.

Mullings, Leith. 1997. *On Our Own Terms: Race, Class, and Gender in the Lives of African American Women.* New York: Routledge.

Mullings, Leith, and Alaka Wali. 2001. *Stress and Resilience: The Social Context of Reproduction in Central Harlem.* New York: Springer.

Murphy, Elizabeth. 1999. "'Breast Is Best': Infant Feeding Decisions and Maternal Deviance." *Sociology of Health and Illness* 21 (2):187–208.

———. 2000. "Risk, Responsibility, and Rhetoric in Infant Feeding." *Journal of Contemporary Ethnography* 29 (3):291–325.

———. 2003. "Expertise and Forms of Knowledge in the Government of Families." *The Sociological Review* 51 (4):433–62.

———. 2004. "Risk, Maternal Ideologies, and Infant Feeding." In *A Sociology of Food and Nutrition: The Social Appetite,* edited by J. Germov and L. Williams. New York: Oxford University Press.

Narayan, Kirin. 1993. "How Native Is a 'Native' Anthropologist?" *American Anthropologist* 95 (3):671–86.

Nathoo, Tasnim, and Aleck Ostry. 2010. "Wet-Nursing, Milk Banks, and Black Markets: The Political Economy of Giving Breastmilk in Canada." In *Giving Breastmilk: Body Ethics and Contemporary Breastfeeding Practices,* edited by A. Bartlett and R. Shaw. Toronto: Demeter Press.

Navarro, Vincente. 2007. *Neoliberalism, Globalization and Inequalities: Consequences for Health and Quality of Life.* Amityville, N.Y.: Baywood Publishing.

Novas, Carlos. 2006. "The Political Economy of Hope: Patients, Organizations, Science and Biovalue." *Biosocieties* 1 (03):289–305.

Ochs, Elinor, and Lisa Capps. 1996. "Narrating the Self." *Annual Review of Anthropology* 25 (1):19–43.

Oddy, Wendy H, and Karen Glenn. 2003. "Implementing the Baby Friendly Hospital Initiative: The Role of Finger Feeding." *Breastfeeding Review: Professional Publication of the Nursing Mothers' Association of Australia* 11 (1):5.

Ong, Aihwa, and Stephen J. Collier, eds. 2005. *Global Assemblages: Technology, Politics and Ethics as Anthropological Problems.* Malden, M.A.: Wiley-Blackwell.

Ortner, Sherry B. 2005. *New Jersey Dreaming: Capital, Culture, and the Class of '58.* Durham, N.C.: Duke University Press.

Pantley, Elizabeth. 2002. *The No-Cry Sleep Solution: Gentle Ways to Help Your Baby Sleep through the Night.* New York: McGraw-Hill.

Parker-Pope, Tara. 2007. "Shhh ... My Child Is Sleeping (in My Bed, Um, with Me)." *New York Times,* 23 October 2007. http://www.nytimes.com/2007/10/23/health/23well.html?pagewanted=all&_r=0 [Accessed 5 October 2012].

Parkes, Peter. 2001. "Alternative Social Structure and Foster Relations in the Hindu Kush: Milk Kinship Allegiance in Former Mountain Kingdoms of Northern Pakistan." *Society For Comparative Study of Society and History* 43(1):4–36.

Parnes, Amie. 2011. "Sarah Palin Slams Michelle Obama over Nursing." *Politico,* 17 February 2011. http://www.politico.com/News/Stories/0211/49758.html [Accessed 20 February 2011].

Pelayo, Rafael, Judith A. Owens, Jodi A. Mindell, and Stephen Sheldon. 2006. "Bed Sharing with Unimpaired Parents Is Not an Important Risk for Sudden Infant Death Syndrome: To the Editor." *Pediatrics* 117 (3): 993.

Peletz, Michael. 2001. "Ambivalence in Kinship since the 1940s." In *Relative Values: Reconfiguring Kinship Studies,* edited by S. Franklin and S. McKinnon. Durham, N.C.: Duke University Press.

Petryna, Adriana. 2002. *Life Exposed: Biological Citizens after Chernobyl.* Princeton, N.J.: Princeton University Press.

———. 2009. *When Experiments Travel: Clinical Trials and the Global Search For Human Subjects.* Princeton, N.J.: Princeton University Press.

Phillip, Barbara L., and Sheina Jean-Marie. 2007. African American Women and Breastfeeding. Washington, DC: Joint Center for Political and Economic Studies.

Pickert, Kate. 2012. "The Man Who Remade Motherhood." *Time* 179 (20):32.

Pleshette, Ann. 2008. "Baby Feeding by Mom's Friends." http://abcnews.go.com/GMA/Parenting/story?id=5459697&page=1; [Accessed 20 April 2011].

Quinn, J.B. 2002. "Baby's Bedding: Is It Creating Toxic Nerve Gasses?" *Midwifery Today* 61 :21–22.

Rapp, Rayna. 1999. *Testing Women, Testing the Fetus: The Social Impact of Amniocentesis in America, Anthropology of Everyday Life.* New York: Routledge.
———. 2001. "Gender, Body, Biomedicine: How Some Feminist Concerns Dragged Reproduction to the Center of Social Theory." *Medical Anthropology Quarterly* 15 (4):466–77.
Reagan, Lisa. 2012. "The Cover Shot Heard 'Round the World." *Pathways to Family Wellness.* http://pathwaysoffamilywellness.org/The-Outer-Womb/the-cover-shot-heard-round-the-world.html [Accessed 12 September 2012].
Reed, Richard K. 2005. *Birthing Fathers: The Transformation of Men in American Rites of Birth.* New Brunswick, N.J.: Rutgers University Press.
Reich, Jennifer A. 2010. "From Maternal Love to Toxic Exposure: State Interpretations of Breastfeeding Mothers in the Child Welfare System." In *Giving Breastmilk: Body Ethics and Contemporary Breastfeeding Practice,* edited by R. Shaw and A. Bartlett. Toronto: Demeter Press.
Richard, Christopher A., and Sarah S. Mosko. 2004. "Mother-Infant Bedsharing Is Associated with an increase in Infant Heart Rate." *Sleep* 27 (3):507–11.
Riordan, Jan. 2005. *Breastfeeding and Human Lactation.* 3rd ed. Sudbury, M.A.: Jones & Bartlett Learning.
Roberts, Dorothy. 1997. *Killing the Black Body: Race, Reproduction, and the Meaning of Liberty.* New York: Vintage.
Rolston, Jessica Smith. 2010. "Risky Business: Neoliberalism and Workplace Safety in Wyoming Coal Mines." *Human Organization* 69 (4):331–42.
Rose, Nikolas. 1996. "Governing 'Advanced' Liberal Democracies." In *Foucault and Political Reason,* edited by A. Barry, T. Osborne, and N. Rose. London: University College London Press.
Rose, Nikolas, and Carlos Novas. 2005. "Biological Citizenship." In *Global Assemblages: Technology, Politics and Ethics as Anthropological Problems,* edited by A. Ong and S.J. Collier. New York: Wiley Online Library.
Rose, Nikolas, Pat O'Malley, and Mariana Valverde. 2006. "Governmentality." *Annual Review of Law and Social Science* 2:83–104.
Rose, Nikolas S. 2007. *Politics of Life Itself: Biomedicine, Power, and Subjectivity in the Twenty-First Century.* Princeton, N.J.: Princeton University Press.
Rosenberg, Kenneth D., Carissa A. Eastham, and Laurin J. Kasehagen. 2008. "Marketing Infant Formula through Hospitals: The Impact of Commercial Hospital Discharge Packs on Breastfeeding." *American Journal of Public Health* 98 (2):290–95.
Rosin, Hanna. 2009. "The Case Against Breast-Feeding." *Atlantic Monthly,* 1 April 2009, http://www.theatlantic.com/Magazine/Archive/2009/04/the-Case-Against-Breast-Feeding/7311/ [Accessed 5 March 2011].
Rothman, Barbara Katz. 1981. "Awake and Aware, or False Consciousness: The Cooptation of Childbirth Reform in America." In *Childbirth: Alternatives to Medical Control,* edited by S. Romalis. Austin: University of Texas Press.

———. 2000. *Recreating Motherhood*. New Brunswick, N.J.: Rutgers University Press.

———. 2008. "New Breast Milk in Old Bottles." *International Breastfeeding Journal* 3(1): 9.

Rubin, Gayle. 1975. "The Traffic in Women: Notes on the 'Political Economy' of Sex." In *Toward an Anthropology of Women*, edited by R. Reiter. New York: Monthly Review Press.

Ryan, Kath, Paul Bissell, and Jo Alexander. 2010. "Moral Work in Women's Narratives of Breastfeeding." *Social Science & Medicine (1982)* 70 (6):951–58.

Salmon, Marylynn. 1994. "The Cultural Significance of Breastfeeding and Infant Care in Early Modern England and America." *Journal of Social History* 247 (23):1–15.

Scheper-Hughes, Nancy. 1993. *Death without Weeping: The Violence of Everyday Life in Brazil*. Berkeley: University of California Press.

Scheper-Hughes, Nancy, and Margaret Lock. 1987. "The Mindful Body: A Prolegomenon to Future Work in Medical Anthropology." *Medical Anthropology* 1 (1):6–41.

Schmied, Virginia, and Lesley Barclay. 1999. "Connection and Pleasure, Disruption and Distress: Women's Experience of Breastfeeding." *Journal of Human Lactation* 15 (4):325–34.

Schmied, Virginia, and Deborah Lupton. 2001. "Blurring the Boundaries: Breastfeeding and Maternal Subjectivity." *Sociology of Health and Illness* 23 (2):234–50.

Schulz, Amy J., and Leith Mullings. 2006. *Gender, Race, Class, & Health*. San Francisco: Jossey-Bass.

Schwartz, Marie Jenkins. 1996. "'At Noon, Oh How I Ran': Breastfeeding and Weaning on Plantation and Farm in Antebellum Virginia and Alabama." In *Discovering the Women in Slavery: Emancipating Perspectives on the American Past*, edited by P. Morton. Athens: University of Georgia Press.

Sears, William, Martha Sears, Robert Sears, and James Sears. 2013. *The Baby Book: Everything You Need to Know About Your Baby from Birth to Age Two, Revised Edition*. New York: Little, Brown and Company.

Shaw, Rhonda. 2004. "Performing Breastfeeding: Embodiment, Ethics and the Maternal Subject." *Feminist Review* 78 (1):99–116.

———. 2010. "Perspectives on Ethics and Human Milk Banking." In *Giving Breastmilk: Body Ethics and Contemporary Breastfeeding Practice*, edited by R. Shaw and A. Bartlett. Toronto: Demeter Press.

Shellenbarger, Sue. 2009. "Can Pumping at Work Get You Fired?" *Wall Street Journal* 31 August 2009. http://blogs.wsj.com/juggle/2009/08/31/can-pumping-at-work-get-you-fired/ [Accessed 5 March 2011].

Shweder, Richard A., Lenee A. Jensen, and Williamm Goldstein. 1995. "Who Sleeps by Whom Revisited: A Method For Extracting the Moral Goods Implicit in Practice." *New Directions for Child Development* (67):21–39.

Simonds, Wendy. 2002. "Watching the Clock: Keeping Time during Pregnancy, Birth, and Postpartum Experiences." *Social Science & Medicine (1982)* 55 (4):559–70.

Smale, Mary. 2001. "The Stigmatisation of Breastfeeding." In *Stigma and Social Exclusion in Healthcare*, edited by C. Carlisle, T. Mason, C. Watkins, and E. Whitehead. New York: Routledge.

Small, Meredith F. 1998. *Our Babies, Ourselves: How Biology and Culture Shape the Way We Parent.* New York: Bantam Dell.

Smith, Jessica Rolston. 2008. "Crafting Kinship At Home and Work: Women Miners in Wyoming." *WorkingUSA: The Journal of Labor and Society* 11 (4):439–58.

Solinger, Rickie. 1998. "Poisonous Choice." In *"Bad" Mothers: The Politics of Blame in Twentieth-Century America*, edited by L. Umansky and M. Ladd-Taylor. New York: New York University Press.

———. 2001. *Beggars and Choosers: How the Politics of Choice Shapes Adoption, Abortion, and Welfare in the United States.* New York: Hill & Wang.

Stearns, Cindy A. 1999. "Breastfeeding and the Good Maternal Body." *Gender and Society* 13 (3):308–25.

———. 2009. "The Work of Breastfeeding." *Women's Studies Quarterly* 37 (3/4):63–80.

———. 2010. "The Breast Pump." In *Giving Breastmilk: Body Ethics and Contemporary Breastfeeding Practice*, edited by R. Shaw and A. Bartlett. Toronto: Demeter Press.

Stearns, Peter N., Perrin Rowland, and Lori Giarnella. 1996. "Children's Sleep: Sketching Historical Change." *Journal of Social History* 30 (2):345–66.

Steger, Brigitte, and Lodewijk Brunt. 2003. *Night-Time and Sleep in Asia and the West: Exploring the Dark Side of Life.* London: Routledge.

Super, Charles M., and Sarah Harkness. 1982. "The Infant's Niche in Rural Kenya and Metropolitan America." In *Cross-Cultural Research at Issue*, edited by L.L. Adler. New York: Academic Press.

Sykes, Karen M. 2009. *Ethnographies of Moral Reasoning: Living Paradoxes of a Global Age.* New York: Palgrave Macmillan.

Taylor, Janelle S. 2000. "Of Sonograms and Baby Prams: Prenatal Diagnosis, Pregnancy, and Consumption." *Feminist Studies* 26 (2):391–418.

Thompson, E.P. 1967. "Time, Work-Discipline, and Industrial Capitalism." *Past and Present* 38 (1):56–97.

Tomori, Cecilia. 2005. "'Listening to the Heart': A Compelling Moral Discourse of Mothering through Breastfeeding in La Leche League International Publications." Ann Arbor: Alfred P. Sloan Center for the Ethnography of Everyday Life and the Department of Anthropology at the University of Michigan.

———. 2009. "Breastfeeding as Men's 'Kin Work' in the United States." *Phoebe: Journal of Gender & Cultural Critiques* 21 (2):31–44.

Townsend, Nicholas W. 2002. *The Package Deal: Marriage, Work, and Fatherhood in Men's Lives.* Philadelphia: Temple University Press.

Traina, Cristina L.H. 2000. "Maternal Experience and the Boundaries of Christian Sexual Ethics." *Signs* 25 (2):369–405.

Trouillot, Michel-Rolph. 2003. *Global Transformations: Anthropology and the Modern World.* New York: Palgrave Macmillan.

Tsianakas, Vicki, and Pranee Liamputtong. 2007. "Infant Feeding Beliefs and Practices among Afgan Women Living in Melbourne, Australia." In *Child Rearing and Infant Care Issues,* edited by P. Liamputtong. Hauppauge, N.Y.: Nova Science Publishers.

Turner, Bryan S. 2008. *The Body & Society: Explorations in Social Theory, Body and Society.* 3rd ed. London: Sage.

U.S. Census Bureau. 2000. "United States 2000 Census." http://www.census.gov/Main/Www/Cen2000/html [Accessed 20 April 2011].

U.S. Consumer Product Safety Commission. 1999. "CPSC Warns Against Placing Babies in Adult Beds; Study Finds 64 Deaths Each Year from Suffocation and Strangulation." 29 September 1999. http://www.cpsc.gov/en/Newsroom/News-Releases/1999/CPSC-Warns-Against-Placing-Babies-in-Adult-Beds-Study-finds-64-deaths-each-year-from-suffocation-and-strangulation/ [Accessed 26 March 2014].

U.S. Department of Health and Human Services. 2011. *The Surgeon General's Call to Action to Support Breastfeeding.* Washington, DC: U.S. Department of Health and Human Services, Office of the Surgeon General.

Ulrich, Laurel Thatcher. 1990. *A Midwife's Tale: The Life of Martha Ballard, Based on Her Diary, 1785–1812.* New York: Vintage.

United States Breastfeeding Committee. 2011. "Workplace Support in Federal Law." http://www.usbreastfeeding.org/Employment/WorkplaceSupport/WorkplaceSupportinFederalLaw/tabid/175/Default.aspx [Accessed 26 March 2014].

Vallone, S.A. 2012. "Hands in Support of Breastfeeding: Manual Therapy." *Supporting Sucking Skills in Breastfeeding Infants*: 253.

Van Esterik, Penny. 1989. *Beyond the Breast-Bottle Controversy.* New Brunswick, N.J.: Rutgers University Press.

———. 2002. "Contemporary Trends in Infant Feeding Research." *Annual Review of Anthropology* 31:257–78.

———. 2012. "Breastfeeding across Cultures: Dealing with Difference." In *Beyond Health, Beyond Choice: Breastfeeding Constraints and Realities,* edited by P.H. Smith, B. Hausman, and M.H. Labbok. New Brunswick, N.J.: Rutgers University Press.

Van Vleet, Krista E. 2008. *Performing Kinship: Narrative, Gender, and the Intimacies of Power in the Andes.* Austin: University of Texas Press.

Venn, Susan, Sara Arber, Robert Meadows, and Jenni Hislop. 2008. "The Fourth Shift: Exploring the Gendered Nature of Sleep Disruption among Couples with Children." *The British Journal of Sociology* 59 (1): 79–97.

Vennemann, Mechtild M., Hans-Werner Hense, Thomas Bajanowski, Peter S. Blair, Christina Complojer, Rachel Y. Moon, and Ursula Kiechl-Kohlendorfer. 2012. "Bed Sharing and the Risk of Sudden Infant Death

Syndrome: Can We Resolve the Debate?" *The Journal of Pediatrics* 160 (1):44–48. E2.
Walker, Marsha. 2007. *Still Selling Out Mothers and Babies: Marketing of Breast Milk Substitutes in the USA.* Weston, M.A.: National Alliance for Breastfeeding Advocacy.
Wall, Glenda. 2001. "Moral Constructions of Motherhood in Breastfeeding Discourse." *Gender & Society* 15 (4):592–610.
Ward, Julia DeJager. 2000. *La Leche League: At the Crossroads of Medicine, Feminism, and Religion.* Chapel Hill: University of North Carolina Press.
Warner, Judith. 2005. *Perfect Madness: Motherhood in the Age of Anxiety.* New York: Riverhead.
Wasson, C., K. Brondo, B. Lemaster, T. Turner, M. Cudhea, K. Moran, I. Adams, A. McCoy, M. Ko, and T. Matsumoto. 2008. *We've Come a Long Way, Maybe: Academic Climate Report of the Committee on the Status of Women in Anthropology.* American Anthropological Association. http://www.aaanet.org/Resources/Departments/Upload/Coswa-Academic-Climate-Report-2008.pdf [Accessed 20 April 2011].
Weber, Max. 1958. *The Protestant Ethic and the Spirit of Capitalism.* New York: Scribner.
Weiner, Lynn Y. 1994. "Reconstructing Motherhood: The La Leche League in Postwar America." *Journal of American History* 80 (4):1357–81.
Welles-Nystrom, Barbara. 2005. "Co-Sleeping as a Window into Swedish Culture: Considerations of Gender and Health Care." *Scandinavian Journal of Caring Sciences* 19 (4):354–60.
Wertz, Richard W., and Dorothy C. Wertz. 1989. *Lying-in: A History of Childbirth in America.* New Haven, C.T.: Yale University Press.
Weston, Kath. 2001. "Kinship, Controversy, and the Sharing of Substance: The Race/Class Politics of Blood Transfusion." In *Relative Values: Reconfiguring Kinship Studies,* edited by S. Franklin and S. McKinnon. Durham, N.C.: Duke University Press.
Whitaker, Elizabeth D. 2000. *Measuring Mamma's Milk: Fascism and the Medicalization of Maternity in Italy.* Ann Arbor: University of Michigan Press.
Whittemore, Robert D., and Elizabeth A. Beverly. 1996. "Mandinka Mothers and Nurslings: Power and Reproduction." *Medical Anthropology Quarterly* 10 (1):45–62.
Wiggs, Luci. 2007. "Are Children Getting Enough Sleep? Implications for Parents." *Sociological Research Online* 12 (5):13.
Wight, Nancy, and James J. McKenna. 2005. *Breastfeeding Is Associated with a Lower Risk of SIDS according to the Academy of Breastfeeding Medicine.* Academy of Breastfeeding Medicine. http://www.liebertpup.com/Prdetails.Aspx?Pr_Id416 [Accessed 20 April 2011].
Wilk, Richard. 2001. "Consuming Morality." *Journal of Consumer Culture* 1 (2):245.
Williams, Mary Elizabeth. 2012. "Why Time's Cover Shocks." *Salon,* 10 May 2012. http://www.salon.com/2012/05/10/why_times_cover_shocks/ [Accessed 5 October 2012].

Williams, Simon J., Robert Meadows, and Sara Arber. 2010. "The Sociology of Sleep." In *Sleep, Health, and Society: From Aetiology to Public Health*, edited by F.P. Cappuccio, M.A. Miller, and S.W. Lockley. Oxford, U.K.: Oxford University Press.

Williams, Simon J. 2005. *Sleep and Society: Sociological Ventures into the (Un) Known*. London: Routledge.

———. 2007. "The Social Etiquette of Sleep: Some Sociological Reflections and Observations." *Sociology* 41 (2):313–28.

———. 2011. "Our Hard Days' Nights." *Contexts: Understanding People in their Social Worlds* 10 (1):26.

Williams, Simon J., and Nick Crossley. 2008. "Introduction: Sleeping Bodies." *Body & Society* 14 (No. 4):1–13.

Williams, Simon J., Pam Lowe, and Frances Griffiths. 2007. "Embodying and Embedding Children's Sleep: Some Sociological Comments and Observations." *Sociological Research Online* 12 (5).

Willinger, Marian, Chia-Wen Ko, Howard J. Hoffman, Ronald C. Kessler, and Michael J. Corwin. 2003. "Trends in Infant Bed Sharing in the United States, 1993–2000." *Archives of Pediatric and Adolescent Medicine* 157:43–49.

Wilson, Alex, and Jessica Boehland. 2005. "Small Is Beautiful: US House Size, Resource Use, and the Environment." *Journal of Industrial Ecology* 9 (1–2):277–87.

Wolf-Meyer, Matthew. 2008. "Sleep, Signification and the Abstract Body of Allopathic Medicine." *Body & Society* 14 (4):93–114.

Wolf, Abraham W., Betsy Lozoff, Sara Latz, and Robert Paludetto. 1996. "Parental Theories in the Management of Young Children's Sleep in Japan, Italy, and the United States." In *Parents' Cultural Belief Systems: Their Origins, Expressions, and Consequences*, edited by S. Harkness and C.M. Super. New York: Guilford Press.

Wolf, Jacqueline H. 2001. *Don't Kill Your Baby: Public Health and the Decline of Breastfeeding in the Nineteenth and Twentieth Centuries*. Columbus: Ohio State University Press.

———. 2003. "Low Breastfeeding Rates and Public Health in the United States." *American Journal of Public Health* 93 (12):2000–2011.

———. 2006. "What Feminists Can Do for Breastfeeding and What Breastfeeding Can Do for Feminists." *Signs: Journal of Women in Culture and Society* 31 (2):397–424.

———. 2008. "Got Milk? Not in Public!" *International Breastfeeding Journal* 3(1):11-14.

———. 2009. *Deliver Me from Pain: Anesthesia and Birth in America*. Baltimore, M.D.: Johns Hopkins University Press.

Wolf, Joan B. 2007. "Is Breast Really Best? Risk and Total Motherhood in the National Breastfeeding Awareness Campaign." *Journal of Health Politics, Policy and Law* 32 (4):595–636.

———. 2011. *Is Breast Best? Taking on the Breastfeeding Experts and the New High Stakes of Motherhood*. New York: New York University Press.

Worthman, Carol M. 2007. "After Dark: The Evolutionary Ecology of Human Sleep." In *Evolutionary Medicine and Health: New Perspectives*, edited by W.R. Trevathan, E.O. Smith, and J.J. McKenna. Oxford, U.K.: Oxford University Press.

———. 2011. "Developmental Cultural Ecology of Sleep." In *Sleep and Development: Familial and Socio-Cultural Considerations*, edited by Mona El-Sheikh. New York: Oxford University Press.

Worthman, Carol M., and Ryan A. Brown. 2007. "Companionable Sleep: Social Regulation of Sleep and Cosleeping in Egyptian Families." *Journal of Family Psychology: Journal of the Division of Family Psychology of the American Psychological Association (Division 43)* 21 (1):124–35.

Wright, Anne L., Mark Bauer, and Clarina Clark. 1993. "Cultural Interpretations and Intracultural Variability in Navajo Beliefs about Breastfeeding." *American Ethnologist* 20:781–96.

Wright, Anne L., and Richard J. Schanler. 2001. "The Resurgence of Breastfeeding at the End of the Second Millennium." *The Journal of Nutrition* 131 (2):421s.

Yanagisako, Sylvia Junko. 2002. *Producing Culture and Capital: Family Firms in Italy.* Princeton, N.J.: Princeton University Press.

Yang, Chang-Kook, and Hong-Moo Hahn. 2002. "Cosleeping in Young Korean Children." *Journal of Developmental & Behavioral Pediatrics* 23 (3):151.

Yang, Lawrence H., Arthur Kleinman, Bruce G. Link, Jo C. Phelan, Sing Lee, and Byron Good. 2007. "Culture and Stigma: Adding Moral Experience to Stigma Theory." *Social Science & Medicine* 64 (7):1524–35.

Yimyam, Susanha, Monica Morrow, and W. Srisuphan. 1999. "Role Conflict and Rapid Socio-Economic Change: Breastfeeding among Employed Women in Thailand." *Social Science & Medicine* 49 (7):957–65.

Young, Iris M. 2005. *On Female Body Experience: "Throwing Like A Girl" and Other Essays.* New York: Oxford University Press.

Yovsi, R.D., and H. Keller. 2003. "Breastfeeding: An Adaptive Process." *Ethos* 31 (2):147–71.

Yovsi, Relindis D., and Heidi Keller. 2007. "The Architecture of Cosleeping among Wage-Earning and Subsistence Farming Cameroonian Nso Families." *Ethos* 35 (1):65–84.

Zeitlyn, Sushila, and Rabela Rowshan. 1997. "Privileged Knowledge and Mothers' 'Perceptions': The Case of Breast-Feeding and Insufficient Milk in Bangladesh." *Medical Anthropology Quarterly* 11 (1):56–68.

Zelizer, Viviana A.R. 1994. *Pricing the Priceless Child: The Changing Social Value of Children.* Princeton, N.J.: Princeton University Press.

Zigon, Jarrett. 2007. "Moral Breakdown and the Ethical Demand: A Theoretical Framework for an Anthropology of Moralities." *Anthropological Theory* 7 (2):131–50.

———. 2008. *Morality: An Anthropological Perspective.* Oxford, U.K.: Berg.

———. 2009. "Hope Dies Last: Two Aspects of Hope in Contemporary Moscow." *Anthropological Theory* 9 (3):253–71.

———. 2010a. "A Disease of Frozen Feelings: Ethically Working on Emotional Worlds in a Russian Orthodox Church Drug Rehabilitation Program." *Medical Anthropology Quarterly* 24 (3):326–43.

———. 2010b. Moral and Ethical Assemblages: A Response to Fassin and Stoczkowski. *Anthropological Theory* 10 (1–2):3–15.

———. 2011a. *HIV Is God's Blessing: Rehabilitating Morality in Neoliberal Russia.* Berkeley: University of California Press.

———. 2011b. A Moral and Ethical Assemblage in Russian Orthodox Drug Rehabilitation. *Ethos* 39 (1):30–50.

Zimmerman, Frederick, and Janice Bell. 2010. "Associations of Television Content Type and Obesity in Children." *American Journal of Public Health* 100 (2):334–40.

# INDEX

**A**
Abbott, Susan, 35
American College of Obstetricians and Gynecologists (ACOG), 110
American Academy of Pediatrics (AAP)
　position on breastfeeding, 64–66
　guidelines' use in childbirth education, 102
　and Sudden Infant Death Syndrome guidelines, 71–75, 134
Apple, Rima, 58–59, 87n7
Asad, Talal, 26–27
attachment parenting. *See under* parenting
Avishai, Orit, 23n30, 27, 114–15, 121
authoritative knowledge. *See under* breastfeeding

**B**
baby-carrying, 105, 109. *See also* sling
Bachelard, Gaston, 171, 179, 181, 185, 203, 204nn3–4
Bachmann, Michele, 242
Bakhtin, Mikhail, 204n4
Ball, Helen, 22n13, 24n39, 24n42, 29–31, 49n39, 71–72, 74–75, 241
Bartlett, Allison, 142n1

bassinet, 2, 30, 73, 169n9
　as a "capitalist morality lesson," 31–32
　in childbirth education courses, 103, 108
　infant sleep plans and, 182–87
　infant sleep practices and, 112, 134–40, 188, 190, 192–95, 197, 200, 220–22, 249–50, 252, 257–60
Basso, Keith, 204n4
bed sharing, 3–6, 9–10, 15, 18, 22n13, 23n32, 25, 29–32
　and adult beds, 186–87, 191–94
　and attachment parenting, 77
　and breastfeeding (*see under* breastfeeding)
　in childbirth education courses, 101–9, 119n16, 152
　in cross-cultural studies, 34–36
　in home birth care, 111
　and independence (*see under* independence)
　and men, 152, 161–63
　moral concerns/ambivalence about, 19, 36–38, 233, 235–37, 240, 244
　and pediatric advice, 3, 132–39
　practices, 2–3, 111–13, 126–27, 133–39, 143n25, 162–63, 189–98, 217–22, 231–33, 235, 238n24, 249–59
　and race, 41, 67–68, 73

and sexuality, 36, 152, 196–97
stigmatization of, 6 (*see also*
   stigmatization)
and Sudden Infant Death
   Syndrome, 6, 30, 68, 71–78,
   102–3, 108–9, 134, 192 (*see
   also under* American Academy
   of Pediatrics)
bedroom, 10, 126, 163, 174,
   206n21, 222, 224–25, 228,
   233, 236, 259
child's bedroom, 171–72, 176–
   80 (*see also* nursery)
moving children out of the
   parental bedroom, 197–201
parents' bedroom, 180–87
separation of parental and child,
   36, 171
and sexuality, 180–82, 196–97
spatial problems of, 191–97
Beidelman, Thomas O., 49–50n45,
   205n18
Ben-Ari, Eyal, 32, 49n32
Benjamin, Regina M., 68–69
Biological anthropology, 3, 10, 29,
   72, 102, 117, 119n24, 240–41
biomedicalization, 7, 22–23n23,
   37, 39, 46
of breastfeeding (*see under*
   breastfeeding)
of childbirth (*see under*
   childbirth)
of sleep (*see under* sleep)
Blum, Linda, 81–84, 88n22, 114,
   141
Bobel, Chris, 88n19, 116–17,
   119n14
body techniques. *See under*
   embodiment
Borst, Charlotte, 87n6, 87n10
Bradley, Robert, 118n4
breasts
   sexualization of, 5, 36, 58, 244
   as normal part of pregnancy and
      breastfeeding, 99, 101
   as source of nourishment, 103
   *See also* breastfeeding; breastmilk

breastmilk, 17, 128, 143n9, 230,
   253
and biocapitalism, 38, 242
in breastfeeding promotion, 4
commercial exploitation of, 38,
   45–46, 54n71, 241–42
and disgust, 5
as equivalent to infant formula,
   141
expression, 125–26, 129, 147,
   155, 157–58, 168n3, 189, 199
   (*see also* breast pump)
as hazardous, 5, 17, 45, 58
and health, 28, 45
insufficient supply of, 28, 126,
   130, 169n13, 199–200, 232
legal protection for expression
   of, 147–48, 168n3, 242
milk kinship, 33 (*see also* kinship)
and neonatal jaundice (*see under*
   jaundice)
and poverty, 28
and sexuality, 21n7, 36
sharing, 34
spouses' role in feeding, 155,
   157–60, 162, 165
substitutes, 64, 66, 88n18 (*see
   also* breastfeeding; breast
   pump; infant formula)
supplementation with infant
   formula (*see under* infant
   formula)
use of in finger-feeding system
   (*see under* breastfeeding)
breast pump, 27, 65–66, 116, 188,
   242, 259
breastfeeding
advocacy, 4, 62–70, 77–78, 80–
   85, 111, 150, 152, 155, 164–
   65, 167, 241–42, 244
assisted by finger-feeder, 124–
   25, 128, 143n9
and authoritative knowledge,
   19, 55–88
bed sharing, 132–42, 161–64,
   187–97, 201–3, 217–24,
   231–33

and biological interrelationship of sleep, 29–30, 75, 79, 102, 241
biomedicalization of, 56–88
in childbirth education, 89–119, 121, 150–53, 155, 167
"choice," 68, 78–88, 90, 106, 111, 116, 127, 242
cluster feeding, 129–31
cross-nursing, 142n1
engorgement, 122–23, 227
exclusive, 4, 24n43, 30, 64, 152, 165, 228, 249–60
and feminism (*see under* feminism)
and health, 4, 7, 18, 20, 28, 41, 45, 57–58, 63–70, 81–85, 88n26, 120–21, 138, 241–44
history, 56–78
and incest, 5–6, 36, 139, 182
and independence (*see under* independence)
and kinship (*see under* kinship)
and La Leche League (*see under* La Leche League)
legal aspects of, 69, 147–48, 242–43
in the media, 3, 4–7, 21, 22n15, 25, 47, 77, 115, 119n21, 130, 244
and men, 125–28, 135, 144–70, 187–94, 195–203, 217–33, 236–37
and "moral work," 124, 141–42
and morality, 5–6, 66, 120–43, 182
as natural, 25–26, 62–63, 77, 80, 100–101, 105, 111–18, 119n14, 148
on-demand, 59, 117
pain during, 2, 123, 124–25, 188, 227
and pediatric advice, 14–15, 64–65, 132, 198–200, 202
and pregnancy, 35
as a "project," 114–15, 121

and religion, 57, 63, 79, 87n4, 146–47
and sexuality, 6, 21, 27, 36, 45, 139, 152, 163, 166, 182, 194, 196–97, 244
sexualization of, 5–6, 36, 58, 80, 82, 101, 182, 244
and skin-to-skin contact, 101, 107
and slavery, 68, 82
and sleep arrangements, 132–43, 162–66, 187–202, 217–37 (*see also* bed sharing)
and social justice, 85
stigmatization of, 20–21, 22n15, 42, 45, 86, 120–31, 145
and Sudden Infant Death Syndrome, 30, 41, 67–68, 70–78, 102–3, 134 (*see also* American Academy of Pediatrics; bed sharing)
and wet-nurses, 34, 56–59, 68, 87n6
Bridges, Khiara, 52nn53–54.
Bourdieu, Pierre, 203n2, 205n18

**C**

capitalism, 3, 18–21, 26, 32, 38–47, 50, 51–52n51, 52–53n56, 53–54n60, 81, 83–84, 90, 115–17, 142, 146, 168, 169n1
biocapitalism, 38, 44–45, 53–54n66, 242 (*see also* breastmilk)
neoliberal capitalism, 21, 38, 44, 83, 116
and time, 208–37, 238nn5–6, 242
Capps, Lisa, 121
Carsten, Janet, 33, 48n21, 48–49n25, 169n5, 203n1
Carter, Pam, 81–82
Caudill, William, 34
childbirth, 39, 51–52n51, 55, 80–81, 123
anesthetics in, 60
biomedicalization of, 39, 69, 84, 101, 185

Cesarean section (C-section), 40, 69, 95, 100–101, 111, 119n11, 153–54, 190, 195, 206n31, 252, 254, 257, 260
education (*see under* childbirth education)
epidural anesthesia, 14, 97, 113, 123, 133, 154, 157,
history of, 42, 56–63, 87n10
hospital birth, 57, 69, 110
home birth, 9, 110–11, 113, 116, 154, 186, 257 (*see also* midwives)
induction of, 40, 123, 142n4, 250–51, 256
"informed choice," 106, 110–11, 116
interventions (biomedical) 40, 100–101
men's roles in, 150–54
and midwives (*see under* midwives)
"natural childbirth" 93, 100–101
and Pitocin, 114, 123, 133, 153, 250, 253–54, 258, 260
practices, 9, 39, 101, 151
as a rite of passage, 39
childbirth education, 42, 89–119, 121, 124
as a consumer good, 89–98, 114–15
men's role in, 150–55
as a rite of passage, 89, 150
childcare, 4, 65, 80, 157, 168, 213
Clarke, Adele, 22–23n23
Clarke, Alison, 179
Colen, Shellee, 40–41
Collier, Stephen J., 43, 53n60, 88n28
Consumer Product Safety Commission, 102–3
consumption, 84, 88n29, 104
and childbirth education (*see under* childbirth education)
ethical consumption,119n15, 119n22

middle-class practices, 10, 20, 38, 42–43, 46, 97, 114, 182–87
of parenting models, 110–18
Co-Sleeper, 2, 103–4, 107, 119n13, 182, 184–85, 187–90, 192–94, 198, 218, 229, 251, 253–56
co-sleeping
bed sharing as a form of, 22n13
outside of beds, 126–27, 187–88
*See also* bed sharing
Craniosacral Therapy (CST), 125, 127
Craven, Christa, 88–89n29, 116
crib, 3, 31–32, 137, 181, 183, 185, 192–93, 195–97, 200, 220–24, 227, 230, 236, 246, 250, 254–60
in childbirth education courses, 103–4, 108–9
in children's bedrooms, 177–78
"crib death," 70
mattresses, 103
and sleep guidelines, 73
and Sudden Infant Death Syndrome, 72
Crook, Thomas, 179, 182
cross-nursing. *See under* breastfeeding
Crossley, Nick, 48n2

**D**
Davis-Floyd, Robbie, 39–40, 86n1, 88n27, 89, 119n19, 209
Department of Health and Human Services Call to Action to Support Breastfeeding, 68
Dettwyler, Katherine, 33, 79
diapering, 12, 156, 177, 192
cloth, 104–5, 111, 113–14, 127
disposable, 112
storage, 177, 192
Di Leonardo, Micaela, 51n50, 145, 148–49
doula, 9, 13, 91, 99, 103, 113, 129–30, 133, 187
birth, 109, 111, 113–14, 124, 250–54, 256, 258

*Index* 293

postpartum, 14, 101
Dudgeon, Matthew, 168
Dykes, Fiona, 39, 169, 209, 238n2, 238n4, 238n6

**E**
Eidelman, Arthur I., 72
Ekirch, Roger, 28
embodiment, 48n2, 62, 79, 86
 body as machine, 39, 169n13, 209
 "body techniques," 26–27
 breastfeeding and sleep as embodied social practice, 3, 16–21, 26–32, 42, 47–48, 48n9, 77, 114, 107, 118, 120, 244
 embodied inequalities, 38–47, 49–51nn45–46, 67–68, 241
 embodied moral dilemmas and ambivalence (*see under* morality)
 embodied morality (*see under* morality)
 embodied moral work (*see under* morality)
 habitus, 26–27, 37, 50–51n46, 221, 223, 233, 237
England, Pam, 118n4
ethnographic study
 description of, 3, 7–20, 24n42, 47, 85, 90, 114–15, 119n21, 120, 142240, 244, 256
 of biomedicine, 85, 86n1
 of breastfeeding and sleep, 28–29, 31–35, 139, 141–42, 169nn5, 169–70n17, 209, 238n2
 of childbirth, 55, 88n29
 of inequality, 52n53
 of men and gender, 144–45, 148–51, 167, 169nn6, 177
 of moral personhood, 51nn47–48
 of morality, 49–50n50
 of social class, 52n56
 of space, 205–6n15
evolution, 29, 75, 79, 102, 241

**F**
feminism, 4, 15
 and attachment parenting, 77
 and breastfeeding, 19, 27, 57, 78–86, 148, 168n2, 215, 240
 and La Leche League, 63, 79–80, 88n19
Faircloth, Charlotte, 141, 88n19
family leave policies, 4, 65, 69, 80, 96, 117, 147, 153, 156–58, 160, 164, 167, 168n3 175, 213–14, 235, 249–50, 252–55, 258–59. *See also* Patient Protection and Affordable Care Act
fatigue. *See under* sleep deprivation
Ferber, Richard, 75–76, 88n20
formula. *See under* infant formula
Foucault, Michel, 44, 55, 142
Franklin, Sarah, 53n65

**G**
Gartner, Lawrence M., 72
Gettler, Lee, 22n13, 24n39, 71–72
gender
 discrimination, 147 (*see also* breastfeeding: legal aspects of)
 division of labor, 125–26, 153, 156–62, 166, 168n2, 169–70n17, 175, 194–95, 213–14, 235–36, 244 (*see also* kinship, kin work)
 and inequality, 38–47, 51n50, 52n53, 67–68, 80–85, 88, 117, 147–48, 175, 241
 and intersectionality, 40–42, 47, 52n53, 85, 87n15
 and kinship (*see under* kinship)
 and "kin work" (*see under* kinship)
 and embodied labor of breastfeeding, 121, 144, 148, 152
 naturalization of, 80–81, 117 (*see also* breastfeeding: as natural)
 and moral labor of breastfeeding stigma, 142 (*see also*

breastfeeding: stigmatization of; morality)
and moral personhood, 121
men's role in childbirth and breastfeeding (*see under* breastfeeding; childbirth)
and space, 174–75
and time, 210, 213–17, 220, 222, 236–37
*See also* breastfeeding; feminism
Giarnella, Lori, 60–61, 76
Ginsburg, Faye, 23n27, 40–41
"global assemblages," 43–46, 53n60, 88n28
Goffman, Ervin, 120, 133, 141
Golden, Janet, 56–59
Gottlieb, Alma, 10–11, 31–32,
Grumet, Jamie Lynn, 22n15, 77

# H
habitus. *See under* embodiment
Hackett, Martine, 67–68
Hall Smith, Paige, 85–86
Han, Sallie, 49n25, 177–78
Hartigan, John, 42
Hausman, Bernice, 79–86, 88n19, 88n22, 88nn24–25, 119n24, 130
Hays, Sharon, 148, 205n16
Heintz, Monica, 49–50n45
Henderson, Jacqueline, 74–75
Hochschild, Arlie Russel, 148
Holt, Emmett, 61, 76
Horowitz, Robert, 118n4
houses
and construction of kinship and personhood, 171–72, 201–3, 203–4nn1–4 (*see also* personhood)
as instantiation of middle class norms, 171–82
and political economy, 172–75
significance of for raising children, 171–87

# I
independence
breastfeeding/bed sharing as challenging norms of, 5–6, 35, 131–33, 138–40, 146, 202–3, 209, 220–36
*See also* personhood
infant feeding, 3–4
and biomedicine, 55–88
and capitalism, 45, 237
in childbirth education, 89
and feminism, 78–86
and history, 56–78
and kinship, 32–38
and morality, 120, 141–42
and race, 42
and stigmatization, 142
*See also* breastfeeding; breastmilk; childbirth education; infant formula
infant formula. 143n6, 143n9, 162, 165, 169n9, 246, 251, 253, 259
and capitalism, 83–84
cultural norm of feeding with, 70–71, 76, 87–88n16, 106–7, 110, 130
feeding, 16, 25, 34
industry, 4, 28, 46–47, 66–70, 88n18, 242–43
and health, 64–67, 80, 87–88n16
history of replacement of breastfeeding with, 58–61, 86
and infant sleep, 61–62, 72
mimicking human breastmilk, 46–47
stigmatization of feeding with, 120, 128–29
supplementation with, 119n12, 189, 209, 243
Infant Sleep Information Source (ISIS), 241
Inhorn, Marcia, 44, 144–46, 166–67, 168n1
Innocenti Declaration, 64–65
International Board Certified Lactation Consultant (IBCLC), 106
intersectionality, 40–42, 47, 52n53, 87n15

## J

jaundice (neonatal), 102, 123, 143n6, 154–55, 169n9
Johansen, Shawn, 170n22
Jordan, Brigitte, 55, 86n1

## K

Kelleher, Christa, 122
kinship, 18, 26, 51nn49–50, 119n25
   construction of through breastfeeding and sleep, 32–38, 47–49n25, 169n5, 220–23, 233, 237, 243
   and gender, 37–41, 49n25, 79–80, 121–22, 142, 144–70
   and the house, 171, 177–78, 203n1,
   "kin work," 49n25, 144–70, 177–78
   and men, 49n25, 142, 144–70, 177–78
"kin work." *See under* kinship
Krieger, Nancy, 87n15
Kukla, Rebecca, 82–83

## L

La Leche League International, 9–10, 88n18, 130, 241
   and attachment parenting (*see under* parenting)
   and companionate marriage, 146–47
   and feminism (*see under* feminism)
   history of, 62–64
Labbok, Miriam, 85–86
lactation. *See under* breastfeeding
lactation consultants, 9, 14, 87–88n16. *See also* International Board Certified Lactation Consultant (IBCLC)
Lambek, Michael, 49–50n45
Lane, Sandra, 52n53
Latch on NYC, 87n13, 242
Layne, Linda, 179
Leavitt, Judith Walzer, 23n30, 56–58
Lock, Margaret, 22–23n23, 23n27, 53n60, 53–54n67

## M

Maher, Vanessa, 48n8
marriage, 3, 61, 149
   companionate, 146–47, 213
Martin, Emily, 38–39, 51–52n51
Marx, Karl, 52n53, 210–11
maternalism, 62–63, 79
Mather, Cotton, 57
Mauss, Marcel, 26–27, 37, 48n2, 50–51n46, 221
MacIntyre, Alasdair, 49–50n45
McKenna, James J., 22n13, 24n39, 29–30, 71–75, 79, 102, 139, 241
middle class, 1, 3, 18, 240
   and the biomedicalization of childbirth, 57
   and the biomedicalization of infant sleep, 60–61
   breastfeeding ideologies, 79
   and childbirth education, 89–98, 110–18
   childhood/children's personhood, 175–80, 187
   comparative ethnographic study of, 41–42, 47, 52–53n56
   consumption (*see under* consumption)
   employment accommodations for breastfeeding, 199–200
   ethnographic study of, 10–11, 14
   fatherhood, 49n25, 144–70
   historical transformations in, 61
   houses and house spaces (*see under* houses)
   models of parenthood, 114–18
   models of personhood, kinship, 20, 26, 31–32, 42, 171, 220–23, 233, 237, 243 (*see also* kinship; personhood)
   models of reproduction, 40
   motherhood, 42, 114–17, 141
   norms for adult beds, 194
   norms of childrearing, 42
   norms of solitary infant sleep, 31–32, 73, 139, 202

sexuality, 180–82
temporality, 208–17
as trendsetters, 8
*See also* consumption; personhood
Midwest, 43, 48–49n25, 51n50, 177, 250
midwives, 59–60, 62, 87n5, 87n10, 88n29, 96
  Certified Practicing Midwife (CPM), 110, 257
  home birth midwives, 99–111, 113, 257
  hospital nurse-midwives, 2, 9, 92, 97, 112, 114, 133
  stigmatization of, 59
  *See also* childbirth
Miller, Daniel, 119n15, 119n25
morality
  anthropological study of, 37–38, 44–45, 49–51nn45–29, 53–54n66
  and breastfeeding (*see under* breastfeeding)
  embodied morality, 49–51nn45–29, 53–54n66, 88n23, 208, 233
  embodied moral dilemmas or ambivalence, 19, 37–38, 233, 235–37, 240
  embodied moral work, 120–44
  and infant formula (*see under* infant formula)
  moral concerns about bed sharing (*see under* bed sharing)
  moral norms of sleep, 138–40
  moral personhood, 51nn47–48, 121
  *See also* stigmatization
Morelli, Gilda, 30, 35
Mothering Magazine, 77, 102, 104
Mullings, Leith, 41, 52n53, 68
Murphy, Elizabeth, 23n36, 120, 128, 141

**N**

neoliberalism, 21, 23n26, 43–45, 51n47, 82–83, 88n29. *See also* capitalism

Nguyen, Vinh Kim, 22–23n23, 53n60
nursery, 3, 48–49n25, 108, 176–79, 192, 206n21, 225
  at hospital, 154
  *See also* bedroom
nursing. *See under* breastfeeding

**O**

Obama, Barack, 242
Obama, Michelle, 242
Ochs, Elinor, 121
Ong, Aihwa, 43
Ortner, Sherry, 42, 52–53n56

**P**

Pack 'n Play portable play yard, 183–84, 187, 194–95, 225, 233, 250, 252, 254–55
parenting, 3, 126–27, 140, 143n10, 146, 148, 152, 202, 218, 225–26, 230
  attachment, 5, 21–22n12, 76–77, 88n19, 103–4, 113, 114, 185
  intensive, 161, 175
  men in, 49n25, 117, 144–70
  "natural mothering," 116–17, 119n14
  "natural parenting," 77, 96, 105, 111–17, 186
The Patient Protection and Affordable Care Act, 65, 168n3, 242
pediatricians, 62, 159. *See also* American Academy of Pediatrics; breastfeeding; sleep
Peletz, Michael, 37, 51n49
personhood
  children's, 20, 31–32, 47, 131, 140, 142, 176–80, 186–203, 208–39
  construction of through breastfeeding and sleep, 32–38, 187–203, 208–39
  construction of through consumption, 42–43, 46–47, 89–98, 110–18, 119n25

fathers', 49n25, 110–18, 144–70, 177–78 (*see also* kinship; "kin work")
and morality (*see under* morality)
mothers', 110–18, 122–43
and space, 171–207
and temporality, 208–39
*See also* parenting
Plath, David W., 34
political economy, 7, 20–21, 26, 28, 30, 38–40, 43, 47, 51n50, 83–84, 86, 90, 175, 240, 243. *See also* capitalism
postpartum depression, 126
pregnancy, 33, 48–49n25, 51–52nn53–54, 56, 66–67, 95, 98–100, 103, 111, 147, 149–51
preeclempsia, 121–23, 142n4
loss, 24n40
Protestant ethic, 53–54n66, 210

**R**
race, 4, 8, 15, 17, 37–39, 41–42, 52n53, 63, 67–68, 73, 81, 85, 88n29, 174–75, 205n15, 243–44
Rapp, Rayna, 23n27, 37–38, 40, 51n48, 53n64
Ratner, Herbert, 63
Reed, Richard, 89, 94, 150–51, 169n6
relatedness. *See under* kinship
reproduction, 15–16, 23n27, 23n30, 37–43
biomedicalization of, 7
stratified reproduction, 40–41
risk, 4
and breastfeeding, 124–30, 141
-based advocacy of breastfeeding, 67–68, 82
of bed sharing, 71–73, 134, 136, 162, 190
and health, 7, 23n26, 44–45, 52n53
and home birth, 110
of Sudden Infant Death Syndrome, 6, 71–73

Roberts, Dorothy, 52n53
Rolston, Jessica Smith, 51n50
Rose, Nikolas, 23n26, 44, 53–54nn65–66
Rosin, Hanna, 82–83, 144, 148
Rothman, Barbara Katz, 46, 81, 119n23
Rowland, Perrin, 60–61, 76
Ryan, Kath, 120, 124, 141–42, 143n29

**S**
Scheper-Hughes, Nancy, 28, 81, 88n24
Sears, William, 77, 88n18, 88n20, 103–4, 109, 185
self-regulation, 133, 140, 146, 209–10, 222, 225–26. *See also* independence
self-reliance, 3, 35, 131, 133. *See also* independence
sexuality
and abuse, 182
and bed sharing (*see under* bed sharing)
and bedrooms (*see under* bedroom)
and breastfeeding (*see under* breastfeeding)
and breastmilk (*see under* breastmilk)
middle class norms of (*see under* middle class)
Shaw, Rhonda, 45, 142n1
Shweder, Richard, 89, 94, 150–51, 169n6
slavery, 52n53, 82
forced wet-nursing in, 68
sleep
and adult beds (*see under* bed sharing)
and bassinets (*see under* bassinet)
and bed sharing (*see under* bed sharing)
biomedicalization of, 60–62, 67–68, 70–78
and co-sleeping (*see under* co-sleeping)

"crying it out," 140, 229–36
cross-cultural studies of, 28–29, 31–32, 34–36
deprivation, 31, 71, 122–23, 126, 132, 136, 161, 164, 188, 195–96, 208, 217, 230–31, 233, 236,
health, 6, 70–78
history of infant, 60–62
and incest, 6, 36, 139, 182
interruptions and, 6, 154, 187, 218, 226
moral norms of, 138–40
pediatricians' advice on infants', 34–35, 56, 61, 68, 70, 102, 129, 132, 134–38, 196, 198–200, 209, 234–35
and room sharing, 34–35, 198, 217, 221–23, 232
and secrecy, 133, 137, 139
"self-soothing," 132
sociological studies of, 29, 48n9, 169–70n17
solitary infant, 31–32, 34–36, 56, 60–62, 68, 70–78, 161, 169–70n17, 198, 202, 235 (*see also* independence)
and Sudden Infant Death Syndrome (*see under* breastfeeding; bed sharing; risk)
training, 74–75, 140, 164, 198, 202, 217, 221–36
uninterrupted (value of), 62, 66, 74–75, 209, 220–21, 224–25, 227, 230
sling, 99, 103, 109, 111–13, 127–28, 192
Snuggle Nest, 185–86, 193, 257
social class, 8, 20, 37, 39, 42–43, 67, 73, 81, 88n29, 97–98, 116–17, 145–46, 168, 187, 202, 204n5, 205n15. *See also* middle class
Solinger, Rickie, 84, 90, 118n2
Spock, Benjamin, 61
Stearns, Peter, 60–61, 76

stigmatization
of African American families, 68
of bed sharing (*see under* bed sharing)
of breastfeeding (*see under* breastfeeding)
of breastfeeding and sleep arrangements, 20–21, 42, 86, 132–43
of "blue collar" labor, 52–53n56
of feeding with infant formula (*see under* infant formula)
of infertility, 145
of midwifery (*see under* midwives)
spouses as mitigating, 145–46, 155, 167
Sudden Infant Death Syndrome (SIDS)
American Academy of Pediatrics guidelines on (*see under* American Academy of Pediatrics)
and bed sharing (*see under* bed sharing)
and breastfeeding (*see under* breastfeeding)
as "crib death," 70
racial disparities, 41, 67–68
risk of (*see under* risk)

T
"technologies of the self," 44, 142
Thompson, E.P., 209–10, 215, 236–37, 238nn5–6
time/temporality, 208–39
Time magazine, 5–6, 22n15, 77
Townsend, Nicholas, 166–67

U
Ulrich, Laurel Thatcher, 87n5

V
Van Esterik, Penny, 80–81, 86, 243
Van Vleet, Krista, 169n5
Volpe, Lane, 49n39, 74

## W

Wali, Alaka, 52n53, 41
Ward, Julia, 63, 87n4, 88n19, 147–47
Watson, John, 61, 76
Weber, Max, 49–50n45, 210
Weiner, Lynn, 62–64
wet-nurse. *See under* breastfeeding
Wight, Nancy, 72–73
White, Gregory, 63
White, Mary, 63
Wilk, Richard, 119n15

Williams, Simon, 28–29, 48n9, 169n17
Wolf, Jacqueline H., 23n30, 58–61, 80, 87n3, 87n10, 146
Wolf, Joan B., 4, 82–84, 87n14
Wolf-Meyer, Matthew, 54n67

## Z

Zelizer, Viviana, 87n12, 205n16
Zigon, Jarett, 37, 49–51nn45–48, 143n29

## Fertility, Reproduction and Sexuality

GENERAL EDITORS:

*Soraya Tremayne*, Founding Director, Fertility and Reproduction Studies Group, and Research Associate, Institute of Social and Cultural Anthropology, University of Oxford.

*Marcia C. Inhorn*, William K. Lanman, Jr. Professor of Anthropology and International Affairs, Yale University.

*Philip Kreager*, Director, Fertility and Reproduction Studies Group, and Research Associate, Institute of Social and Cultural Anthropology and Institute of Human Sciences, University of Oxford.

Volume 1
**Managing Reproductive Life: Cross-Cultural Themes in Fertility and Sexuality**
Edited by Soraya Tremayne

Volume 2
**Modern Babylon? Prostituting Children in Thailand**
Heather Montgomery

Volume 3
**Reproductive Agency, Medicine and the State: Cultural Transformations in Childbearing**
Edited by Maya Unnithan-Kumar

Volume 4
**A New Look at Thai AIDS: Perspectives from the Margin**
Graham Fordham

Volume 5
**Breast Feeding and Sexuality: Behaviour, Beliefs and Taboos among the Gogo Mothers in Tanzania**
Mara Mabilia

Volume 6
**Ageing without Children: European and Asian Perspectives on Elderly Access to Support Networks**
Edited by Philip Kreager and Elisabeth Schröder-Butterfill

Volume 7
**Nameless Relations: Anonymity, Melanesia and Reproductive Gift Exchange between British Ova Donors and Recipients**
Monica Konrad

Volume 8
**Population, Reproduction and Fertility in Melanesia**
Edited by Stanley J. Ulijaszek

Volume 9
**Conceiving Kinship: Assisted Conception, Procreation and Family in Southern Europez**
Monica M. E. Bonaccorso

Volume 10
**Where There Is No Midwife: Birth and Loss in Rural India**
Sarah Pinto

Volume 11
**Reproductive Disruptions: Gender, Technology, and Biopolitics in the New Millennium**
Edited by Marcia C. Inhorn

Volume 12
**Reconceiving the Second Sex: Men, Masculinity, and Reproduction**
Edited by Marcia C. Inhorn, Tine Tjørnhøj-Thomsen, Helene Goldberg, and Maruska la Cour Mosegaard

Volume 13
**Transgressive Sex: Subversion and Control in Erotic Encounters**
Edited by Hastings Donnan and Fiona Macgowan

Volume 14
**European Kinship in the Age of Biotechnology**
Edited by Jeanette Edwards and Carles Salazar

Volume 15
**Kinship and Beyond: The Genealogical Model Reconsidered**
Edited by Sandra Bamford and James Leach

Volume 16
**Islam and New Kinship: Reproductive Technology and the Shariah in Lebanon**
Morgan Clarke

Volume 17
**Childbirth, Midwifery and Concepts of Time**
Edited by Christine McCourt

Volume 18
**Assisting Reproduction, Testing Genes: Global Encounters with the New Biotechnologies**
Edited by Daphna Birenbaum-Carmeli and Marcia C. Inhorn

Volume 19
**Kin, Gene, Community: Reproductive Technologies among Jewish Israelis**
Edited by Daphna Birenbaum-Carmeli and Yoram S. Carmeli

Volume 20
**Abortion in Asia: Local Dilemmas, Global Politics**
Edited by Andrea Whittaker

Volume 21
**Unsafe Motherhood: Mayan Maternal Mortality and Subjectivity in Post-War Guatemala**
Nicole S. Berry

Volume 22
**Fatness and the Maternal Body: Women's Experiences of Corporeality and the Shaping of Social Policy**
Edited by Maya Unnithan-Kumar and Soraya Tremayne

Volume 23
**Islam and Assisted Reproductive Technologies: Sunni and Shia Perspectives**
Edited by Marcia C. Inhorn and Soraya Tremayne

Volume 24
**Militant Lactivism?: Infant Feeding and Maternal Accountability in the UK and France**
Charlotte Faircloth

Volume 25
**Pregnancy in Practice: Expectation and Experience in the Contemporary US**
Sallie Han

Volume 26
**Nighttime Breastfeeding: An American Cultural Dilemma**
Cecília Tomori

Volume 27
**Globalized Fatherhood**
Edited by Marcia C. Inhorn, Wendy Chavkin, and José-Alberto Navarro

Volume 28
**Cousin Marriages: Between Tradition, Genetic Risk and Cultural Change**
Edited by Alison Shaw and Aviad Raz

Volume 29
**Achieving Procreation: Childlessness and IVF in Turkey**
Merve Demircio lu Göknar

Volume 30
**Thai in Vitro: Gender, Culture and Assisted Reproduction**
Andrea Whittaker

Volume 31
**Assisted Reproductive Technologies in the Third Phase: Global Encounters and Emerging Moral Worlds**
Edited by Kate Hampshire and Bob Simpson

Volume 32
**Parenthood between Generations: Transforming Reproductive Cultures**
Edited by Siân Pooley and Kaveri Qureshi

Volume 33
**Patient-Centred IVF: Bioethics and Care in a Dutch Clinic**
Trudie Gerrits

Volume 34
**Conceptions: Infertilities and Procreative Technologies in India**
Aditya Bharadwaj

Volume 35
**The Online World of Surrogacy**
Zsuzsa Berend